New Frontiers in Liver Transplantation

New Frontiers in Liver Transplantation

Edited by Duke Todd

hayle
medical

New York

Hayle Medical,
750 Third Avenue, 9th Floor,
New York, NY 10017, USA

Visit us on the World Wide Web at:
www.haylemedical.com

ISBN: 978-1-63241-764-0

The publisher's policy is to use permanent paper from mills that operate a sustainable forestry policy. Furthermore, the publisher ensures that the text paper and cover boards used have met acceptable environmental accreditation standards.

Printed in China.

Cataloging-in-Publication Data

New frontiers in liver transplantation / edited by Duke Todd.
p. cm.
Includes bibliographical references and index.
ISBN 978-1-63241-764-0
1. Liver--Transplantation. 2. Liver--Transplantation--Technique. 3. Liver--Surgery.
4. Transplantation of organs, tissues, etc. I. Todd, Duke.
RD546 .N48 2019
617.556 205 92--dc23

Table of Contents

Preface

Over the recent decade, advancements and applications have progressed exponentially. This has led to the increased interest in this field and projects are being conducted to enhance knowledge. The main objective of this book is to present some of the critical challenges and provide insights into possible solutions. This book will answer the varied questions that arise in the field and also provide an increased scope for furthering studies.

The replacement of a diseased liver with a healthy liver is known as liver transplantation. Liver transplantation is used as a treatment option for acute liver failure and end-stage liver disease. Orthotopic transplantation is a common and effective technique used for liver transplantation. The transplantation surgery usually takes 4 to 18 hours. The common requirements for a liver donor include good health, a blood type which is compatible with the recipient, having an age of 20-60 years, and being of similar or larger size than the recipient. Liver transplantation involves a few complications, such as infection, bleeding, possibility of blood clots, painful incision and prolonged recovery. This book brings forth some of the most innovative concepts and elucidates the unexplored aspects of liver transplantation. It studies, analyzes and upholds the pillars of liver transplantation and its utmost significance in modern times. The extensive content of this book provides the readers with a thorough understanding of the subject.

I hope that this book, with its visionary approach, will be a valuable addition and will promote interest among readers. Each of the authors has provided their extraordinary competence in their specific fields by providing different perspectives as they come from diverse nations and regions. I thank them for their contributions.

Editor

1

Oral Cavity Metastasis of Hepatocellular Carcinoma following Liver Transplantation

Nicolás Goldaracena,[1] Mariela Barreto,[2] Gabriel Casas,[2] Margarita Anders,[3] Ricardo Mastai,[3] and Lucas McCormack[1]

[1] *Liver Surgery and Transplantation Unit, Hospital Alemán of Buenos Aires, Avenne Pueyrredón 1640, Buenos Aires 1118AAT, Argentina*
[2] *Pathology Service, Hospital Alemán of Buenos Aires, Avenne Pueyrredón 1640, Buenos Aires 1118AAT, Argentina*
[3] *Hepatology Service and Liver Transplantation Unit, Hospital Alemán of Buenos Aires, Avenne Pueyrredón 1640, Buenos Aires 1118AAT, Argentina*

Correspondence should be addressed to Lucas McCormack, lmccormack@hospitalaleman.com

Academic Editors: D. Capone, G. Forrest, M. R. Moosa, and M. Sadeghi

Liver transplantation (LT) remains the only cure for hepatocellular carcinoma (HCC) in many cases. Over many years, most centers have applied the Milan criteria for selecting cirrhotic patients with HCC for LT. In a new era where several transplant groups are pushing the limits of transplanting HCC outside Milan criteria as an aggressive approach with promising results, we present interesting images of a patient that presented a unique and rare site of HCC metastasis after 36 months of liver transplantation.

1. Introduction

Over many years, most centers have applied the Milan selection criteria for cirrhotic patients with hepatocellular carcinoma (HCC). However, several groups from different countries have challenged these restrictive criteria with promising results [1]. This more aggressive approach could result in higher rates of tumor recurrence that should carefully be assessed in these patients with advanced HCC within the liver. We report here a case with an unusual site of tumor recurrence after liver transplantation (LT) that should be known as a potential site of metastasis.

2. Case Report

A 58-year-old male patient with liver cirrhosis due to hepatitis C virus (HCV) infection and alcohol consumption with HCC beyond Milan criteria underwent LT at our unit. The pathological study of the liver specimen revealed multiple well-differentiated HCC with a major nodule of 6,6 cm in diameter without vascular invasion (T3aN0M0). After LT the patient received tacrolimus and mycophenolate as immunosuppression regimen. During follow-up, he never experienced HCV recurrence. In addition, any episodes of rejection or opportunistic infections needing specific treatment were detected.

Follow-up images and tumoral markers showed no tumoral recurrence until 36 months after LT when he was admitted to our hospital presenting with a 2 cm in diameter bleeding oral mass localized in the retromolar trigonum (Figure 1(a)). The bleeding stopped by local compression, and a biopsy of the lesion was taken. The pathological study of the oral lesion demonstrated mucosal infiltration by a poor-differentiated carcinoma (Figures 1(b) and 1(c)). Immunohistochemistry was performed and the lesion was positive for Heppar 1 and CD34 (Figure 2). With the morphological features and the immunohistochemical profile the oral lesion was diagnosed as a metastatic HCC.

After diagnosing the oral lesion as a metastatic HCC a PET-CT was performed showing no other metastatic

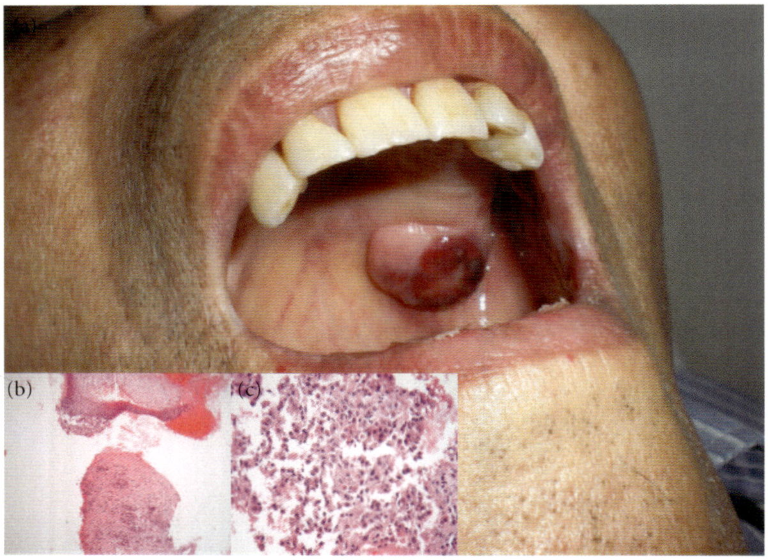

Figure 1: (a) Patient oral cavity showing 2 cm exophytic mass in the left retromolar trigonum; biopsy from the oral mass (hematoxylin and eosin stain) demonstrates infiltration by carcinoma of nodular and glandular pattern, consisting of atypical cuboidal cells with slightly acidophilic granular cytoplasm. (b) Magnification × 40. (c) Magnification × 100.

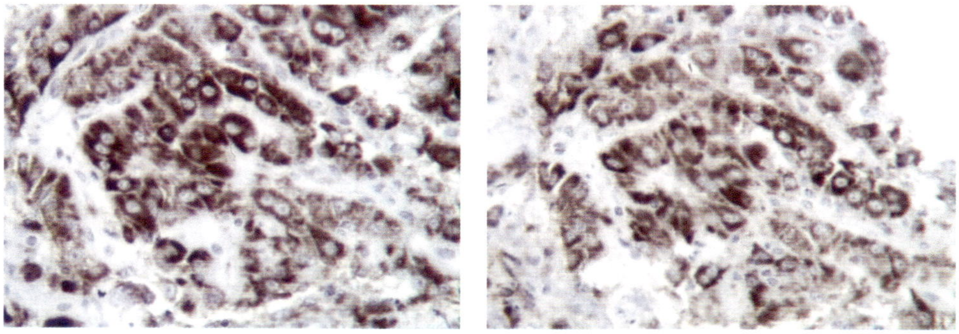

(a) (b)

Figure 2: Immunohistochemistry showing expression of Heppar 1 and CD34 on the tumor biopsy: (a) expression of Heppar 1 (magnification × 400) and (b) expression of CD34 (magnification × 400).

disease elsewhere. Alpha-fetoprotein levels were still normal. His immunosuppression was switched to sirolimus, and he started treatment with sorafenib 400 mg/12 hs.

3. Discussion

To the best of our knowledge, this is the first case of a metastatic HCC to the oral cavity after LT reported in English literature. Surprisingly, this was the only site of metastasis after 36 months of LT due to HCC beyond Milan criteria.

In patients transplanted due to HCC on a cirrhotic liver the most frequent site of metastasis is the transplanted liver. Other sites in which HCC metastases most frequently occur are the lungs, adrenal glands, and bones. Interestingly, the PET-CT did not show any metastasis elsewhere, assuming that its long-term recurrence first appeared at a distant location and not in the new liver, as expected. Metastases from HCC to the oral cavity have only been reported occasionally but only in patients with disseminated disease that did not receive a LT [2].

Most cases of metastatic HCC in the oral cavity involve the mandible and gingival presenting either as exophytic tumors or as intraosseous lesions [3]. Usually, the symptoms caused by this type of metastatic lesions are pain, dysphagia, and bleeding among others. In our case, the oral metastasis presented as a gingival exophytic bleeding mass without bone involvement.

When oral metastasis appears, the prognosis is very poor. therefore these lesions are treated with surgery, radiotherapy, or sorafenib to relieve symptoms and improve the quality of life [4]. Unfortunately, in the setting of a patient with immunosuppression with sirolimus after LT, data is lacking in the literature.

Abbreviations

HCC: Hepatocellular carcinoma
LT: Liver transplantation
HCV: Hepatitis C virus.

References

[1] M. Weber and P. A. Clavien, "Hepatocellular carcinoma and liver transplantation: entering the area after the Milan and University of California at San Francisco criteria?" *Liver Transplantation*, vol. 14, no. 7, pp. 911–914, 2008.

[2] A. Chin, T. S. Liang, and A. J. Borislow, "Initial presentation of hepatocellular carcinoma as a mandibular mass: case report and review of the literature," *Oral Surgery, Oral Medicine, Oral Pathology, Oral Radiology, and Endodontics*, vol. 86, no. 4, pp. 457–460, 1998.

[3] P. Marker and P. P. Clausen, "Metastases to the mouth and jaws from hepatocellular carcinomas. A case report," *International Journal of Oral and Maxillofacial Surgery*, vol. 20, no. 6, pp. 371–374, 1991.

[4] Y. Nagao, A. Cho, H. Yamamoto et al., "Hepatocellular carcinoma with pharyngeal metastasis: report of a case," *Surgery Today*, vol. 38, no. 11, pp. 1060–1062, 2008.

2

Delayed Gastric Emptying after Living Donor Hepatectomy for Liver Transplantation

Hanjay Wang,[1] Adam D. Griesemer,[1] Ronald F. Parsons,[2] Jay A. Graham,[3] Jean C. Emond,[1] and Benjamin Samstein[1,4]

[1] *Center for Liver Disease and Transplantation, Department of Surgery, Columbia University Medical Center, New York, NY 10032, USA*
[2] *Department of Surgery, Emory University School of Medicine, Atlanta, GA 30322, USA*
[3] *Department of Surgery, Montefiore Medical Center, Bronx, NY 10467, USA*
[4] *New York Presbyterian Hospital/Columbia, PH Room Floor 14, Room 202, 622 West 168th Street, New York, NY 10032, USA*

Correspondence should be addressed to Benjamin Samstein; bs212@columbia.edu

Academic Editor: Piero Boraschi

Delayed gastric emptying is a significant postoperative complication of living donor hepatectomy for liver transplantation and may require endoscopic or surgical intervention in severe cases. Although the mechanism of posthepatectomy delayed gastric emptying remains unknown, vagal nerve injury during intraoperative dissection and adhesion formation postoperatively between the stomach and cut liver surface are possible explanations. Here, we present the first reported case of delayed gastric emptying following fully laparoscopic hepatectomy for living donor liver transplantation. Additionally, we also present a case in which symptoms developed after open right hepatectomy, but for which dissection for left hepatectomy was first performed. Through our experience and these two specific cases, we favor a neurovascular etiology for delayed gastric emptying after hepatectomy.

1. Introduction

Delayed gastric emptying (DGE) complicates living donor hepatectomy for liver transplantation in 2% of patients and is almost exclusively associated with left-sided hepatectomy [1, 2]. Symptoms include nausea, vomiting, bloating, and epigastric discomfort, which typically resolve with conservative treatment, but severe cases may require endoscopic or surgical intervention. Because living donors are generally healthy prior to surgery, postoperative DGE is an important complication to recognize, treat, and prevent. Understanding the mechanism of posthepatectomy DGE is therefore essential.

Here, we present two cases of DGE that developed after hepatectomy for living donor liver transplantation, including the first reported example of this complication following laparoscopic hepatectomy. Importantly, we also present a case in which DGE developed after an open right hepatectomy, but for which dissection for a left hepatectomy was first performed. All patient data was reviewed under IRB-approved study protocol IRB-AAAM5707. Through our experience, we favor a neurovascular etiology as the primary cause of DGE after hepatectomy.

2. Case 1

KS, a 31-year-old woman with mild gastroesophageal reflux disease requiring no home medications, presented for planned open left hepatectomy (our preferred technique at the time) for liver donation. During the procedure, a replaced left hepatic artery was visualized and dissected to the level of its origin from the left gastric artery. To completely mobilize the replaced artery, neurovascular branches supplying the lesser curvature of the stomach were divided. Upon examination of the hepatic hilum, a standard left hepatic artery was found, as well as a small segment-4 artery from the proximal right hepatic artery. These additional arteries were not seen on preoperative imaging. Due to concern for increased risk of

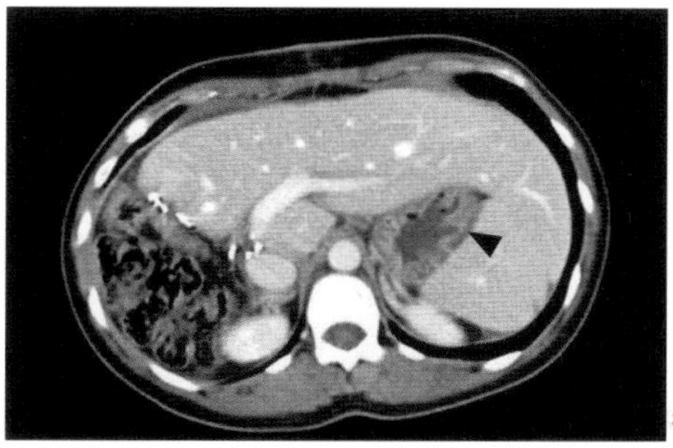

FIGURE 1: Computed tomography scan of the abdomen with intravenous contrast for patient KS, one month following open right hepatectomy. There is no evidence of adhesion formation between the stomach and cut liver surface. The stomach (black arrow) is far removed from the cut surface of the liver.

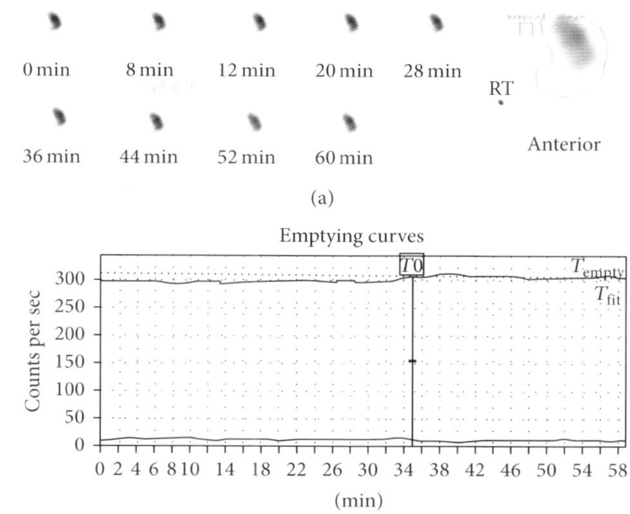

Parameter	99 m technetium
Emptying	1%
Emptying beginning ($T0$)	35 min
Emptying ending	59 min
T 1/2	978 min
$T0 \rightarrow T$ 1/2	943 min

(b)

FIGURE 2: Gastric emptying study for patient KS following open right hepatectomy. (a) Gastric emptying was observed for 60 minutes with intermittent imaging. The region of interest is indicated at right by a line drawn around the activity within the stomach in the anterior view. (b) The emptying curves over 60 minutes (T_{empty}—solid; T_{fit}—dotted) are shown. The half-emptying time (T 1/2) was calculated using the geometric mean. Gastric emptying time was markedly prolonged, with absent emptying during the 60-minute period.

graft failure, the decision was made to convert to a right hepatectomy. The operation proceeded without complications. After removal of the right lobe graft, omentum and colon were placed in the resection bed, and Seprafilm adhesion barrier was applied to the cut liver surface. During the first postoperative week, the patient complained of nausea, heartburn, reflux, and nonbilious vomiting. The patient gradually improved with medical management including a proton pump inhibitor, sucralfate, and metoclopramide, and she was discharged home on postoperative day (POD) 9. On POD 31, the patient was readmitted for severe nausea, bilious vomiting, and burning epigastric pain. A computed tomography (CT) scan of the abdomen did not suggest bowel obstruction or adhesion formation between the stomach and cut liver surface (Figure 1). Endoscopy revealed retained food products in the stomach, and a gastric emptying study demonstrated absent emptying over one hour (Figure 2). Following initial improvement with medical management as described above, the patient experienced worsening emesis on POD 43 with solid food trial. During repeat endoscopy, 200 units of botulinum toxin were injected at the pylorus. Afterward, the patient experienced no further emesis and tolerated oral medications. An upper gastrointestinal series with small bowel follow-through showed no abnormalities. The patient was discharged home on POD 49. She underwent a repeat gastric emptying study one week after discharge, which showed marked improvement and normal gastric emptying (Figure 3). In subsequent follow-up, she reports feeling well and eating normally. She is currently over four years postdonation.

3. Case 2

IS, a healthy 46-year-old woman, underwent a totally laparoscopic full left hepatectomy for liver donation, using our previously described technique [3]. A replaced left hepatic artery was visualized during the procedure. To have a larger arterial orifice, branches to the lesser curvature of the stomach were taken and the artery was divided at the level of the left gastric artery. The operation proceeded without complications. The patient had a postoperative course notable for mild heartburn and bloating, controlled with a proton pump inhibitor and H2 receptor antagonist, and was discharged home on POD 6. On POD 10, the patient was readmitted for nausea, epigastric pain, and heartburn. A gastric emptying study demonstrated marked delay suggesting gastroparesis (Figure 4). Endoscopy revealed a deformity of the gastric antrum and food residue within the stomach. 40 units of botulinum toxin were injected into the deformed area of the stomach, and the patient reported prompt improvement of her symptoms. A subsequent abdominal CT scan showed passage of contrast through the small bowel. In addition, there was no evidence on CT scan to suggest a structural etiology for DGE, such as adhesion formation between the stomach and cut liver surface (Figure 5). The patient was discharged home on POD 18. Currently, she is over 6 months postdonation and reports feeling well and eating normally but continues to take a proton pump inhibitor for heartburn.

4. Discussion

Postoperative DGE occurs in 2% of all living liver donors and is primarily associated with left-sided hepatectomy [1, 2],

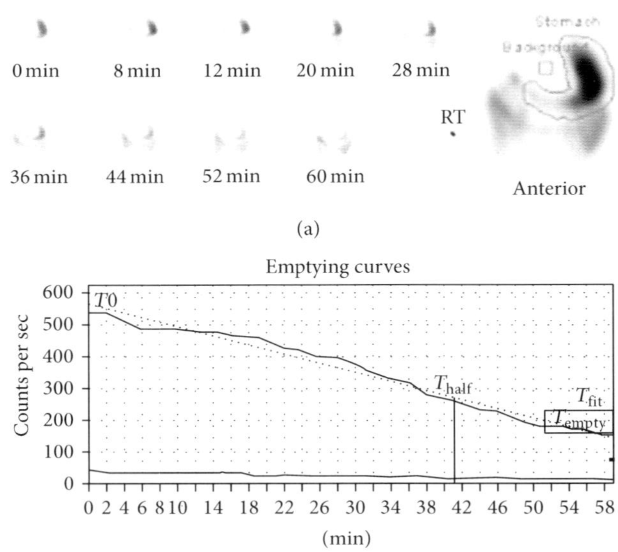

Parameter	99 m technetium
Emptying	75%
Emptying beginning ($T0$)	2 min
Emptying ending	59 min
T 1/2	41 min
$T0 \rightarrow T$ 1/2	39 min

(b)

Figure 3: Gastric emptying study for patient KS following intrapyloric botulinum toxin injection. (a) Gastric emptying was observed for 60 minutes with intermittent imaging. The region of interest is indicated at right by a line drawn around the activity within the stomach in the anterior view. (b) The emptying curves over 60 minutes (T_{empty}—solid; T_{fit}—dotted) are shown. The half-emptying time (T 1/2) was calculated using the geometric mean. Gastric emptying time was normal with 75% emptying over 60 minutes and a half-emptying time of 41 minutes.

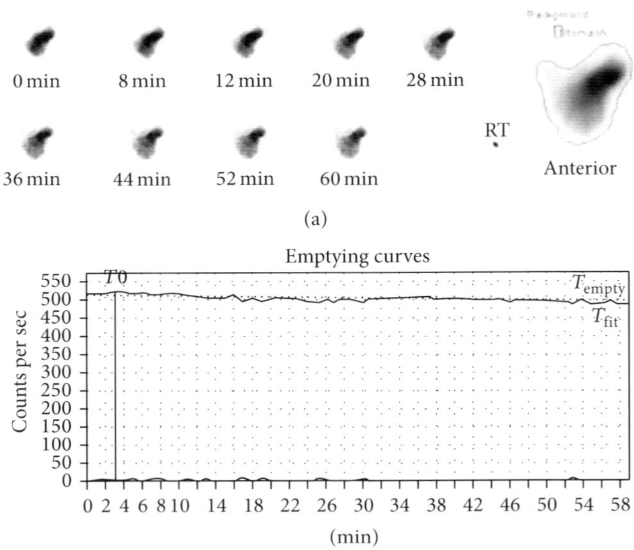

Parameter	99 m technetium
Emptying	4%
Emptying beginning ($T0$)	3 min
Emptying ending	59 min
T 1/2	627 min
$T0 \rightarrow T$ 1/2	624 min

(b)

Figure 4: Gastric emptying study for patient IS following laparoscopic left hepatectomy. (a) Gastric emptying was observed for 60 minutes with intermittent imaging. The region of interest is indicated at right by a line drawn around the activity within the stomach in the anterior view. (b) The emptying curves over 60 minutes (T_{empty}—solid; T_{fit}—dotted) are shown. The half-emptying time (T 1/2) was calculated using the geometric mean. Gastric emptying time was markedly delayed, with no definitive evidence of radiotracer passing into the duodenum during the 60-minute period.

although Kim et al. reported six cases (1.2%) in a series of 500 right-sided liver donors [4]. The mechanism of posthepatectomy DGE remains unknown. One hypothesis involves adhesion formation between the stomach and cut liver surface. After a left-sided hepatectomy, the stomach may twist and fall into the resection bed. As a result, the dislocated stomach may contact the raw surface of the remaining liver and ultimately become fixed via adhesions. Gastric obstruction may develop due to disruption of motility at the points of adhesion, leading to symptoms of DGE.

Direct visualization of gastrohepatic adhesions after left-sided hepatectomy for living liver donation has been documented via surgical reexploration in two cases by Umeshita et al. [1] and one by Kinoshita et al. [5]. All three patients reportedly experienced resolution of symptoms after lysis of adhesions. In addition, some studies have suggested that wrapping the liver with greater omentum [5] or suturing the greater omentum to the peritoneum [6, 7] may decrease the risk of posthepatectomy DGE by preventing contact between the stomach and cut liver surface. Several other studies, however, found no significant effect using the same and/or different techniques to prevent adhesions [8–12]. Overall, the majority of these studies are small, single-center, nonrandomized trials, and the collective data is ambiguous.

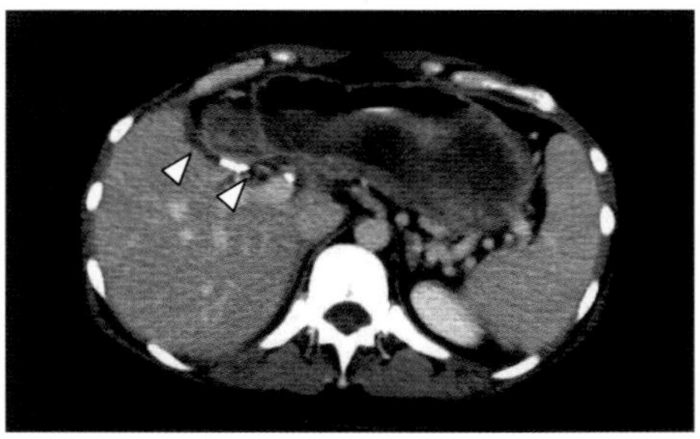

Figure 5: Computed tomography scan of the abdomen with intravenous contrast for patient IS, two weeks following laparoscopic left hepatectomy. There is no evidence of a structural etiology for delayed gastric emptying, including adhesion formation between the stomach and cut liver surface (white arrows).

The cases of KS and IS add insight to our understanding of posthepatectomy DGE. To our knowledge, the case of IS represents the first report of DGE following laparoscopic hepatectomy for living donor liver transplantation. Laparoscopic abdominal surgeries generally result in fewer adhesions compared to open procedures [13]. Indeed, one study involving pigs found that, compared to open resection of the hepatic left lateral segment, laparoscopic resection resulted in a marked decrease in postoperative adhesions [14]. Despite not using an adhesion barrier in the case of IS, we did not find evidence of postoperative adhesions between the stomach and cut liver surface on CT scan.

The case of KS is particularly noteworthy in the fact that we initially performed the dissection for a left hepatectomy but ultimately used a right lobe graft. As a result, the resection bed was far removed from the stomach, and the cut liver surface was faced away from the stomach. The absence of apposition significantly decreases the probability of adhesion formation between the stomach and the cut surface of the liver. Indeed, we did not find evidence of postoperative gastrohepatic adhesions on CT scan for KS.

An alternative hypothesis for the cause of posthepatectomy DGE involves injury to branches of the anterior vagal trunk coursing through the gastrohepatic ligament, which is typically divided during dissection and mobilization of the liver [15]. In particular, injury to the nerves of Latarjet, the vagal efferents that innervate the gastric antrum and pylorus, may compromise antral contractility and pyloric relaxation, ultimately resulting in delayed emptying and retention [16]. Symptom onset during the immediate postoperative period after hepatectomy is consistent with a neurovascular etiology. Moreover, in the cases of both KS and IS, the injection of botulinum toxin into the pylorus promptly led to symptom resolution. Botulinum toxin, which blocks the release of acetylcholine into neuronal synapses, decreases pyloric muscle activity when injected locally and has been reported to reduce symptoms in gastroparesis patients [17]. The efficacy of intrapyloric botulinum toxin injection in the cases of KS and IS indicates that impaired pyloric relaxation may contribute to posthepatectomy DGE, and our observation is consistent with the possibility that injury to vagal nerve branches innervating the pylorus may be the cause.

Notably, both of our cases involved a replaced left hepatic artery, an anatomical variant in which the left hepatic artery arises not from the proper hepatic artery as in normal anatomy but from the left gastric artery. In the context of performing a left hepatectomy for liver donation, a replaced left hepatic artery requires surgeons to perform a more extensive dissection of the gastrohepatic ligament in order to prepare the arterial graft from the left gastric artery. Greater dissection within this area increases the risk of vagal nerve injury and may therefore increase the risk of DGE. To our knowledge, the relationship between replaced vascular anatomy and risk of DGE after hepatectomy has not yet been investigated, but several groups have previously suggested that increased manipulation of the hepatic hilum may result in higher risk of DGE after surgery [8, 9, 18]. The presence of a replaced left hepatic artery in both cases of KS and IS required us to thoroughly dissect the gastrohepatic ligament and take down neurovascular branches to the lesser curvature of the stomach, a process that may have contributed to the onset of DGE in the immediate postoperative period.

Overall, based on our experience and specifically the cases of KS and IS, we favor the hypothesis that extensive dissection of the gastrohepatic ligament may increase the risk of posthepatectomy DGE due to increased risk of damage to vagal branches in the area. Further studies involving larger case collections and multicenter experiences are required to elucidate the true mechanism underlying the development of DGE after living donor hepatectomy.

Acknowledgment

The authors thank Mark A. Hardy, M.D., for his guidance and suggestions.

References

[1] K. Umeshita, K. Fujiwara, K. Kiyosawa et al., "Operative morbidity of living liver donors in Japan," *The Lancet*, vol. 362, no. 9385, pp. 687–690, 2003.

[2] A. Taketomi, H. Kayashima, Y. Soejima et al., "Donor risk in adult-to-adult living donor liver transplantation: impact of left lobe graft," *Transplantation*, vol. 87, no. 3, pp. 445–450, 2009.

[3] B. Samstein, D. Cherqui, F. Rotellar et al., "Totally laparoscopic full left hepatectomy for living donor liver transplantation in adolescents and adults," *The American Journal of Transplantation*, vol. 13, no. 9, pp. 2462–2466, 2013.

[4] S.-J. Kim, G.-H. Na, H.-J. Choi, Y.-K. Yoo, and D.-G. Kim, "Surgical outcome of right liver donors in living donor liver transplantation: single-center experience with 500 cases," *Journal of Gastrointestinal Surgery*, vol. 16, no. 6, pp. 1160–1170, 2012.

[5] A. Kinoshita, M. Takatsuki, M. Hidaka, A. Soyama, S. Eguchi, and T. Kanematsu, "Prevention of gastric stasis by omentum patching after living donor left hepatectomy," *Surgery Today*, vol. 42, no. 8, pp. 816–818, 2012.

[6] H. Yoshida, Y. Mamada, N. Taniai et al., "Fixation of the greater omentum for prevention of delayed gastric emptying after left-sided hepatectomy: a randomized controlled trial," *Hepato-Gastroenterology*, vol. 52, no. 65, pp. 1334–1337, 2005.

[7] H. Yoshida, Y. Mamada, N. Taniai et al., "Fixation of the greater omentum for prevention of delayed gastric emptying after left hepatectomy with lymphadenectomy for cholangiocarcinoma," *Journal of Hepato-Biliary-Pancreatic Surgery*, vol. 14, no. 4, pp. 392–396, 2007.

[8] T. Oida, K. Mimatsu, A. Kawasaki, H. Kanou, Y. Kuboi, and S. Amano, "Fixation of the round ligament to the peritoneum and wrapping of the cut surface of the liver for prevention of early delayed gastric emptying after hepatic lateral segmentectomy," *Langenbeck's Archives of Surgery*, vol. 395, no. 6, pp. 655–659, 2010.

[9] T. Igami, H. Nishio, T. Ebata, Y. Yokoyama, G. Sugawara, and M. Nagino, "Using the greater omental flap to cover the cut surface of the liver for prevention of delayed gastric emptying after left-

sided hepatobiliary resection: a prospective randomized controlled trial," *Journal of Hepato-Biliary-Pancreatic Sciences*, vol. 18, no. 2, pp. 176–183, 2011.

[10] A. Nanashima, S. Tobinaga, T. Abo et al., "Usefulness of omental wrapping to prevent biliary leakage and delayed gastric emptying in left hepatectomy," *Hepato-Gastroenterology*, vol. 59, no. 115, pp. 847–850, 2012.

[11] C. S. Park, S. Hwang, C. S. Ahnm et al., "A comparative study regarding the effect of an intraperitoneal anti-adhesive agent application in left-liver living donors," *Korean Journal of Hepato-Biliary-Pancreatic Surgery*, vol. 18, no. 1, pp. 26–28, 2014.

[12] H. Uchiyama, K. Shirabe, H. Nakagawara et al., "Revisiting the safety of living liver donors by reassessing 441 donor hepatectomies: is a larger hepatectomy complication-prone?" *American Journal of Transplantation*, vol. 14, no. 2, pp. 367–374, 2014.

[13] C. N. Gutt, T. Oniu, P. Schemmer, A. Mehrabi, and M. W. Büchler, "Fewer adhesions induced by laparoscopic surgery?" *Surgical Endoscopy*, vol. 18, no. 6, pp. 898–906, 2004.

[14] S. E. Burpee, M. Kurian, Y. Murakame, S. Benevides, and M. Gagner, "The metabolic and immune response to laparoscopic vs open liver resection," *Surgical Endoscopy*, vol. 16, no. 6, pp. 899–904, 2002.

[15] J. F. Renz and J. P. Roberts, "Long-term complications of living donor liver transplantation," *Liver Transplantation*, vol. 6, no. 6, pp. S73–S76, 2000.

[16] R. A. Hejazi, H. P. Parkman, and R. W. McCallum, "Postsurgical gastroparesis," in *Gastroparesis: Pathophysiology, Presentation and Treatment*, H. P. Parkman and R. W. McCallum, Eds., Clinical Gastroenterology, pp. 191–203, Humana Press, New York, NY, USA, 2012.

[17] R. Coleski, M. A. Anderson, and W. L. Hasler, "Factors associated with symptom response to pyloric injection of botulinum toxin in a large series of gastroparesis patients," *Digestive Diseases and Sciences*, vol. 54, no. 12, pp. 2634–2642, 2009.

[18] A. C. A. Tannuri, N. E. M. Gibelli, L. R. S. Ricardi et al., "Living related donor liver transplantation in children," *Transplantation Proceedings*, vol. 43, no. 1, pp. 161–164, 2011.

3

Concurrent Hepatic Artery and Portal Vein Thrombosis after Orthotopic Liver Transplantation with Preserved Allografts

Arshad Khan,[1] P. Park,[1,2] Jose Oberholzer,[1] Ivo Tzvetanov,[1] Raquel Garcia Roca,[1] Ron C. Gaba,[3] Enrico Benedetti,[1] and Hoonbae Jeon[1,4]

[1] *Department of Surgery, College of Medicine, University of Illinois at Chicago, Chicago, IL 60612, USA*
[2] *Department of Surgery, Korea University Guro Hospital, 80 Guro-dong, Guro-gu, Seoul 152-703, Republic of Korea*
[3] *Department of Radiology, College of Medicine, University of Illinois at Chicago, Chicago, IL 60612, USA*
[4] *Division of Transplantation, Department of Surgery, College of Medicine, University of Illinois at Chicago, CSB Suite 402, MC 958, 840 South Wood Street, Chicago, IL 60612, USA*

Correspondence should be addressed to Hoonbae Jeon; jeonhb@uic.edu

Academic Editors: P. Boraschi, D. Conti, and Y. Sugawara

In contrast to early HAT, late HAT has an insidious clinical presentation. Nevertheless, biliary and vascular reconstructions in this late setting are unlikely to improve outcome. Patent portal flow makes an important contribution to the viability of liver in case of late HAT while the allograft reconstitutes intrahepatic arterial flow through neovascularization. Concurrent HAT with PVT without immediate graft necrosis is extremely rare, and allograft and patient survival are seemingly impossible without retransplantation. In fact, hepatopetal arterial and portal venous neovascularization are known albeit obscure phenomena that can preserve posttransplant hepatic function under the extenuating circumstances of complete interruption of blood flow to the graft. We describe two such cases that developed combined HAT and PVT more than six months after OLT with perfect preservation of graft function. The survival of allografts in our cases was due to extensive hepatopetal arterial and portal venous collateralization. Simultaneous HAT and PVT after OLT are rare events and almost uniformly fatal, if they occur early. Due to paucity of such cases, however, underlying mechanisms and etiology remain elusive, and despite radiological diagnosis of these complications, there is no way to predict these events in the wake of stable graft function.

1. Introduction

The critical determinants of a successful liver transplant procedure are establishment of uncompromised inflow and adequate venous outflow. However, the postoperative course can be marred by vascular complications involving the HA and PV which are associated with high morbidity and mortality [1].

Although HAT and PVT occur infrequently, they pose a major threat to patient and graft survival and present formidable challenges for prevention and treatment. HAT has an incidence of 4–15% and when present in isolation may lead to acute graft failure and biliary destruction requiring retransplantation in most cases. Mortality may be as high as 27–58% and may increase to 73% when retransplantation is not carried out [2].

PVT complicates 2% of liver transplants and also can be fatal. It can present as portal hypertension, elevated transaminases, and acute graft failure [3]. While an increase in HA flow routinely accompanies a decrease in PV flow, the opposite does not characteristically occur and presents important implications in case of vascular compromise.

In the event of hepatic artery compromise the portal vein is the main source of hepatic blood flow and the liver responds by extracting greater amount of oxygen from portal blood and inducing neovascularization while viability is maintained by portal blood flow. Isolated portal vein thrombosis has been shown to cause hepatic infarction in the absence of arterial compromise [4].

If not recognized in timely manner, PVT leads to graft failure and retransplantation or patients death [5].

However, the biliary ductal system is solely supplied by HA via peribiliary plexus (PBP). Recent reports have indicated important contribution by portal circulation, as ischemic type biliary lesions (ITBL) develop in patients with a patent hepatic artery and thrombosed PV, implying altered microcirculation in PBP in face of intact arterial supply. This suggests that portal blood flow, while not only supplying hepatocytes, may make an important contribution to the biliary microcirculation and that compromised portal venous blood supply alone can predispose to the development of ITBL which necessitates retransplantation in 50% of such cases [6]. Thus, the HA and PV interplay in a harmonious way to preserve the hepatic viability when arterial or venous flow is jeopardized.

Given this fact it can be easily conceived that concurrent early HAT and PVT will have a devastating effect on biliary ductal system and hepatocytes necessitating transplantation. This notion is supported by few case reports in the literature showing prohibitive mortality in combined HAT and PVT [7]. There is not much information about the outcome of late concurrent HAT and PVT on the allograft due to extreme paucity of such cases in the literature.

With this in mind, we herein present two unique cases of concurrent late HAT and PVT in which patients survived many years after transplantation with normal graft function. The survival of the allograft in the present cases was due to extensive hepatopetal arterial and portal venous neovascularization.

2. Case Reports

Case 1. A 47-year-old female with a diagnosis of unresectable hilar cholangiocarcinoma had undergone biliary stents placement, neoadjuvant chemoradiation, brachytherapy, and maintenance chemotherapy according to the Mayo protocol. She subsequently underwent OLT. Concomitant pancreatoduodenectomy with native hepatectomy was performed to completely excise the distal bile duct possibly bearing malignancy and to approach the nonirradiated segment of the portal vein. The anastomosis of the portal vein was performed at the level of confluence between superior mesenteric and splenic veins in end-to-end fashion. The hepatic artery was reconstructed through an infrarenal aortic conduit using a donor iliac artery and the common hepatic artery of the recipient was ligated to avoid anastomosis to irradiated inflow vessel. After that, the continuity of pancreatobiliary and gastrointestinal tracts was restored.

On the 7th postoperative day, acute PVT was diagnosed on duplex US and triple phase CT, with subsequent confirmation by mesenteric angiography. Portal vein thrombectomy and anastomotic revision were urgently performed. There was no evidence of ischemic damage to the allograft. A thorough evaluation for hypercoagulable condition did not reveal any abnormalities and empirical anticoagulation with warfarin was started.

Six months after transplantation, the patient presented to the hospital with vague diffuse abdominal pain despite all normal laboratory values and therapeutic INR of 2.5 on warfarin, and surveillance DUS discovered PVT and lack of extra hepatic arterial flow. On CT, despite totally obstructive HAT and PVT, the graft liver was well enhanced without perfusion defect or infarcted area. Angiography revealed multiple arterial collaterals supplying the graft. Collaterals from right intercostal arteries, a right adrenal artery, and jejunal branches from superior mesenteric artery were confirmed with angiogram as shown in Figures 1(a), 1(b), and 1(c). Three years after transplantation, the patient remains alive and well with stable allograft function and no complication.

Case 2. A 66-year-old male underwent OLT for alcoholic cirrhosis. Operation was done in a piggy bag fashion without venovenous bypass. Bile duct continuity was restored by duct-to-duct anastomosis. Patient had an uneventful postoperative course and two years later developed cyclosporine induced kidney failure for which he received a living donor kidney transplant. The patient also had recurrent episodes of lower extremity DVT and was on warfarin therapy. Six years later he was admitted to undergo colonoscopy for bleeding per rectum and warfarin therapy was withheld in preparation for colonoscopy. Simultaneously patient developed some derangement of liver function and underwent duplex ultrasonography and MRI of liver, which revealed a homogenous hepatic lesion at the dome of liver, intrahepatic portal vein thrombosis, and patency of hepatic artery but a slurring of systolic upstroke. Tumor markers were normal (AFP = 5.4 mcg/L, CEA = 0.6 mcg/L). Thrombophilic workup was unrevealing. Biopsy of the liver lesion revealed normal liver architecture and no rejection. In view of extensive portal vein thrombosis as shown in Figures 2(a) and 2(b), a catheter directed thrombolysis with TPA was done with only partial improvement in flow which was short lasting and was complicated by progressive thrombosis of PV. The thrombolysis was followed by mild transaminitis and a pseudoaneurysm formation in the right lobe of liver. In order to delineate this anatomically a celiac angiogram was done which revealed complete occusion of common hepatic artery of the aloograft. Innumerable small collaterals arising from gastroepiploic artery and gastroduodenal artery were seen supplying the liver reconstituting intrahepatic arterial supply as shown in Figures 2(c) and 2(d). Serial multiple follow-up DUS and MRI confirmed the blockage of dual blood supply to liver. During this entire course the liver function stayed completely normal. Three years after dual thrombosis, the patient is alive and well with stable allograft function and no complication.

3. Discussion

Complete devascularization of the native liver is difficult to achieve due to the dual blood supply and number of collaterals which develop in case of vascular interruption. Total hepatectomy at the time of transplant disrupts these collaterals; however, allograft may survive only on the portal flow while arterial collaterals develop over few weeks [8]. When the complete dearterialization of native liver is achieved experimentally, extensive necrosis is not averted

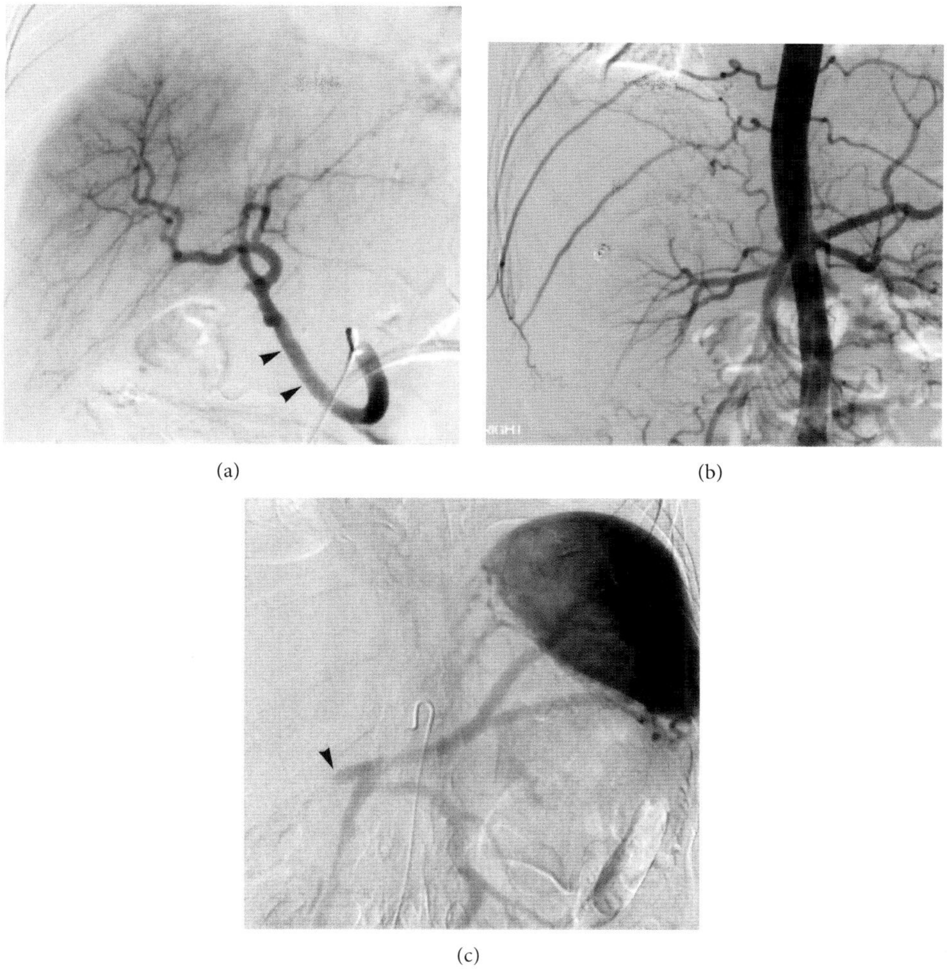

FIGURE 1: Digital subtraction angiogram (DSA) (a) shows patent iliac artery to hepatic artery graft (arrowheads). Digital subtraction aorta gram (b) demonstrates lack of iliac artery to hepatic artery graft opacification, indicating occlusion. Delayed venous phase imaging (c) reveals concurrent proximal portal vein occlusion (arrowhead).

by intact portal circulation [9] and an anecdotal series has shown death rate in excess of 50% with accidental hepatic artery ligation [10]. In contrast, a recent report in which the hepatic artery was ligated for HA rupture following liver transplantation found that all 6 patients with HA ligation were alive, though some patients required adjunctive procedures [11]. Another anecdotal report by Tygstrup et al. showed that, with occlusion of the proper hepatic artery, extraction of oxygen from the portal venous blood increased, thereby compensating for the loss of the arterial supply. They concluded that, under ordinary circumstances, the hepatic artery could be ligated with impunity [12].

The foregoing data have made it clear that an effective compensatory mechanism of increased oxygen extraction from the portal venous blood is ordinarily sufficient to maintain hepatic viability. It suggested that many of the fatalities which have followed interruption of the HA are probably due to factors which either have further increased hepatic oxygen needs or have reduced the volume of portal flow like fever, atelectasis, cardiac failure, and shock.

Similarly in case of interruption of portal blood flow due to PVT, which accounts for two-thirds of total liver blood flow, the liver allograft has the tendency to survive in most of the cases due to arterial buffer response and rapid development of collaterals, which become apparent in several days, reconstituting the intrahepatic blood flow [13].

We believe that the predisposing factors for vascular thrombosis in our first patient were generalized hypercoagulable state due to previous malignancy, the presence of aortohepatic conduit, and surgical reconstruction of portal vein and portal venous thrombectomy as shown by others [3, 14]. Of note, because of the increased risk of post-transplant vascular complications due to preoperative radiotherapy, aortohepatic conduit using cadaveric iliac artery graft was recommended to avoid late arterial complications. Nonetheless, any modification of portal vein reconstruction has not been recommended because large veins are less damaged by irradiation [15]. It has been reported that infrarenal aortohepatic conduit is an effective option for reconstruction of the hepatic artery of the transplant liver

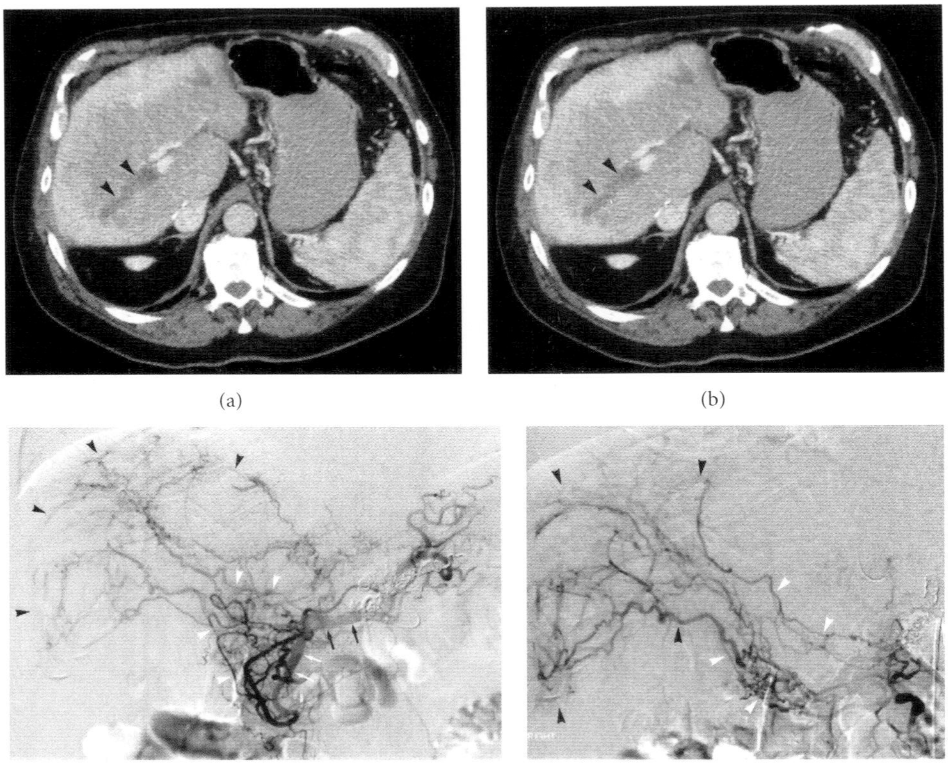

(a) (b) (c) (d)

FIGURE 2: Axial contrast enhanced CT scan image (a) reveals right-sided intrahepatic portal vein thrombosis (arrowheads). Thrombus (arrowhead) extends into main portal vein on more caudal image (b). Subtracted common hepatic arteriogram (a) demonstrates chronic proper hepatic artery occlusion with transplant liver perfusion (black arrowheads) via mature pancreaticoduodenal collateral vessels (white arrowheads). Black and white arrows delineate common hepatic artery and gastroduodenal artery, respectively. Selective gastroduodenal arteriogram (b) better demonstrates mature pancreaticoduodenal collateral vessels (white arrowheads), which result in transplant liver perfusion (black arrowheads).

and the long-term graft survival is comparable to that of control group, despite the higher incidence of HAT [16]. The second patient had percutaneous biopsy of the liver and subsequently TAE of hepatic pseudoaneurysm as a sequel of biopsy. We believe that TAE of pseudoaneurysm resulted in traumatizing hepatic artery resulting in increased periarterial inflammation, friability, and predisposition to thrombosis as has been reported previously [3]. Furthermore, during these invasive procedures accidental cannulation of portal vein changed the hemodynamics of portal system and these treatments triggered thrombosis similar to a previous report [17]. It is difficult to know the pathophysiology and effects of concurrent HA and PVT on morbidity and mortality following OLT due to paucity of such cases. After extensive search we are able to retrieve cases as shown in Table 1.

In our two cases, the concurrent HA and PVT were detected during the follow-up and the liver function was pristine. The blood flow to the liver was reconstituted by various portal and arterial collaterals. Neovascularization of the ischemic liver is an obscure phenomenon and various mechanisms have been proposed. Some ascribe a role to angiogenic properties of omentum and mesentery [20]. Others proposed opening and dilatation of vasa vasorum along the hepatic artery and capillaries and venules around the portal vein. Since during the implantation of liver all of these connections are severed, it has been proposed that this neovascularization may occur de novo and the precise mechanisms are not fully understood. Experiments of hepatic ischemia in murine model lead to upregulation of VEGF, a key factor which triggers neovascularization. Moreover exogenous recombinant VEGF can induce angiogenesis in a host [21]. Furthermore, correlation between prolonged hepatic hypoxia and angiogenesis was found by Panaro et al. implying an association between the HAT and neovascularization [22]. In the transplant setting, ischemic liver could trigger an enzymatic cascade for angiogenesis leading to neovascularization from surrounding arterial and venous territories [21].

In the present two cases we opine that neovascularization might have been triggered by the ischemic liver late in the posttransplant period as the liver got ischemic or the neovascularization might have occurred time ahead of the dual thrombosis permitting the survival of allografts. Robustness of the collateral circulation was elucidated by angiography in both of these cases. Neovascularized hepatic allografts that had suffered late HAT and PVT may survive, though

Table 1: Depiction of cases with concurrent HAT and PVT in the literature.

Author (year)	Number of patients/type	Indications for transplant	Type of transplant	HAT and PVT in relation to transplant	Treatment	Outcome
Langnas et al. (1991) [1]	3/2 children, 1 adult	Biliary atresia 2, cholangiocarcinoma 1	CLTx	Within a week	Adult Re-Tx, 1st child Re-Tx, 2nd child observation	2 deaths, 1 child in vegetative state at 4 years
Kaneko et al. (2004) [7]	4/2 children, 2 adults	Biliary atresia 1, Wilson's disease 1, PBC 1, primary hyperoxaluria 1	LDLTx	Within a week	3 thrombectomy, 1 RE-Tx	4 deaths
Haque et al. (2009) [18]	1 adult	Wilson's disease 1	CLTx	12 years	Conservative	Alive at one year after the event
Ayala et al. (2011) [19]	1 adult	NA	CLTx	NA	NA	NA
Present series (2013)	2 adults	Cholangiocarcinoma 1, alcoholic cirrhosis 1	CLTx	6 months 6 years	Conservative	Alive with normal liver function at 3 years

CLTx: cadaveric liver transplant, LDLTx: living donor liver transplant, Re-Tx: retransplantation, NA: not available.

there remains an increased risk of development of ischemic cholangiopathy [22].

4. Conclusion

Concurrent HAT and PVT early in the aftermath of OLT are devastating complications leading to loss of allograft and necessitating retransplantation. However if the event occurs late, simple observation may suffice provided that the robustness of collateral circulation and reconstitution of intrahepatic blood flow are elucidated angiographically. Nonetheless, these allografts should have more rigorous surveillance due to high risk of ischemic cholangiopathy.

Abbreviations

HAT: Hepatic artery thrombosis
PVT: Portal vein thrombosis
OLT: Orthotopic liver transplantation
TAE: Transarterial embolization
HA: Hepatic artery
PV: Portal vein
PBP: Peribiliary plexus
ITBL: Ischemic type biliary lesions
DUS: Doppler ultrasound
DVT: Deep venous thrombosis.

References

[1] A. N. Langnas, W. Marujo, R. J. Stratta, R. P. Wood, and B. W. Shaw Jr., "Vascular complications after orthotopic liver transplantation," *The American Journal of Surgery*, vol. 161, no. 1, pp. 76–83, 1991.

[2] A. G. Tzakis, R. D. Gordon, B. W. Shaw Jr., S. Iwatsuki, and T. E. Starzl, "Clinical presentation of hepatic artery thrombosis after liver transplantation in the cyclosporine era," *Transplantation*, vol. 40, no. 6, pp. 667–671, 1985.

[3] J. P. Duffy, J. C. Hong, D. G. Farmer et al., "Vascular complications of orthotopic liver transplantation: experience in more than 4,200 patients," *Journal of the American College of Surgeons*, vol. 208, no. 5, pp. 896–903, 2009.

[4] A. Gladysz-Polak, W. G. Polak, P. Jazwiec et al., "Favorable resolution of hepatic infarctions in transplanted liver after portal vein thrombosis treated by surgical thrombectomy: a case report," *Transplantation Proceedings*, vol. 38, no. 9, pp. 3135–3137, 2006.

[5] J. Lerut, A. G. Tzakis, K. Bron et al., "Complications of venous reconstruction in human orthotopic liver transplantation," *Annals of Surgery*, vol. 205, no. 4, pp. 404–414, 1987.

[6] W. R. R. Farid, J. de Jonge, J. C. Slieker et al., "The importance of portal venous blood flow in ischemic-type biliary lesions after liver transplantation," *American Journal of Transplantation*, vol. 11, no. 4, pp. 857–862, 2011.

[7] J. Kaneko, Y. Sugawara, J. Togashi, Y. Kishi, N. Akamatsu, and M. Makuuchi, "Simultaneous hepatic artery and portal vein thrombosis after living donor liver transplantation," *Transplantation Proceedings*, vol. 36, no. 10, pp. 3087–3089, 2004.

[8] S. Bengmark and K. Rosengren, "Angiographic study of the collateral circulation to the liver after ligation of the hepatic artery in man," *The American Journal of Surgery*, vol. 119, no. 6, pp. 620–624, 1970.

[9] H. Stridbeck, L. E. Lorelius, and S. R. Reuter, "Collateral circulation following repeated distal embolization of the hepatic

artery in pigs," *Investigative Radiology*, vol. 19, no. 3, pp. 179–183, 1984.

[10] R. R. Graham and D. Cannell, "Accidental ligation of the hepatic artery," *British Journal of Surgery*, vol. 20, no. 80, pp. 566–579, 1933.

[11] E. Boleslawski, A. F. Bourse, S. Truant et al., "Hepatic artery ligation for the arterial rupture following liver transplantation: a reasonable option," *American Journal of Transplantation*, vol. 13, no. 4, pp. 1055–1062, 2013.

[12] N. Tygstrup, K. Winkler, K. Mellemgaard, and M. Andreassen, "Determination of the hepatic arterial blood flow and oxygen supply in man by clamping the hepatic artery during surgery," *The Journal of Clinical Investigation*, vol. 41, pp. 447–454, 1962.

[13] J. M. Henderson, G. T. Gilmore, G. J. Mackay, J. R. Galloway, T. F. Dodson, and M. H. Kutner, "Hemodynamics during liver transplantation: the interactions between cardiac output and portal venous and hepatic arterial flows," *Hepatology*, vol. 16, no. 3, pp. 715–718, 1992.

[14] Y. Kishi, Y. Sugawara, Y. Matsui, N. Akamatsu, and M. Makuuchi, "Late onset portal vein thrombosis and its risk factors," *Hepato-Gastroenterology*, vol. 55, no. 84, pp. 1008–1009, 2008.

[15] H. T. J. Mantel, C. B. Rosen, J. K. Helmbach et al., "Vascular complications after orthotopic liver transplantation after neoadjuvant therapy for hilar cholangiocarcinoma," *Liver Transplantation*, vol. 13, no. 10, pp. 1372–1381, 2007.

[16] D. Nikitin, L. W. Jennings, T. Khan et al., "Twenty years of follow-up of aortohepatic conduits in liver transplantation," *Liver Transplantation*, vol. 14, no. 10, pp. 1486–1490, 2008.

[17] K. Yamashita, H. Tsukuda, Y. Mizukami et al., "Hepatic infarction with portal thrombosis," *Journal of Gastroenterology*, vol. 32, no. 5, pp. 684–688, 1997.

[18] M. Haque, P. A. Schumacher, A. Harris et al., "Late acute celiac and hepatic artery thrombosis with portal vein thrombosis resulting in hepatic infarction 12 years post orthotopic liver transplantation," *Annals of Hepatology*, vol. 8, no. 4, pp. 396–399, 2009.

[19] R. Ayala, J. Martínez-López, T. Cedena et al., "Recepient and donor thrombophilia and the risk of portal venous thrombosis and hepatic artery thrombosis in liver recipients," *BMC Gastroenterology*, vol. 11, no. 1, article 130, 2011.

[20] J. W. Yedlicka Jr., J. Halloran, W. D. Payne et al., "Angiogenesis after hepatic arterial occlusion in liver transplant patients," *Journal of Vascular and Interventional Radiology*, vol. 2, no. 2, pp. 235–240, 1991.

[21] Y. Tsurui, M. Sho, Y. Kuzumoto et al., "Dual role of vascular endothelial growth factor in hepatic ischemia-reperfusion injury," *Transplantation*, vol. 79, no. 9, pp. 1110–1115, 2005.

[22] F. Panaro, B. Gallix, H. Bouyabrine et al., "Liver transplantation and spontaneous neovascularization after arterial thrombosis: 'the neovascularized liver'," *Transplant International*, vol. 24, no. 9, pp. 949–957, 2011.

4

Point of Care Perioperative Coagulation Management in Liver Transplantation and Complete Portal Vein Thrombosis

Cristiano Piangatelli,[1] Lucia Faloia,[2] Claudia Cristiani,[1] Ilaria Valentini,[1] and Marco Vivarelli[3]

[1] *Division of Anaesthesia and Resuscitation, Department of Emergency, Ospedali Riuniti, Via Conca 71, 60020 Ancona, Italy*
[2] *Department of Emergency, Anesthesia and Resuscitation Unit, Università Politecnica delle Marche, Via Conca 71, 60020 Ancona, Italy*
[3] *Department of Liver Surgery and Transplantation, Ospedali Riuniti, Via Conca 71, 60020 Ancona, Italy*

Correspondence should be addressed to Lucia Faloia; luciafaloia@libero.it

Academic Editors: C. Costa and S. Faenza

Liver transplantation (LT) is a serious hemostatic challenge in patients with portal vein thrombosis (PVT). Advances in monitoring systems have improved surgery in this setting. We report the successful application of a point-of-care (POC) rotational viscoelastic thromboelastometry-guided (TEM) testing system (ROTEM) which allowed management of coagulation during LT in a 64-year-old cirrhotic patient with a model for end-stage liver disease (MELD) score of 16. Perioperatively, the patient showed complete PVT, hepatomegaly, splenomegaly, recanalization of the umbilical vein, and portosystemic shunt. Macroscopic liver and spleen adherences with collateral circulation were evident. Coagulation factors and fibrinolysis were assessed preoperatively and at graft reperfusion to evaluate the need of hemostatic therapy. Based on ROTEM findings, the patient received 16 g of human fibrinogen concentrate, half preoperatively (with prothrombin complex concentrate 2000 IU, tranexamic acid 1 g, and platelets 2 IU), and two doses of 4 g before and after graft reperfusion; we achieved normalization of all monitored parameters. No ischemia-reperfusion syndrome was present. Postoperatively portal vein flux at Color-Doppler ultrasonography was normal. After a 3-day ICU stay, the patient was moved to the Department of Surgery and discharged on day 14. The postoperative course was uneventful and did not require any further haemostatic therapy.

1. Introduction

Chronic liver disease affects hemostasis via three predominant mechanisms: reduced synthesis of coagulation factors and inhibitors, thrombocytopenia and/or thrombocytopathy, and altered fibrinolysis. Liver transplantation (LT) is a serious haemostatic challenge faced by patients with chronic liver disease [1], as the risk of coagulopathic bleeding adds to surgical bleeding. In liver cirrhosis, portal hypertension may induce the formation of collateral vessels that drain portal blood directly into the general circulation, bypassing the liver and causing congestion of the portal area [2]. This situation may dramatically increase surgical bleeding during LT. Portal vein thrombosis (PVT) may decrease the portal flow worsening portal hypertension [3], a condition which shows an incidence of 2–26% in patients with end-stage liver disease which are candidates to LT [4] and who demonstrate exacerbate bleeding during hepatectomy.

LT is always a complex surgical procedure; its complexity increases even more in patients with PVT [5] and in the past PVT used to be considered an absolute contraindication for surgery [6]. However, the advancement in surgical techniques in the last two decades allows now for successfully performing LT in these difficult patients also.

2. A Case Report

We describe a point-of-care (POC) system used to successfully manage intraoperative coagulation in a 64-yearold man with hepatitis C virus- (HCV-) related liver cirrhosis and

PVT undergoing LT. Our technique assessed the need of prophylactic intraoperative administration of coagulation factor concentrates based on a thromboelastometry-guided (TEM) viscoelastic testing.

The patient had a model for end-stage liver disease (MELD) score of 16 and was listed for cadaveric liver transplantation. At a perioperative abdominal computer tomography with contrast, the patient showed a complete portal vein thrombosis, hepatomegaly, splenomegaly, recanalization of the umbilical vein, and portosystemic shunt. We obtained normalization of all parameters, respect ROTEM reference values [7] (Table 1). A point-of-care (POC) rotational TEM device (ROTEM, Tem International GmbH, Munich, Germany) was used to perform EXTEM and FIBTEM assays. Coagulation factors and fibrinolysis were performed preoperatively, immediately before graft reperfusion to assess the need of administration of hemostatic therapy, and repeated after 20 min from reperfusion.

The patient received general anesthesia and routine vascular accesses were inserted: the right jugular vein was cannulated with a high-flow trilumen catheter (AVA Edwards Lifesciences, Irvine, CA, USA), and a Swan-Ganz catheter (Edwards Lifesciences, Irvine, CA, USA) was inserted. The right femoral artery was cannulated and a peripheral high-flow catheter was placed in the right arm.

Blood temperature was continuously monitored and maintained at >36°C with forced-air and fluid-warming devices.

After surgical opening of the peritoneum and aspiration of ascites, liver and spleen macroscopic adherences with collateral circulation were evident. The clinical picture was indicative of a potential important surgical bleeding, which could be worsened by a concomitant hepatic insufficiency related bleeding. Perioperatively, ROTEM findings suggested an increased clotting time (CT), a reduction in α angle, probably due to a hypofibrinogenemia supported by the value of the maximum clot firmness (MCF) assessed with FIBTEM test, and a modest fibrinolysis, according to the value of EXTEM ML30%. On the basis of these values, which are shown in Table 1, preoperatively the patient received in this order 8 g human fibrinogen concentrate (Haemocomplettan P, CSL Behring, Marburg, Germany), 2,000 IU prothrombin complex concentrate (Human Complex Kedrion Biopharma, Castelvecchio Pascoli, Italy), 2 IU platelet concentrate, and 1 g tranexamic acid.

Immediately after therapy, the TEM tests were repeated and showed normalization of parameters without any evidence of pathological clot lysis (see Table 1). Warm ischaemia time was approximately 35 min, fully consistent with usual practice (approximately 35 min).

ROTEM testing performed before reperfusion of the graft showed low levels of blood fibrinogen leading to the administration of a first 4 g dose of fibrinogen. Measurements were repeated 20 mins after reperfusion and values resulting indicated a reduced strength and/or stability of the clot; thus, a further dose of 4 g fibrinogen concentrate was administered. We obtained normalization of all parameters (Table 1). In total the patient received 8 g of fibrinogen concentrate. No ongoing bleeding was present at the time of fibrinogen administration. Arterial and biliary anastomosis were completed concurrently. No evidence of an ischaemia-reperfusion syndrome—a heparin effect of coagulation disorders after reperfusion—was apparent.

The patient was awakened and extubated as soon as the surgical intervention was concluded, as previously described [8]. After 12 hours from transplant, 100 mg daily ASA was started to reduce the risk of hepatic artery thrombosis. Portal vein flux measured with Color-Doppler ultrasonography during the patient's stay in intensive care unit (ICU) was normal. After a 3-day ICU stay, the patient was moved to the Department of Surgery and discharged on day 14 from surgery. The postoperative course was uneventful and did not require further haemostatic therapy.

3. Discussion

Coagulation disorders in liver cirrhosis are well documented. The hemostatic profile of a patient with chronic liver failure typically includes thrombocytopenia, reduced levels of coagulation factors and inhibitors, and unbalanced fibrinolysis [9]. In addition, LT is a challenging surgical procedure and is often associated with extensive bleeding. This surgery has the highest risk of hemorrhage due to the difficult removal of the native liver consequent to adherences and collateral vessels. Portal thrombosis may worsen portal hypertension, thus increasing bleeding during hepatectomy. The intraoperative bleeding can be even more worsened by a deficit of coagulation factors and lower force on coagulum, which are secondary to low levels of fibrinogen and/or platelet.

Viscoelastic testing enables dynamic assessment of clotting in whole blood and provides information on the procoagulant, anticoagulant, and fibrinolytic pathways, thus being a perioperative invaluable tool in LT [10–14]. The successful use of a POC-based ROTEM-guided algorithm for perioperative coagulation management of liver transplantation was previously described by Goerlinger et al. [14]. In contrast, several studies have demonstrated a poor correlation between alterations in conventional laboratory coagulation tests (PT, INR and aPTT) and any bleeding tendency caused by the rebalancing of procoagulant and anticoagulant factors in chronic liver failure [15].

In this case we adopted a restrictive transfusion strategy, associated with limited intraoperative blood loss, which allowed a correction of the CT with a prothrombin complex with coagulation factors (factors II, VII, IX, and X) that contain, also, natural inhibitors (such as proteins C and S).

In our case, we used a POC ROTEM System to identify and treat haemocoagulative alterations. Lisman and Leebeek [15] demonstrated in cirrhotic patients undergoing surgery that the hemostatic balance was preserved, with extremely low reserve. In fact, our patient showed hypofibrinogenemia, causing a reduced clot strength for limited interaction between fibrinogen and platelets.

Thrombocytopenia is present in cirrhotic patients due to splenic sequestration; as a consequence the action of intraoperative administration of platelets is short; moreover, platelet

Table 1: Preoperative ROTEM parameters before and after haemostatic therapy and perioperative values at graft reperfusion and after two rounds of haemostatic therapy.

ROTEM parameters assessed	Range of normal values	Preoperative values		Peri-operative values at graft reperfusion		
		Before therapy	After therapy*	Before reperfusion	After the 1st 4 g dose of fibrinogen concentrate	After the 2nd 4 g dose of fibrinogen concentrate (20 min from reperfusion)
EXTEM clotting time, CT (s)	42–74	28	54	42	43	43
EXTEM maximum clot firmness, mCF (mm)	49–71	35	65	36	50	61
EXTEM maximum lysis 30 min post CT, ML_{30} (%)	0–18	5	0	0	1	0
EXTEM α-angle (°)	63–81	28	70	40	66	72
FIBTEM maximum clot firmness, MCF (mm)	9–25	6	16	6	9	15

*Fibrinogen concentrate 8 g, prothrombin complex concentrate 2000 IU, tranexamic acid 1 g, and platelets 2 IU. EXTEM: extrinsic thromboelastometry assay incorporating recombinant tissue factor as activation enhancer; FIBTEM: fibrinogen thromboelastometry assay based on the EXTEM assay and incorporating cytochalasin D as platelet inhibitor; EXTEM α-angle (°): angle between the baseline and target to the clotting curve through the 2 mm point, it represents kinetic of platelet and fibrin polymerization.

infusion after the graft reperfusion causes an active translocation of platelets into sinusoidal and Disse's space with intrahepatic microthrombosis [16]. Platelets, moreover, are the blood component with the higher risk to induce TRALI (transfusion-related acute lung injury) due to the presence of many surface antigens [17]. Therefore, the administration of fibrinogen allows an improvement of the strength of the clot, also in the patients with low platelet count as shown by Lang et al. [18].

In summary, in the reported case we have demonstrated that optimizing coagulation through goal-directed, TEM-guided use of coagulation factor concentrates before and during surgery can reduce coagulopathic bleeding and subsequent PRCB and FFP (fresh frozen plasma) transfusion requirements in patients with PVT submitted to LT.

Acknowledgments

The authors thank the patient who has given his informed consent for the publication of this paper and Dr. AR Silini Ph.D. for linguistic assistance.

References

[1] L. N. Roberts, R. K. Patel, and R. Arya, "Haemostasis and thrombosis in liver disease," *British Journal of Haematology*, vol. 148, no. 4, pp. 507–521, 2010.

[2] H. Cichoz-Lach, K. Celiński, M. Słomka, and B. Kasztelan-Szczerbińska, "Pathophysiology of portal hypertension," *Journal of Physiology and Pharmacology*, vol. 59, supplement 2, pp. 231–238, 2008.

[3] D. Zhang, J. Hao, and N. Yang, "Protein C and D-dimer are related to portal vein thrombosis in patients with liver cirrhosis," *Journal of Gastroenterology and Hepatology*, vol. 25, no. 1, pp. 116–121, 2010.

[4] P. Bhangui, C. Lim, C. Salloum et al., "Caval inflow to the graft for liver transplantation in patients with diffuse portal vein thrombosis: a 12-Year experience," *Annals of Surgery*, vol. 254, no. 6, pp. 1008–1016, 2011.

[5] J. Hoekstra and H. L. A. Janssen, "Vascular liver disorders (II): portal vein thrombosis," *Netherlands Journal of Medicine*, vol. 67, no. 2, pp. 46–53, 2009.

[6] Y.-F. Tao, F. Teng, Z.-X. Wang et al., "Liver transplant recipients with portal vein thrombosis: a single center retrospective study," *Hepatobiliary and Pancreatic Diseases International*, vol. 8, no. 1, pp. 34–39, 2009.

[7] K. Görlinger, C. Jambor, A. A. Hanke et al., "Perioperative coagulation management and control of platelet transfusion by point-of-care platelet function analysis," *Transfusion Medicine and Hemotherapy*, vol. 34, no. 6, pp. 396–411, 2007.

[8] G. Biancofiore, M. L. Bindi, A. M. Romanelli et al., "Fast track in liver transplantation: 5 Years' experience," *European Journal of Anaesthesiology*, vol. 22, no. 8, pp. 584–590, 2005.

[9] T. Lisman and R. J. Porte, "Rebalanced hemostasis in patients with liver disease: evidence and clinical consequences," *Blood*, vol. 116, no. 6, pp. 878–885, 2010.

[10] J. Trzebicki, E. Flakiewicz, M. Kosieradzki et al., "The use of thromboelastometry in the assessment of hemostasis during orthotopic liver transplantation reduces the demand for blood products," *Annals of Transplantation*, vol. 15, no. 3, pp. 19–24, 2010.

[11] S.-C. Wang, J.-F. Shieh, K.-Y. Chang et al., "Thromboelastography-guided transfusion decreases intraoperative blood transfusion during orthotopic liver transplantation: randomized clinical trial," *Transplantation Proceedings*, vol. 42, no. 7, pp. 2590–2593, 2010.

[12] M. Coakley, K. Reddy, I. Mackie, and S. Mallett, "Transfusion triggers in orthotopic liver transplantation: a comparison of the thromboelastometry analyzer, the thromboelastogram, and conventional coagulation tests," *Journal of Cardiothoracic and Vascular Anesthesia*, vol. 20, no. 4, pp. 548–553, 2006.

[13] A. Stancheva, L. Spassov, and K. Tzatchev, "Correlation between rotation thrombelastometry ROTEM analysis and standard haemostatic parameters during liver transplantation," *Clinical Laboratory*, vol. 57, no. 5-6, pp. 407–413, 2011.

[14] K. Goerlinger, D. Dirkmann, A. Hanke, F. Dusse, and M. Hartmann, "ROTEM-based algorithm for point-of-care coagulation management in visceral surgery and liver transplantation: experience of eight years and 829 LTX," *Liver Transpantation*, vol. 14, supplement 1, pp. S203–S204, 2008.

[15] T. Lisman and F. W. G. Leebeek, "Hemostatic alterations in liver disease: a review on pathophysiology, clinical consequences, and treatment," *Digestive Surgery*, vol. 24, no. 4, pp. 250–258, 2007.

[16] D. Sindram, R. J. Porte, M. R. Hoffman, R. C. Bentley, and P. A. Clavien, "Synergism between platelets and leukocytes in inducing endothelial cell apoptosis in the cold ischemic rat liver: a Kupffer cell-mediated injury," *The FASEB Journal*, vol. 15, no. 7, pp. 1230–1232, 2001.

[17] G. Liumbruno, F. Bennardello, A. Lattanzio, P. Piccoli, and G. Rossetti, "Recommendations for the transfusion of plasma and platelets," *Blood Transfusion*, vol. 7, no. 2, pp. 132–150, 2009.

[18] T. Lang, K. Johanning, H. Metzler et al., "The effects of fibrinogen levels on thromboelastometric variables in the presence of thrombocytopenia," *Anesthesia and Analgesia*, vol. 108, no. 3, pp. 751–758, 2009.

5

ABO-Incompatible Living Donor Liver Transplantation from Hepatitis B Core Antibody Positive Donor to Hepatitis C Liver Cirrhosis Recipient

Akira Umemura, Hiroyuki Nitta, Akira Sasaki, Takeshi Takahara, Yasushi Hasegawa, and Go Wakabayashi

Department of Surgery, Iwate Medical University, 19-1 Uchimaru, Morioka 020-8505, Japan

Correspondence should be addressed to Akira Umemura; aumemura@iwate-med.ac.jp

Academic Editor: Yasuhiko Sugawara

Herein, we describe an extremely rare experience of a patient with liver cirrhosis from hepatitis C virus (LC-HCV) who underwent an ABO-incompatible living donor liver transplantation (ABO-I-LDLT) using a hepatitis B core antibody (HBc-Ab) positive donor's liver graft. A 47-year-old Japanese woman with end stage LC-HCV, as a recipient, was preoperatively administered rituximab, mycophenolate mofetil, and steroids without plasma exchange. A routine ABO-I-LDLT procedure was applied using her daughter's HBc-Ab positive liver graft. Prophylaxis of the hepatitis B virus (HBV) infection using hepatitis B immunoglobulin (HBIG) and entecavir had been properly administered. Three months after the ABO-I-LDLT, HCV hepatitis relapsed. To date, this patient has been under antiviral therapy and prophylaxis of HBV infection using HBIG, while entecavir has been continued. The cognitions and techniques with regard to ABO-I-LDLT, prophylaxis of HBV cross infection, various patterns of immunosuppression, and antiviral therapy for HCV relapse are indispensable in managing a transplant recipient. According to the prophylaxis of HBV cross infection under ABO-I-LDLT, it may be very important to keep the HBs-Ab titer higher than usual for HBV naïve recipients, because severe systemic immunosuppression can cause *de novo* hepatitis.

1. Introduction

Liver cirrhosis by hepatitis C virus (LC-HCV) is a common indication for living donor liver transplantation (LDLT), with the advancement of surgical procedures and antiviral therapies [1]. According to the hepatitis B core antibody (HBc-Ab) positive donor in LDLT, liver grafts can be safely used for hepatitis B surface antigen (HBs-Ag) negative recipients under the administration of prophylaxis using hepatitis B immunoglobulin (HBIG) and entecavir [2]. However, although ABO-incompatible LDLT (ABO-I-LDLT) in adults has not exhibited satisfactory graft survival rates and incidences of complications [3], the employment of plasma exchange (PE), portal vein infusion therapy (PVIT), and immunosuppressive treatment targeted to B cells using rituximab has dramatically improved the outcome [4–6].

In Japan, however, the number of deceased donor liver transplantations (DDLT) has gradually increased since the enforcement of a new law on organ transplantation in 2010, but LDLT is still the most frequent treatment option for patients with end-stage liver disease because of the organ shortage [4, 7]. Patients with end-stage liver disease commonly give up if living donors are not available, and given this unique social context in Japan, we describe our extremely rare experience with an LC-HCV patient who underwent ABO-I-LDLT using an HBc-Ab positive donor's liver graft.

2. Case Report

A 47-year-old Japanese woman with a history of transfusion during labor was diagnosed with LC-HCV and administered liver supporting therapy for several years. After noticing a distension of her abdomen and icteric skin, she was referred to our clinic to consider LDLT. Physical examination revealed the accumulation of ascites, jaundice, and edema of her lower extremities. Routine laboratory investigations

Table 1: Preoperative blood type, HBV and HCV marker status of the recipient and the living donor.

	Recipient	Donor
	Blood type	
	O Rh (+)	A Rh (+)
	Viral marker	
HBs-Ag (IU/mL)	<0.05	0.1
HBs-Ab (mIU/mL)	6.5	859.7
HBc-Ab (S/CO)	<1.0	99.9
HBe-Ag (S/CO)	<0.5	0.1
HBe-Ab (%)	<35	>100
HCV-Ab (COI)	98.4	0.1
HCV-CA (fmol/L)	14,569.2	—
HCV-RNA (log IU/mL)	6.7	—
HCV genotype	1b	—

Abbreviations: HBs-Ag, hepatitis B surface antigen; HBs-Ab, hepatitis B surface antibody; HBc-Ag, hepatitis B core antigen; HBc-Ab, hepatitis B core antibody; HBe-Ag, hepatitis B envelope antigen; HBe-Ab, hepatitis B envelope antibody; HCV-Ab, hepatitis C virus antibody; HCV-CA, hepatitis C virus core antigen, HCV-RNA, hepatitis C virus ribonucleic acid.

Table 2: Preoperative estimations of the recipient's standard liver volume and donor's graft volume.

	Recipient	Donor
	Physical findings	
Height (cm)	163	166
Body weight (kg)	79.8	59.0
BSA (m^2)	1.87	1.66
SLV (mL)	1325	
	CT volumetry	
WLV (mL)		1150
Right lobe (mL)		683
GV/WLV (%)		59.4
GV/RBW (%)		0.86
GV/SLV (%)		51.5

Abbreviations: BSA, body surface area; SLV, standard liver volume; CT, computed tomography; WLV, whole liver volume; GV, graft volume; RBW, recipient body weight.

showed a serum total bilirubin (T-Bil) of 4.6 mg/dL, aspartate aminotransferase (AST) of 50 IU/L, alanine aminotransferase (ALT) of 35 IU/L, albumin of 3.3 g/dL, a prothrombin time-international normalized ratio (PT-INR) of 1.36, and platelet count of $3.7 \times 10^4/\mu L$ and her initial Child-Pugh and model for end-stage liver disease scores were 11 and 16, respectively.

This patient's viral marker status is summarized in Table 1. These data revealed that she had not been previously exposed to hepatitis B virus (HBV). After her admission, we attempted to choose a living donor candidate among her relatives; however, there was no living donor candidate who could meet the general selection criteria of our institution.

A 22-year-old daughter of the patient who underwent a living donor workup was excluded as a donor candidate due to her ABO incompatibility and prior infection with HBV. However, there were no other patient matches that were living donors. Our procedure of ABO-I-LDLT and clinical research of this case have been approved by our institutional ethics committee. After a detailed explanation and informed consent, the patient agreed to undergo ABO-I-LDLT using an HBc-Ab positive liver graft, and her daughter was used as a living donor.

According to the preoperative estimation of the donor, routine laboratory investigations showed only normal liver function; the donor's blood type and viral marker status are summarized in Table 1. In addition, liver imaging studies using enhanced and drip infusion cholecystocholangiography computed tomography (CT) showed no significant anatomical variations or abnormalities, and the preoperative liver needle biopsy did not show any noticeable pathological changes. The right lobe volume of the donor was estimated to be 59.4% of the whole liver volume on CT volumetry, while the graft volume (GV)/recipient body weight and GV/standard liver volume were 0.86% and 51.5%, respectively (Table 2). For these reasons, a right lobe graft was chosen for transplantation into the patient.

Two weeks before the operation, 375 mg/m^2 of rituximab (anti-CD20 antibody) was administered to the recipient. Therefore, the CD19- and CD20-positive B cell counts promptly descended under sensitivity. As the isoagglutinin titers of anti-A and anti-B were 32 × and 16 ×, respectively, preoperative PE was not performed. This patient was also treated with 500 mg of mycophenolate mofetil (MMF) and 5 mg of prednisolone for one week until LDLT.

The routine LDLT procedure was applied for both the donor and the recipient. An intraoperative liver wedge biopsy of the donor revealed no evidence of steatosis, cholecystitis, or overt HBV infection. Immediately following total hepatectomy and splenectomy, 20,000 IU of HBIG was infused into the recipient. A double-lumen catheter was inserted through the portal vein via the ileocolic vein to employ PVIT after vessel and bile duct reconstructions.

Perioperative data and treatments of the recipient are shown in Figure 1. Following LDLT, an additional 375 mg/m^2 of rituximab was administered to the recipient, and steroids, MMF, and tacrolimus were administered. PVIT was also employed for 7 days using prostaglandin E1 and gabexate mesilate. In addition to the routine postoperative treatment, the CD19- and CD20-positive B cell counts, isoagglutinin titers of anti-A and anti-B, and HBs-Ab were frequently monitored. According to prophylaxis of the HBV cross infection, 2000 IU of HBIG was properly administered so that the HBs-Ab was over 300 mIU/mL, and 0.5 mg of entecavir (guanosine analogue) was also added starting from 2 weeks after the LDLT.

Sudden elevations in the hepatic enzymes were observed around the 7th postoperative day, without any impeded blood flow, including outflow block; therefore, acute rejection was highly suspected. As temporal dose increments of steroid and MMF were appropriately administered, liver function gradually improved. The patient recovered progressively without any other complications, and the protocol liver biopsy on postoperative day 30 revealed no evidence of rejection, HCV

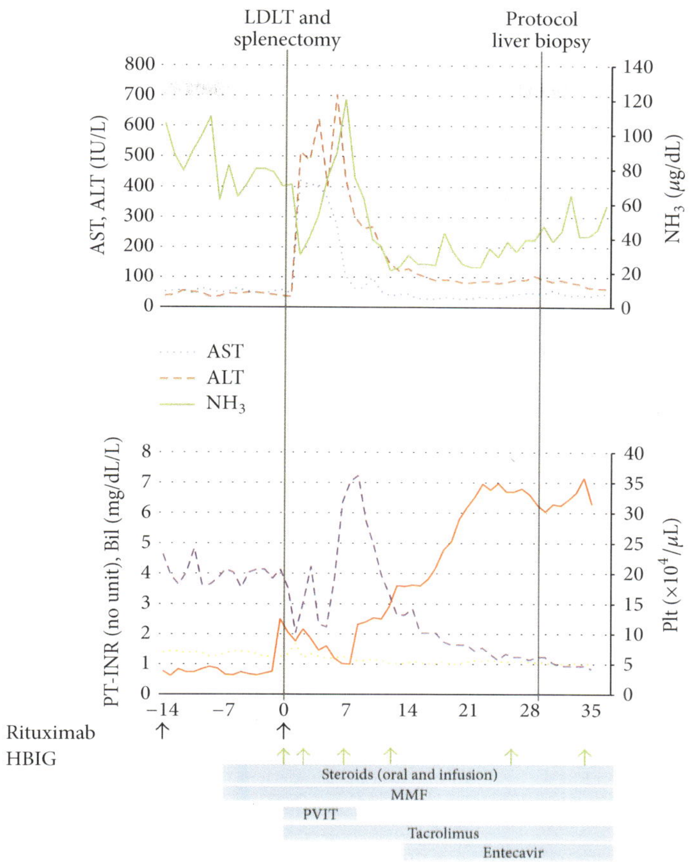

Day	−14	−7	−1	1	7	14	21	28	35
CD19 B cell (%)	16.5	13.3	0.8	<0.1	<0.1	<0.1	<0.1	<0.1	<0.1
CD20 B cell (%)	19.5	15.0	<0.1	<0.1	<0.1	<0.1	<0.1	<0.1	0.1
Isoagglutinin titers									
Anti-A	64 ×	64 ×	32 ×	16 ×	2 ×	2 ×	2 ×	2 ×	4 ×
Anti-B	64 ×	64 ×	16 ×	16 ×	4 ×	2 ×	4 ×	2 ×	4 ×
HBs-Ab (mIU/mL)	—	6.5	6.2	312.4	711.8	631.1	427.3	631.1	410.6

FIGURE 1: Major treatments, events, and laboratory results in the clinical course. Panel shows a timeline of the recipient's clinical course until discharge, with arrows indicating points of administration of rituximab and HBIG. Periods of steroids, MMF, PVIT, tacrolimus, and entecavir are indicated by the gray bars. Results of CD19- and CD20-positive B cell count, isoagglutinin titers of anti-A and anti-B, and HBs-Ab are shown below the graph.

relapse, and HBV infection. She was discharged from the hospital on postoperative day 39.

During the outpatient followup, MMF and tacrolimus were converted to mizoribine and cyclosporine from the viewpoint of the inhibition of HCV ribonucleic acid (HCV-RNA) replication and possibility of administration of pegylated interferon-α 2a (PEG-IFN-α 2a) therapy [8, 9]. She was followed every two weeks and administered liver biopsies every month to monitor for HCV relapse due to severe immunosuppression for ABO-I-LDLT. Three months after the ABO-I-LDLT, routine laboratory investigations and liver biopsy specimens showed HCV relapse. The hepatitis C virus core antigen and HCV-RNA at that time were 79,107.2 fmol/L and 7.8 Log IU/mL, respectively. The patient was promptly started on PEG-IFN-α 2a therapy with ribavirin and prednisolone for immunosuppression, which was gradually tapered. To date, she has been under antiviral therapy and prophylaxis of HBV infection using HBIG, and the entecavir has been continued.

3. Discussion

Although an ABO-I-LDLT was conducted, the HBc-Ab positive donor's liver graft and antiviral therapy for HCV relapse after LDLT are very important topics for transplant surgeons, since these problems have not been completely resolved to date [1–6]. With regard to DDLT in Japan, ABO incompatibility and the possibility of HBV cross infection are strictly considered when the Japan Organ Transplant Network determines the recipient for rare deceased liver grafts. However, with regard to LDLT, when these factors are duplicated between the recipient and the living donor, transplant surgeons must be well acquainted with treatments of ABO-I-LDLT, prophylaxis of HBV cross infection, and antiviral therapy for HCV relapse. We were unable to find any reports about ABO-I-LDLT from an HBc-Ab positive donor to an HCV recipient in the literature.

With regard to ABO-I-LDLT, Tanabe et al. [4, 5] and Egawa et al. [6] reported that triplet treatment consisting of PE, PVIT, and rituximab has dramatically improved the outcome of ABO-I-LDLT. In addition, the recent development of immunosuppression, especially antimetabolites and calcineurin inhibitors, has markedly decreased antibody-mediated rejection [3, 4, 10]. In this case, since the CD19- and CD20-positive B cell counts and isoagglutinin titers of anti-A and anti-B were very low before ABO-I-LDLT, a perioperative PE was never performed.

One of the current efforts to overcome the organ shortage in Japan is based on the use of liver grafts that are from living donors that are HBc-Ab positive [2]. However, the liver grafts from HBc-Ab positive donors are currently main sources of *de novo* hepatitis due to HBV cross infection after LDLT; therefore, HBs-Ag negative recipients should receive appropriate prophylaxis [2, 11–13]. Although the combination of HBIG and lamivudine or entecavir is often used [11, 12], Chotiyaputta et al. [13] reported that entecavir monotherapy without HBIG is sufficient in preventing HBV cross infection in HBs-Ag negative recipients of HBc-Ab positive donor liver grafts. In this case, not entecavir monotherapy but a combination of HBIG infusion and entecavir was administered because the risk of HBV cross infection was thought to be higher from the viewpoint of severe immunosuppression accompanied by ABO-I-LDLT. In addition, the HBs-Ab titer was also kept higher than usual. However, to correctly answer this question, a well-planned study should be performed to definitively determine the nature of the relationship between these prophylactic agents and incidences of *de novo* hepatitis due to HBV cross infection in ABO-I-LDLT from HBc-Ab positive living donors to HBs-Ag negative recipients.

4. Conclusion

We herein described our extremely rare experience with an LC-HCV patient who underwent ABO-I-LDLT using an HBc-Ab positive donor's liver graft. In such a case, in addition to the routine LDLT procedure and postoperative management, cognitions, and techniques about ABO-I-LDLT, the prophylaxis of HBV cross infection, various patterns of immunosuppressive drugs, and antiviral therapy for HCV relapse are indispensable in the management of the recipient. Particularly according to prophylaxis of HBV cross infection under ABO-I-LDLT, it may be very important to keep the HBs-Ab titer higher than usual for HBV naïve recipients, because severe systemic immunosuppression can cause *de novo* hepatitis.

Acknowledgments

The authors would like to thank Dr. Naoko Ito, Dr. Hidenori Itabashi, Dr. Hirokatsu Katagiri, and Dr. Shoji Kanno for helpful discussions.

References

[1] N. Akamatsu and Y. Sugawara, "Living-donor liver transplantation and hepatitis C," *HPB Surgery*, vol. 2013, Article ID 985972, 13 pages, 2013.

[2] E. Cholongitas, G. V. Papatheodoridis, and A. K. Burroughs, "Liver grafts from anti-hepatitis B core positive donors: a systematic review," *Journal of Hepatology*, vol. 52, no. 2, pp. 272–279, 2010.

[3] J. Wu, S. Ye, X. Xu, H. Xie, L. Zhou, and S. Zheng, "Recipient outcomes after ABO-incompatible liver transplantation: a systematic review and meta-analysis," *PLoS ONE*, vol. 6, no. 1, Article ID e16521, 2011.

[4] M. Tanabe, S. Kawachi, H. Obara et al., "Current progress in ABO-incompatible liver transplantation," *European Journal of Clinical Investigation*, vol. 40, no. 10, pp. 943–949, 2010.

[5] M. Tanabe, M. Shimazu, G. Wakabayashi et al., "Intraportal infusion therapy as a novel approach to adult ABO-incompatible liver transplantation," *Transplantation*, vol. 73, no. 12, pp. 1959–1961, 2002.

[6] H. Egawa, S. Teramukai, H. Haga, M. Tanabe, M. Fukushima, and M. Shimazu, "Present status of ABO-incompatible living donor liver transplantation in Japan," *Hepatology*, vol. 47, no. 1, pp. 143–152, 2008.

[7] S. Sakamoto, H. Uchida, I. Hamano et al., "Impact of the current organ allocation system for deceased donor liver transplantation on the outcomes of pediatric recipients: a single center experience in Japan," *Pediatric Surgery International*, vol. 29, no. 11, pp. 1109–1114, 2013.

[8] K. Naka, M. Ikeda, K.-I. Abe, H. Dansako, and N. Kato, "Mizoribine inhibits hepatitis C virus RNA replication: effect of combination with interferon-α," *Biochemical and Biophysical Research Communications*, vol. 330, no. 3, pp. 871–879, 2005.

[9] S. Eguchi, M. Takatsuki, A. Soyama et al., "Intentional conversion from tacrolimus to cyclosporine for HCV-positive patients on preemptive interferon therapy after living donor liver transplantation," *Annals of Transplantation*, vol. 12, no. 4, pp. 11–15, 2007.

[10] V. Raut and S. Uemoto, "Management of ABO-incompatible living-donor liver transplantation: past and present trends," *Surgery Today*, vol. 41, no. 3, pp. 317–322, 2011.

[11] G. V. Papatheodoridis, V. Sevastianos, and A. K. Burroughs, "Prevention of and treatment for hepatitis B virus infection after liver transplantation in the nucleoside analogues era," *American Journal of Transplantation*, vol. 3, no. 3, pp. 250–258, 2003.

[12] D. Shouval and D. Samuel, "Hepatitis B immune globulin to prevent hepatitis B virus graft reinfection following liver transplantation: a concise review," *Hepatology*, vol. 32, no. 6, pp. 1189–1195, 2000.

[13] W. Chotiyaputta, S. J. Pelletier, R. J. Fontana, and A. S. F. Lok, "Long-term efficacy of nucleoside monotherapy in preventing HBV infection in HBsAg-negative recipients of anti-HBc-positive donor livers," *Hepatology International*, vol. 4, no. 4, pp. 707–715, 2010.

6

Anti-Erythropoietin Antibody Associated Pure Red Cell Aplasia Resolved after Liver Transplantation

Annie K. Hung,[1] Jennifer Guy,[2] Caroline M. Behler,[3] and Eugene E. Lee[1]

[1] *Department of Internal Medicine, California Pacific Medical Center, San Francisco, CA 94115, USA*
[2] *Department of Hepatology, California Pacific Medical Center, San Francisco, CA 94115, USA*
[3] *Department of Hematology Oncology, California Pacific Medical Center, San Francisco, CA 94115, USA*

Correspondence should be addressed to Annie K. Hung; hungah@sutterhealth.org

Academic Editor: Piero Boraschi

Patients undergoing antiviral therapy for chronic hepatitis C often develop anemia secondary to ribavirin and interferon. Recombinant erythropoietin has been used to improve anemia associated with antiviral therapy and to minimize dose reductions, which are associated with decreased rates of sustained virologic response. A rare potential side effect of recombinant erythropoietin is anti-erythropoietin antibody associated pure red cell aplasia. In chronic kidney disease patients with this entity, there have been good outcomes associated with renal transplant and subsequent immunosuppression. In this case, a chronic liver disease patient developed anti-erythropoietin associated pure red cell aplasia and recovered after liver transplantation and immunosuppression. It is unclear whether it is the transplanted organ, the subsequent immunosuppression, or the combination that contributed to the response. In conclusion, anti-erythropoietin associated pure red cell aplasia is a serious complication of erythropoietin therapy, but this entity should not be considered a contraindication for solid organ transplantation.

1. Introduction

Pure red cell aplasia (PRCA) is a rare normochromic, normocytic anemia with near to complete absence of erythroblasts in the bone marrow. Current standard diagnostic criteria of this condition include a decrease in red cell count of about 1% per day, reticulocyte count below 1%, and the absence of major changes in white cell count, platelet count, and differential leukocyte count [1]. Elevated serum transferrin saturation and ferritin can also be seen and reflect decreased utilization of iron stores given the absence of erythropoiesis. Confirmation of the diagnosis requires bone marrow examination which should demonstrate normal cellularity with myeloid cells and megakaryocytes, but less than 1% erythroblasts with occasionally up to 5% proerythroblasts or basophilic erythroblasts [1]. Congenital PRCA is rare and includes Diamond Blackfan anemia. There are many causes of acquired PRCA which include parvovirus B19, lymphoproliferative disorders, systemic autoimmune disease, production of erythropoietin-neutralizing antibodies, and drugs such as chloramphenicol [2].

Since their introduction in 1989, erythropoiesis stimulating agents (ESA) have been used widely to improve anemia in those with chronic renal failure [1]. After prolonged use, patients can develop anti-erythropoietin antibodies which also have neutralizing capacity for endogenous erythropoietin, leading to PRCA. This is a rare entity with the estimated overall exposure-adjusted incidence of 0.02–0.03 per 10,000 patient-years [3]. It is associated with a minimum exposure to ESA for 3 weeks, usually occurring after 6 to 8 months [3]. Most cases have been associated with subcutaneous administration [1]. Incidence of antibody-mediated PRCA from intravenous administration is exceedingly rare [3].

Combinations of interferon and ribavirin have long been the standard of treatment for chronic hepatitis C. A common side effect of interferon is bone marrow suppression which can affect granulocytes, erythrocytes, and megakaryocytes [4]. Ribavirin has been known to cause a dose dependent hemolysis, by triggering intracellular ATP depletion leading to cell membranes that are more prone to oxidative damage [5]. When undergoing treatment with combination

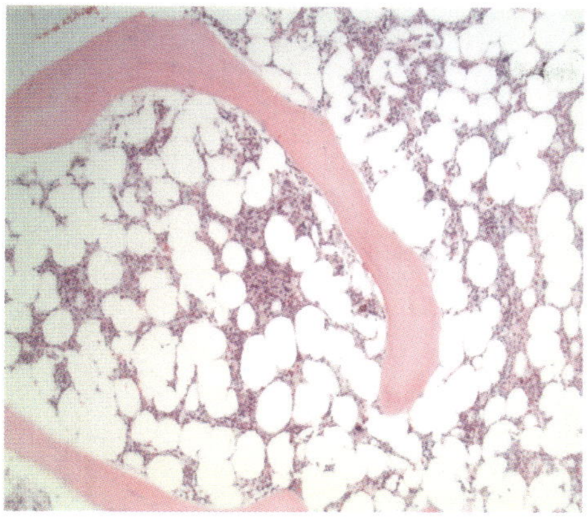

FIGURE 1: Bone marrow showing hypocellularity and trilineage hematopoiesis, without increased blasts. No increased fibrosis or dysplastic changes are seen.

therapy of ribavirin and interferon, dose reductions are often necessary because of anemia [4]. In severe cases, antiviral therapy has to be discontinued [4]. Studies have also demonstrated an association between dose reductions and decreased sustained virologic response (SVR) [6]. Large randomized trials have shown that administration of epoetin alfa in hepatitis C patients receiving interferon and ribavirin therapy helped with anemia, resulting in fewer dose reductions, and improved quality of life [7, 8].

2. Case Report

A 66-year-old African American man underwent treatment for chronic hepatitis C while awaiting liver transplantation due to hepatocellular carcinoma. He was started on triple therapy with telaprevir 750 mg every 8 hours, ribavirin 1000 mg daily, and pegylated interferon 180 mcg subcutaneously weekly. Two weeks into treatment, he developed anemia with drop in hemoglobin to 10 g/dL, from his baseline of 13 g/dL. The anemia was attributed to ribavirin and thus the dose was reduced to 400 mg twice daily. He was also started on epoetin alfa 40,000 units subcutaneously per week.

He underwent a thorough work-up for his anemia including parvovirus serologies, upper endoscopy and colonoscopy, hemoglobin electrophoresis, iron studies, folate, vitamin B12, HIV, ANA, and RPR which were all negative. Because of persistent anemia, his ribavirin dose was again decreased to 200 mg daily. His epoetin alfa dose was increased to 60,000 units per week without any substantial response. After 5 months of recombinant erythropoietin therapy, he became transfusion dependent, requiring 2 to 3 units of packed red blood cells every 3 to 4 weeks, receiving over 30 units over a 7-month period. Because of his severe anemia, ribavirin and peg interferon were both discontinued.

A bone marrow biopsy showed absence of reticulocytes, along with 15% cellularity, with trilineage hematopoiesis (Figure 1). There were no dysplastic findings or increase in fibrosis, but he did have increased marrow stores. Because he had been treated with erythropoietin without much increase in his blood count and remained transfusion dependent, an assay to detect anti-erythropoietin antibodies was sent and found to be positive. The assay showed neutralizing capacity of 21.4 mcg per mL, predominantly IgG1 with minor component of IgG2 and IgG4. Epoetin alfa was immediately discontinued. The patient was felt to have pure red cell aplasia due to anti-erythropoietin antibodies. The hypocellularity seen on bone marrow examination was thought to be related to interferon and ribavirin therapy. He was started on rituximab 375 mg per meters squared intravenously weekly and received 4 treatments. However, after cessation of epoetin alfa and antiviral therapy, as well as completion of rituximab, he continued to be transfusion dependent. The included graph depicts his fluctuating hemoglobin levels throughout the course of his illness (Figure 2).

The patient was listed for liver transplantation for hepatocellular carcinoma but had become inactive because of his anemia. He had uncomplicated Child-Pugh class A cirrhosis with no history of portal hypertension. Despite his anemia, he had completed an adequate course of antiviral therapy and had sustained virologic response at 6 months, presumed to be cured of hepatitis C. Based on lesions measuring 3.6 cm and 1.7 cm, he was also within the Milan criteria. The decision was made to undergo orthotopic liver transplantation. It was also felt that chronic immunosuppression after transplantation would help his anemia. He underwent transplantation without complications. Immunosuppressive therapy was started with tacrolimus, mycophenolate, and prednisone. After liver transplantation and chronic immunosuppression, his anemia improved with stable hemoglobin and reticulocyte levels. Ten weeks after transplantation, his hemoglobin was greater than 10.0 g/dL. He has not required any further transfusions. Repeat titer did not detect anti-erythropoietin antibodies.

3. Discussion

Most cases of antibody associated PRCA have occurred in patients with chronic kidney disease. The majority of these cases were associated with a preparation of epoetin alfa marketed outside the United States (Eprex/Erypo) [3]. Following concerns for transmission of Creutzfeldt-Jacob disease, human serum albumin was removed from Eprex and replaced by polysorbate 80 and glycine [3]. It has been proposed that the polysorbate 80 formulation was less stable, causing aggregation of epoetin alfa molecules especially at increased temperatures, increasing immunogenicity [3]. Another hypothesis proposes that leachates from uncoated rubber syringe stoppers in prefilled syringes could have also increased immunogenicity, leading to antibody formation [3]. Because of the concern for increasing immunogenicity, the subsequent formulations of Eprex replaced uncoated rubber stoppers with fluororesin-coated stoppers and the polysorbate was removed [3].

Although antibody associated PRCA is a serious complication of recombinant erythropoietin therapy, screening for the presence of anti-erythropoietin antibodies is not justified without clinical suspicion [9]. The 2012 Kidney Disease: Improving Global Outcomes guidelines suggest testing for anti-erythropoietin antibodies after exposure of at least 8

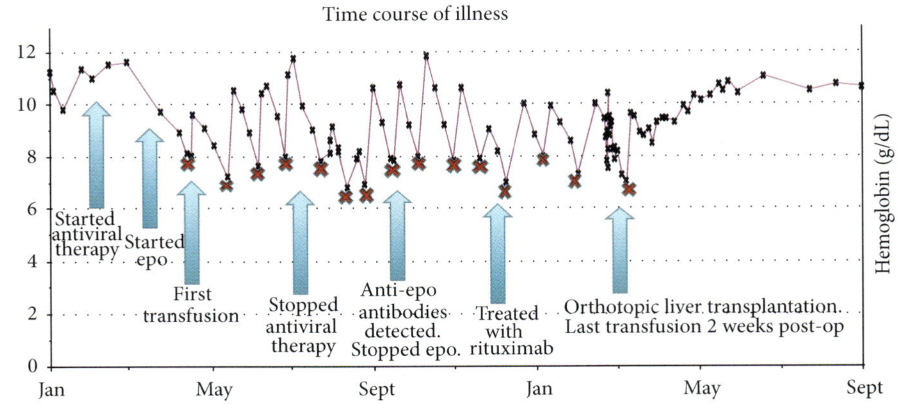

Figure 2: A graph of fluctuating hemoglobin levels throughout time course of illness. The patient experienced a drop in hemoglobin shortly after starting antiviral therapy. Despite dose reduction and discontinuation of antivirals, he was transfusion dependent. Packed red cell transfusions are marked by the red X. After orthotopic liver transplantation, hemoglobin levels increased without any further transfusion requirements. He has continued to have sustaining hemoglobin levels >10 g/dL.

weeks to an ESA, decline in hemoglobin level of >0.5 to 1.0 g/dL per week, or transfusion requirement of at least 1 to 2 units per week, normal white blood cell and platelet count, and absolute reticulocyte count <10,000/microL [9]. The most accurate test to detect anti-erythropoietin antibodies is the radioimmunoprecipitation assay, but it is time consuming and difficult to automate [10]. Enzyme-linked immunosorbent assays are not as accurate but are widely available [11].

The therapeutic recommendations for antibody associated PRCA are cessation of ESA therapy, correction of anemia with blood transfusions as needed, and prompt initiation of immunosuppressive therapy [3]. Typical starting doses for immunosuppressive therapies are 0.5–1.0 mg/kg/day for corticosteroids and 200 mg/day for cyclosporine [3]. In a retrospective review of 47 patients with erythropoietin-induced PRCA, all patients developed this entity after receiving epoetin alfa (Eprex, Ortho Biotech) [12]. Median delay between initiation of erythropoietin treatment and start of pure red cell aplasia was 11 months [13]. Recovery rates were between 56% and 88% in patients treated with corticosteroids, cyclophosphamide, or cyclosporine [13]. However, there were 6 patients who underwent kidney transplant who all recovered from transfusion dependence within 1 month [13]. In other reports from Europe and Canada in 1999 and 2000, several patients with antibody associated PRCA also underwent renal transplantation after failing immunosuppressive regimens and had rapid clinical recovery [11]. In several countries, policies were changed to make patients with antibody associated PRCA a higher priority on waiting lists for kidney transplantation [14]. The data is limited, but kidney transplantation appears to be an effective treatment for this condition [14]. However, it is unclear whether the transplanted organ or the subsequent immunosuppression is the therapeutic agent.

There have been several reports of PRCA associated with chronic hepatitis C and its treatment. Most cases are antibody-mediated and associated with epoetin alfa. In one case, a 65-year-old woman developed antibodies after epoetin alfa treatment for anemia induced by ribavirin and interferon for hepatitis C therapy and was treated successfully with rituximab [13]. In a similar case, a 50-year-old man developed antibody associated PRCA after receiving epoetin alfa for anemia secondary to ribavirin and interferon and was treated successfully with danazol [15]. There are also several cases in the literature of patients with chronic hepatitis C who developed PRCA but did not receive recombinant erythropoietin [14]. Anti-erythropoietin antibodies were not tested in these patients, but the etiology of the PRCA was thought to be the hepatitis C virus itself versus drug induced by either ribavirin or interferon [14].

There is limited literature on PRCA and liver transplant. As far as we know, there are no other cases of this entity resolving after liver transplantation. There have been documented cases of PRCA secondary to parvovirus B19 infection after liver transplant and immunosuppression which responded well to immunoglobulin [16]. Interestingly, there is a case reported of a patient who underwent liver transplantation, started antiviral therapy for hepatitis C with ribavirin and interferon, received recombinant erythropoietin for anemia, but developed anti-erythropoietin antibody-mediated PRCA while on immunosuppression [17]. As mentioned above, immunosuppression should minimize antibody production, but in this patient increased immunogenicity caused by interferon therapy may have led to antibody associated PRCA [17].

The question of rechallenging patients who have recovered from antierythropoietin mediated PRCA is controversial. There have been multiple case reports of patients who have been successfully treated with immunosuppressive therapy and then rechallenged with another epoetin [18]. Rechallenging should be considered if anti-erythropoietin antibodies are around or below the limit of detection and with careful monitoring of reticulocyte and hemoglobin levels [19]. If a patient is rechallenged, administration should be intravenous [19].

Peginesatide is a synthetic dimeric peptidic ESA which activates the human erythropoietin receptor but its primary amino acid sequence is unrelated to human erythropoietin. Thus, it does not induce an immune response against endogenous erythropoietin, decreases the risk of antibody-mediated PRCA, and has been proposed as an alternative to immunosuppression [20]. Based on two randomized controlled trials (EMERALD 1 and EMERALD 2), peginesatide was approved by the US FDA for treatment of anemia in hemodialysis patients [20]. Shortly after FDA approval, peginesatide was recalled [20]. As of now, the application of peginesatide to treat antibody-mediated PRCA is not clear.

4. Conclusion

Antibody associated PRCA is a rare but serious complication of recombination erythropoietin therapy. It should be considered when a patient continues to be anemic despite treatment with recombinant erythropoietin products. A wide range of immunosuppressive therapies as well as kidney transplantation have been associated with clinical recovery of this entity. There are still many unanswered questions regarding the root causes of antibody associated PRCA, as well as the long term outcomes of patients with this entity who have undergone solid organ transplantation with liver and kidney.

Abbreviations

ESA: Erythropoiesis stimulating agents
PRCA: Pure red cell aplasia
SVR: Sustained virologic response
ATP: Adenosine triphosphate.

Acknowledgments

The authors would like to thank all the staff in our various departments for their valuable support.

References

[1] N. Casadevall, D. Cournoyer, J. Marsh et al., "Recommendations on haematological criteria for the diagnosis of epoetin-induced pure red cell aplasia," *European Journal of Haematology*, vol. 73, no. 6, pp. 389–396, 2004.

[2] K.-U. Eckardt and N. Casadevall, "Pure red-cell aplasia due to anti-erythropoietin antibodies," *Nephrology Dialysis Transplantation*, vol. 18, no. 5, pp. 865–869, 2003.

[3] I. C. MacDougall, S. D. Roger, A. de Francisco et al., "Antibody-mediated pure red cell aplasia in chronic kidney disease patients receiving erythropoiesis-stimulating agents: new insights," *Kidney International*, vol. 81, no. 8, pp. 727–732, 2012.

[4] M. Peck-Radosavljevic, M. Wichlas, M. Homoncik-Kraml et al., "Rapid suppression of hematopoiesis by standard or pegylated interferon-alpha," *Gastroenterology*, vol. 123, no. 1, pp. 141–151, 2002.

[5] L. De Franceschi, G. Fattovich, F. Turrini et al., "Hemolytic anemia induced by ribavirin therapy in patients with chronic hepatitis C virus infection: role of membrane oxidative damage," *Hepatology*, vol. 31, no. 4, pp. 997–1004, 2000.

[6] J. G. McHutchison, M. Manns, K. Patel et al., "Adherence to combination therapy enhances sustained response in genotype-1-infected patients with chronic hepatitis C," *Gastroenterology*, vol. 123, no. 4, pp. 1061–1069, 2002.

[7] N. H. Afdhal, D. T. Dieterich, P. J. Pockros et al., "Epoetin alfa maintains ribavirin dose in HCV-infected patients: a prospective, double-blind, randomized controlled study," *Gastroenterology*, vol. 126, no. 5, pp. 1302–1311, 2004.

[8] P. J. Pockros, M. L. Shiffman, E. R. Schiff et al., "Epoetin alfa improves quality of life in anemic HCV-infected patients receiving combination therapy," *Hepatology*, vol. 40, no. 6, pp. 1450–1458, 2004.

[9] International Society of Nephrology, "KDIGO clinical practice guidelines for anemia in chronic kidney disease," *Kidney International Supplements*, vol. 2, no. 4, pp. 279–335, 2012.

[10] J. Rossert, N. Casadevall, and K.-U. Eckardt, "Anti-erythropoietin antibodies and pure red cell aplasia," *Journal of the American Society of Nephrology*, vol. 15, no. 2, pp. 398–406, 2004.

[11] C. L. Bennett, D. Cournoyer, K. R. Carson et al., "Long-term outcome of individuals with pure red cell aplasia and antierythropoietin antibodies in patients treated with recombinant epoetin: a follow-up report from the Research on Adverse Drug Events and Reports (RADAR) Project," *Blood*, vol. 106, no. 10, pp. 3343–3347, 2005.

[12] D. Verhelst, J. Rossert, N. Casadevall, A. Krüger, K.-U. Eckardt, and I. C. Macdougall, "Treatment of erythropoietin-induced pure red cell aplasia: a retrospective study," *The Lancet*, vol. 363, no. 9423, pp. 1768–1771, 2004.

[13] C. M. Behler, N. A. Terrault, J. E. Etzell, and L. E. Damon, "Rituximab therapy for pure red cell aplasia due to anti-epoetin antibodies in a woman treated with epoetin-alfa: a case report," *Journal of Medical Case Reports*, vol. 3, article 7335, 2009.

[14] C.-S. Chang, S.-L. Yan, H.-Y. Lin, F.-L. Yu, and C.-Y. Tsai, "Pure red cell aplasia caused by pegylated interferon-α-2a plus ribavirin in the treatment of chronic hepatitis C," *World Journal of Gastroenterology*, vol. 17, no. 16, pp. 2155–2158, 2011.

[15] R. T. Stravitz, H. Chung, R. K. Sterling et al., "Antibody-mediated pure red cell aplasia due to epoetin alfa during antiviral therapy of chronic hepatitis C," *The American Journal of Gastroenterology*, vol. 100, no. 6, pp. 1415–1419, 2005.

[16] T.-B. Liang, D.-L. Li, J. Yu et al., "Pure red cell aplasia due to parvovirus B19 infection after liver transplantation: a case report and review of the literature," *World Journal of Gastroenterology*, vol. 13, no. 13, pp. 2007–2010, 2007.

[17] J. M. Schecter, J. G. Mears, B. Alobeid, and P. J. Gaglio, "Anti-erythropoietin antibody-mediated pure red cell aplasia in a living donor liver transplant recipient treated for hepatitis C virus," *Liver Transplantation*, vol. 13, no. 11, pp. 1589–1592, 2007.

[18] I. C. Macdougall, A. Roche, J. Rossert, N. Casadevall, P. Francois, and D. M. Kemeny, "Re-challenging patients who developed pure red cell aplasia with epoetin: can it be done?" *Nephrology Dialysis Transplantation*, vol. 19, no. 11, pp. 2901–2905, 2004.

[19] J. Rossert, I. Macdougall, and N. Casadevall, "Antibody-mediated pure red cell aplasia (PRCA) treatment and re-treatment: multiple options," *Nephrology Dialysis Transplantation*, vol. 20, no. 4, pp. iv23–iv26, 2005.

[20] S. Fishbane, B. Schiller, F. Locatelli et al., "Peginesatide in patients with anemia undergoing hemodialysis," *The New England Journal of Medicine*, vol. 368, no. 4, pp. 307–319, 2013.

7

Intracardiac Thrombosis during Adult Liver Transplantation

Marina Moguilevitch and Carlene Broderick

Department of Anesthesiology, Montefiore Medical Center, Albert Einstein College of Medicine, Bronx, NY 10463, USA

Correspondence should be addressed to Marina Moguilevitch; mmoguile@montefiore.org

Academic Editors: M. R. Moosa, Y. Sugawara, and R. Zhang

Intracardiac thrombosis (ICT) and pulmonary embolism (PE) during adult liver transplantation are rare but potentially lethal complications. They are often overlooked because of significant diagnostic challenges. The combination of hemodynamic compromise and transesophageal echocardiography (TEE) findings allows for correct diagnosis. A large variety of putative risk factors for ICT and PE have been suggested, but these events are considered to be multifactorial. There are different proposed treatment modalities for these devastating complications. Unfortunately, in spite of growing knowledge in this area, intraoperative and postoperative mortalities remain very high. The retrospective nature of the study of these events makes the case reports extremely valuable.

1. Introduction

Orthotopic liver transplantation (OTL) is a major surgical procedure which usually involves significant blood loss secondary to coagulation disturbances typical of end stage liver disease. In addition, hyperfibrinolysis can occur intraoperatively, leading to more bleeding complications.

In contrast to bleeding coagulopathies, intraoperative thrombotic complications are less frequently encountered but deserve special attention because of possible life threatening events.

We are reporting a case of intracardiac thrombosis during OLT presented as a sudden cardiac arrest during the neohepatic stage.

Patient's family permission was obtained to publish this case report.

2. Case Presentation

A 67-year-old, 78 kg, 176 cm man with a history of hypertension, diabetes mellitus, and decompensated liver disease secondary to hepatitis C virus (HCV) with portal hypertension, ascites, and hepatic encephalopathy presented for retransplantation with an MELD score of 31. He had undergone liver transplantation 18 months previously that was complicated by a severe recurrence of HCV infection, partially responding to therapy with interferon and ribavirin.

Relevant laboratory studies revealed 82 g/L hemoglobin, 129.6 μmol/L creatinine, 165.87 μmol/L total bilirubin, 2.7 INR, 26.7 sec. prothrombin time (PT), 56 sec. partial thromboplastin time (PTT), $59{,}000 \times 10^9$/L platelets. Preoperative dobutamine stress test demonstrated normal left and right ventricular functions without evidence of ischemia.

After preoxygenation, anesthesia was induced with 2 mg midazolam, 250 mcg fentanyl, 60 mg propofol, and 10 mg vecuronium. After intubation, two additional 16 g peripheral intravenous catheters, a radial arterial catheter and an 8.5 French introducer with pulmonary artery catheter, were placed. The dissection phase was complicated by significant blood loss, leading to transfusion of multiple units of blood, fresh frozen plasma, and cryoprecipitate. Venovenous bypass (VVB) with a heparin-coated circuit was initiated because the patient was not able to tolerate caval cross-clamping. There was no significant or prolonged hemodynamic instability after graft reperfusion. Ninety minutes after discontinuation of VVB, a sudden precipitous drop of the blood pressure with concomitant elevations of central venous pressure and pulmonary artery pressure was noticed. This circulatory collapse

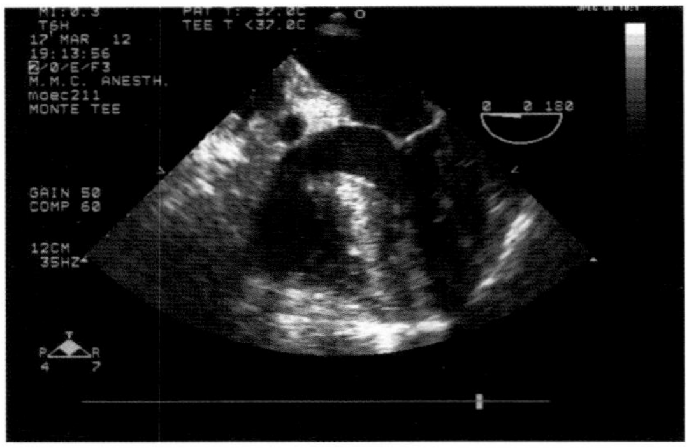

Figure 1: Transesophageal echocardiogram showing thrombus in the left ventricle.

led to pulseless electrical cardiac activity. CPR protocol was initiated (including infusions of epinephrine, vasopressin, and norepinephrine). A transesophageal echo probe was placed, and the study revealed a dilated right ventricle and a collapse of the left ventricle with a thrombus fluctuating under the aortic valve (Figure 1). No thrombus was seen in the pulmonary vessels.

The resuscitation efforts were unsuccessful, and the decision was made to administer tissue plasminogen activator (t-PA) 50 mg intravenously. Shortly after t-PA administration, the thrombus in the left ventricle dissolved and right ventricle function normalized. Unfortunately, dissolution of the thrombus did not lead to the restoration of normal hemodynamics despite the administration of high doses of pressors. After eighty minutes, resuscitation efforts were stopped.

3. Discussion

Since the first report of a thromboembolic event during OLT has been published in 1988 [1], pulmonary thromboembolism (PTE) and ICT have been major causes of intraoperative morbidity and mortality during adult OLT. The incidence of reported PTE and ICT ranges from 1.2% [2] to 6.2% [3]. A review of the literature [4, 5] failed to identify the etiology of this condition; treatment recommendations are inconsistent.

The hemostatic system is a balance between coagulation, anticoagulation, and fibrinolysis. Liver transplantation poses potential massive blood loss due to the patient's preexisting hypocoagulable state, collateral circulation caused by portal hypertension, and major surgery involving multiple vascular anastomoses. Recently, it has been shown that the balance between pro- and antithrombotic factors synthesized by the liver may be reset to a lower level in patients with chronic liver disease [6]. Liver failure causes a reduction of both pro- and anticoagulative factors production. Therefore, under normal conditions, the patients with liver disease do not bleed spontaneously. Bleeding can be caused by additional factors like infection, vascular abnormality, portal hypertension, or mechanical distraction during invasive procedures.

Any disturbance in the delicate balance between coagulation, anticoagulation, and fibrinolysis can lead to fatal bleeding or thrombotic complication. It is known that the defect in platelet number and function is balanced by the elevated plasma concentration of von Willebrand factor (vWf) and factor VIII, which are not synthesized by the liver. Moreover, we can see a decrease in the production of all procoagulant factors synthesized by the liver as well as of anticoagulant proteins: protein C, protein S, protein Z, antithrombin, and heparin factor II. In addition, the synthesis of all proteins involved in fibrinolysis is decreased in patients with liver disease. The levels of tissue plasminogen activator (tPA) and plasminogen activator inhibitor (PAI-1) are elevated, secondary to reduced clearance by the liver. PAI-1 and tPA have extrahepatic origin. Moreover, coagulation tests like PT measures only procoagulant factors, and INR was developed and validated only for those patients on anticoagulation therapy.

The complexity of hemostatic problems in patients with end stage liver disease (ESLD) undergoing liver transplantation and the inability of routine tests to reflect defects in the pro- and anticoagulant system make the anesthetic care of these patients more challenging.

There have been multiple attempts to identify risk factors and diagnostic predictors for potentially fatal thrombotic complications during OLT. The most recent retrospective review [5] analyzed 495 consecutive, isolated OLTs from deceased donors. The standard technique was VVB without antifibrinolytic prophylaxis. Among the preoperative recipient risk factors were an increased incidence of portal hypertension with ascites, low serum albumin levels, and preoperative hospitalization especially with ventilator support. In terms of intraoperative factors, the group with thrombotic complications had higher baseline pulmonary artery pressures, more hemodynamic instability, increased level of serum lactate, and a flat-line thromboelastogram (TEG). The diagnostic criteria for PTE and ICT were the combination of hemodynamic compromise and TEE findings of intravascular or intracardiac thrombosis. Heparin, tissue plasminogen (tPA), and hemodynamic support with vasoactive drugs were the medications of choice to treat this potentially lethal complication. Intraoperative and in-hospital mortalities after thrombotic complications reached 30% and 45%, respectively.

ICT remains a highly lethal and multifactorial complication, which is still very difficult to prevent and treat.

References

[1] A. A. Navalgund, Y. Kang, J. B. Sarner, J. S. Jahr, and R. Gieraerts, "Massive pulmonary thromboembolism during liver transplantation," *Anesthesia and Analgesia*, vol. 67, no. 4, pp. 400–402, 1988.

[2] E. Gologorsky, A. M. De Wolf, V. Scott, S. Aggarwal, M. Dishart, and Y. Kang, "Intracardiac thrombus formation and pulmonary thromboembolism immediately after graft reperfusion in 7

patients undergoing liver transplantation," *Liver Transplantation*, vol. 7, no. 9, pp. 783–789, 2001.

[3] A. B. Lerner, E. Sundar, F. Mahmood, T. Sarge, D. W. Hanto, and P. J. Panzica, "Four cases of cardiopulmonary thromboembolism during liver transplantation without the use of antifibrinolytic drugs," *Anesthesia and Analgesia*, vol. 101, no. 6, pp. 1608–1612, 2005.

[4] N. Warnaar, I. Q. Molenaar, S. D. Colquhoun et al., "Intraoperative pulmonary embolism and intracardiac thrombosis complicating liver transplantation: a systematic review," *Journal of Thrombosis and Haemostasis*, vol. 6, no. 2, pp. 297–302, 2008.

[5] T. Sakai, T. Matsusaki, F. Dai et al., "Pulmonary thromboembolism during adult liver transplantation: incidence, clinical presentation, outcome, risk factors, and diagnostic predictors," *British Journal of Anaesthesia*, vol. 108, no. 3, pp. 469–477, 2012.

[6] M. Senzolo, P. Burra, E. Cholongitas, and A. K. Burroughs, "New insights into the coagulopathy of liver disease and liver transplantation," *World Journal of Gastroenterology*, vol. 12, no. 48, pp. 7725–7736, 2006.

8

Early Introduction of Everolimus Immunosuppressive Regimen in Liver Transplantation with Extra-Anatomic Aortoiliac-Hepatic Arterial Graft Anastomosis

Emanuele Felli, Giovanni Vennarecci, Marco Colasanti, Roberto Santoro, Edoardo de Werra, Andrea Scotti, Mirco Burocchi, Giovanni B. Levi Sandri, Alessandra Campanelli, Pasquale Lepiane, and Giuseppe M. Ettorre

Digestive and Transplant Liver Surgery Unit, S. Camillo Hospital, Piazza Carlo Forlanini 1, 00151 Rome, Italy

Correspondence should be addressed to Emanuele Felli; e.felli@hotmail.com

Academic Editor: Yasuhiko Sugawara

Liver transplantation is the treatment of choice for patients with acute and chronic end-stage liver disease, when no other medical treatment is possible. Despite high rates of 1- to 5-year survival, long-term adverse effects of immunosuppressant agents remain of major concern. Current research and clinical efforts are made to develop immunosuppressant agents that minimize adverse effects along with a low rate of graft rejection. Tailoring immunosuppressive therapy to individual patients by the use of proliferation signal inhibitors seems to be the best way to minimize toxicity and increase efficacy. Recently everolimus has been introduced in clinical practice; among its adverse effects an increased incidence of arterial graft thrombosis in renal transplants, vascular anastomosis leakage, impaired wound healing, and thrombotic microangiopathy have been reported. We present the case of a 54-year-old patient submitted to liver transplantation for end-stage liver disease treated by an extra-anatomic aortoiliac-hepatic arterial graft anastomosis and early postoperative introduction of everolimus for acute renal failure. Postoperative period was characterized by two abdominal collections and reactivation of cytomegalovirus infection that were treated by percutaneous drainage and antiviral therapy, respectively; the patient is well after 8-month followup with patency of the arterial conduit and no leakage.

1. Introduction

Liver transplantation is the treatment of choice for patients with acute and chronic end-stage liver disease when no other medical treatment is possible [1]. Despite high rates of 1- to 3-year survival, major concerns remain over long-term adverse effects of immunosuppressant agents, such as diabetes, dyslipidemia, renal insufficiency, hypertension, and osteoporosis, all of which compromise quality of life and long-term patient survival [2–4]. The current clinical challenge is to develop regimens that maintain high rates of transplantation success while minimizing unwanted and harmful metabolic and other effects. It appears increasingly likely that efficacy and toxicity may be balanced by tailoring immunosuppressive therapy to individual patients by the use of proliferation signal inhibitors. These agents, which include the macrolide semisynthetic derivative of rapamycin, everolimus, appear to be well tolerated especially when used at lower dosages. Among side effects of everolimus episodic arterial graft thrombosis that has been described in renal transplant patients during the first postoperative month are vascular anastomosis leakage, impaired wound healing, and thrombotic microangiopathy. We report the case of a 54-year-old patient that was submitted to liver transplantation in our unit for HCV and alcohol abuse cirrhosis, with MELD score of 40 treated by an extra-anatomic aortoiliac-hepatic arterial graft anastomosis and early postoperative introduction of everolimus immunosuppressive regimen for acute renal failure.

2. Case Report

We present the case of a 54-year-old patient affected by HCV and alcohol abuse cirrhosis with end-stage liver disease with acute liver failure due to spontaneous bacterial peritonitis and MELD score of 40 submitted to our unit for orthotopic liver transplantation. In his past medical history we found blood hypertension controlled by medications, alcohol abuse, past heroin addiction, and chronic HCV infection.

The graft was procured by cadaveric donor. Cold ischemia time was 8 hours. Caval anastomosis was performed between the patient hepatic veins and the donor inferior vena cava; initially an end-to-end arterial anastomosis was performed between the donor celiac trunk and the patient common hepatic artery after the incision of a diaphragmatic median arcuate ligament; the biliary anastomosis was end-to-end protected by a T-Kehr tube. No temporary portocaval anastomosis was performed. Hemodynamic instability was present throughout the operation with consistent hypotension non-responsive to medical treatment. Blood loss was 7000 mL with 5 packed red blood cells and 26 fresh frozen plasma transfused. Operative time was 10 hours. Arterial Doppler in the end of the operation showed a good flow with a RI index in the normal range. In the second postoperative day the patient was reoperated on for hemorrhagic shock secondary to hemoperitoneum. No evident cause of bleeding was found in the second operation. The final arterial Doppler was not satisfactory with a low flow and arterial graft hypopulsatility. Then, an extra-anatomic arterial by-pass using cadaveric iliac artery graft was performed with an end-to-end anastomosis between the common hepatic artery and the donor iliac artery in the proximal side and a side-to-end anastomosis between the distal abdominal aorta and the donor iliac artery (Figure 1). Arterial Doppler at the end of the second operation was normal. Early immunosuppression in our institution is based on the combination of tacrolimus, corticosteroids, and mycophenolate mofetil, and this regimen was applied to the presented patient. In the first postoperative week the patient developed acute renal insufficiency and so we decided to make an early switch to everolimus. Daily arterial Doppler showed normal flow, with good patency of the arterial graft. In the postoperative period two intra-abdominal collections developed, all drained percutaneously, along with cytomegalovirus reactivation treated by antiviral agents. After eight-month followup the patient is well with good patency of the arterial graft and normal liver function.

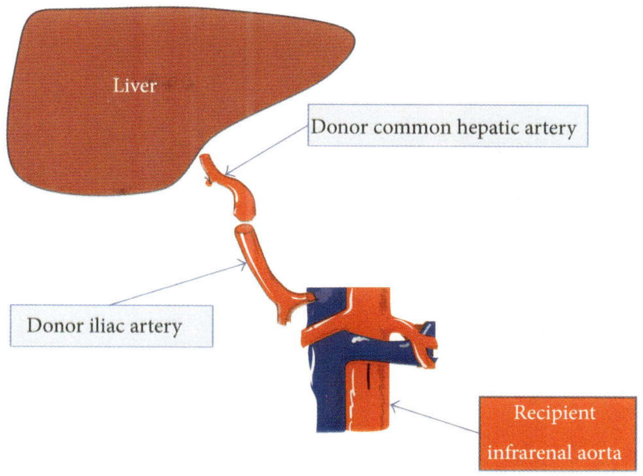

Figure 1: Schematic representation of the arterial conduit between the donor common hepatic artery and recipient infrarenal aorta.

3. Discussion

Everolimus, a proliferation signal inhibitor, prevents allograft rejection in rodent and nonhuman primate models of allotransplantation. It exerts its immunosuppressive effect by inhibiting the proliferation and thus clonal expansion of antigen-activated T cells which is driven by T cell specific interleukins. Everolimus inhibits an intracellular signalling pathway which is triggered upon binding of these T cell growth factors to their respective receptors and which normally leads to cell proliferation. Its application in human transplantation has been already described; among its adverse effects arterial graft thrombosis has been reported in renal transplants within the first month of transplantation. In the phase III, randomised, controlled, open-label study (H2304) [5], reduced tacrolimus exposure and everolimus were administered to HCV positive and HCV negative patients starting approximately 4 weeks after transplantation, investigated versus standard tacrolimus exposure. A third arm in study H2304 with complete withdrawal of tacrolimus at 4 months after transplantation was terminated early because it has been associated with an increased risk of acute rejections. In the 12-month analysis, the incidence of the composite endpoint (biopsy proven acute rejection, graft loss, or death) was lower in everolimus + reduced tacrolimus arm compared to the tacrolimus control arm. The reduction in glomerular filtration rate was less substantial at 12 months and at 24 months. We decided to introduce everolimus in the patient immunosuppressive treatment in relation to the acute postoperative renal insufficiency, thus minimizing anticalcineurin renal damage. Impaired wound healing, thrombotic microangiopathy, vascular leakage, and intra-abdominal collections, especially lymphocele, have been described as adverse effects of everolimus treatment. In this case it is difficult to relate the two abdominal collections that appeared in the postoperative period to the use of everolimus because of the multiple operations and the intra- and postoperative complications. In conclusion we present the case of early introduction of everolimus treatment in the setting of a difficult liver transplantation that was not associated with arterial thrombosis, vascular leakage, wound healing alteration, and microangiopathy.

References

[1] R. H. Wiesner, J. Rakela, M. B. Ishitani et al., "Recent advances in liver transplantation," *Mayo Clinic Proceedings*, vol. 78, no. 2, pp. 197–210, 2003.

[2] M. Vilatoba, J. L. Contreras, and D. E. Eckhoff, "New immunosuppressive strategies in liver transplantation: balancing efficacy and toxicity," *Current Opinion in Organ Transplantation*, vol. 8, no. 2, pp. 139–145, 2003.

[3] F. Conti, E. Morelon, and Y. Calmus, "Immunosuppressive therapy in liver transplantation," *Journal of Hepatology*, vol. 39, no. 5, pp. 664–678, 2003.

[4] G. T. Everson, J. F. Trotter, M. Kugelmas, and L. Forman, "Immunosuppression in liver transplantation," *Minerva Chirurgica*, vol. 58, no. 5, pp. 725–740, 2003.

[5] P. de Simone, F. Nevens, L. de Carlis et al., "Everolimus with reduced tacrolimus improves renal function in de novo liver transplant recipients: a randomized controlled trial," *The American Journal of Transplantation*, vol. 12, no. 11, pp. 3008–3020, 2012.

9

Chronic Hepatitis E Infection Resulting in Graft Failure in a Liver Transplant Tourist

Hui-Hui Tan,[1] Hoe-Nam Leong,[2] Boon-Huan Tan,[3] Lynette Lin-Ean Oon,[4] Kiat-Hon Lim,[4] Jason Pik-Eu Chang,[1] and Chee-Kiat Tan[1]

[1] *Liver Transplant Service, Department of Gastroenterology & Hepatology, Singapore General Hospital, Singapore 169608*
[2] *Department of Infectious Diseases, Singapore General Hospital, Singapore 169608*
[3] *Defence Science Organisation, Singapore 118230*
[4] *Department of Pathology, Singapore General Hospital, Singapore 169608*

Correspondence should be addressed to Hui-Hui Tan, tan.hui.hui@sgh.com.sg

Academic Editors: B. H. Ozdemir, M. Sadeghi, and Y. Sato

Hepatitis E, usually an acute hepatitis in the immunocompetent, has a chronic form described in immunocompromised hosts. We report the clinical course and outcome of an adult liver transplant recipient whose posttransplant period was complicated by chronic hepatitis E, Epstein-Barr virus infection, and cellular rejection of the graft.

1. Introduction

Hepatitis E virus (HEV) infection is known to be transmissible via various routes. A chronic form of persistent HEV has been described in immunocompromised hosts, especially in transplant recipients who are on immunosuppression. We describe an adult liver transplant (LT) recipient whose post-LT course was complicated by chronic HEV, Epstein-Barr viremia (EBV), and acute cellular graft rejection resulting in management dilemmas and ultimately graft failure and mortality.

2. Case Report

Mr. X was a 48-year-old Chinese male with chronic hepatitis B virus infection and multifocal hepatocellular carcinoma that was beyond standard criteria, precluding LT. In early November 2009, he approached a center in another country as a transplant tourist and received a deceased liver graft. Postoperatively, he was discharged with tacrolimus 1mg bid, mycophenolate mofetil 750 mg bid, and prednisolone 20 mg od.

He returned to us 3 weeks later to continue post-LT care at our center. He was noticed to be deeply jaundiced with a mixed cholestatic-hepatitic picture on his liver tests (see Table 1 and Figure 1).

Serology and blood polymerase chain reaction (PCR) were positive for Epstein-Barr virus (EBV) and hepatitis E virus (HEV) genotype 3. Liver tissue was also positive for EBV by PCR. Serology and blood PCR were negative for cytomegalovirus, herpes simplex virus, hepatitis B virus, hepatitis C virus, parvovirus, and human herpes virus 6. Liver tissue was negative for viral inclusions. He was treated with acyclovir for EBV infection with demonstrable reduction in serum EBV viral load by PCR.

Doppler imaging of the graft confirmed patent graft vessels. Magnetic resonance imaging was suggestive of an anastomotic biliary stricture, and this led to successful endoscopic deployment of a biliary stent across the stricture. However, despite regular stent changes per 3 months with good bile outflow, his liver tests did not improve and he remained deeply jaundiced. A liver biopsy was performed in December 2009 that demonstrated moderate acute cellular rejection (rejection activity index score 5) (Figure 2(a)). This was treated with pulse methylprednisolone. Repeat biopsy performed 2 weeks later confirmed good histological response of the acute cellular rejection to steroid pulses (Figure 2(b)). However, liver function tests did not improve,

TABLE 1: Serial liver tests for patient Mr. X.

(a)

Date	Oct-09	24 Nov-09	28 Nov-09	4 Dec-09	12 Dec-09
Event	pre-OLT	OLT 3 Nov-09	ERCP 26 Nov-09	Liver biopsy	Liver biopsy 11 Dec-10 ERCP 11 Dec-10
Bilirubin (Normal: 3–24 umol/L)	14	246	298	453	458
Alkaline phosphatase (Normal 32–103 U/L)	224	319	244	251	138
Alanine transaminase (Normal: 7–36 U/L)	22	129	151	285	169
Aspartate transaminase (Normal: 15–33 U/L)	43	138	172	407	164
γ-Glutamyl transferase (Normal: 11–63 U/L)	—	192	126	100	77

(b)

Date	17 Dec-09	Feb-10	Mar-10	Apr-10
Event	ERCP 14 Dec-10	Liver biopsy	ERCP stent change	2 weeks prior to demise
Bilirubin (Normal: 3–24 umol/L)	471	438	457	662
Alkaline phosphatase (Normal 32–103 U/L)	128	277	372	951
Alanine transaminase (Normal: 7–36 U/L)	163	257	121	168
Aspartate transaminase (Normal: 15–33 U/L)	137	207	128	264
γ-Glutamyl transferase (Normal: 11–63 U/L)	67	227	207	180

and a third liver biopsy in February 2010 demonstrated only lymphocytic portal and lobular hepatitis with marked cholestasis, without acute or chronic graft rejection (Figure 3). Metavir fibrosis score was 1/4. No atypical mononuclear infiltrate was seen in the biopsy specimen. There was no evidence of lymphoproliferative disease in any of the liver histologies nor on serial radiologic imaging.

His graft function continued to deteriorate with HEV RNA detectable up to 6 months after LT. He was admitted in April 2010 with jaundice, ascites, peripheral oedema, and constitutional symptoms. Graft failure with disseminated bacterial and fungal infection led to his demise soon after (6 months post-LT).

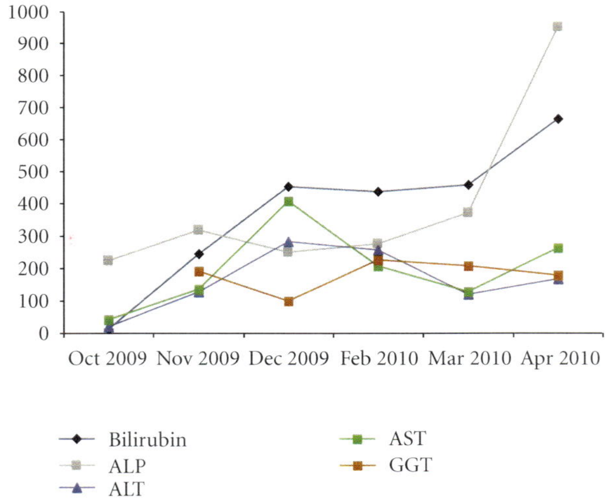

FIGURE 1: Serial liver tests for patient Mr. X. Bilirubin (Normal: 3–24 umol/L), ALP: Alkaline phosphatase (Normal: 32–103 U/L), ALT: alanine transaminase (Normal: 7–36 U/L), AST: aspartate transaminase (Normal: 15–33 U/L), GGT: γ-glutamyl transferase (Normal: 11–63 U/L).

3. Discussion

HEV is an RNA virus, transmissible by the fecal-oral route, usually through contaminated food and water. However, it is now recognized that in the viremic phase, HEV transmission may be blood borne as well [1–5]. It is endemic in several developing countries [6], but not in Singapore. Phylogenetic analysis classifies HEV into 4 genotypes [7, 8]. Genotype 1

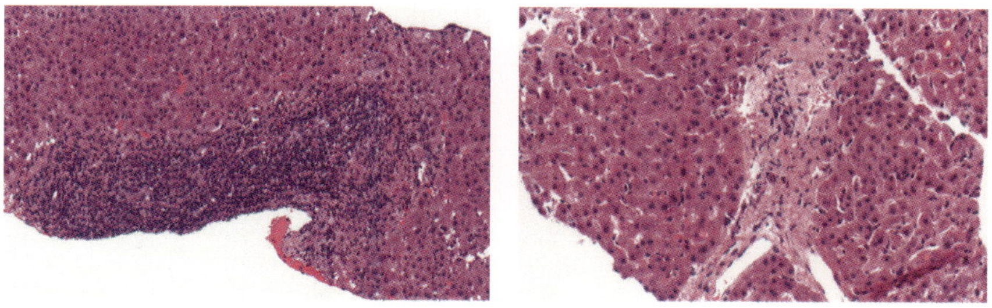

(a) Marked portal inflammation with bile duct damage, endothelialitis, and mixed lymphoplasmacytic infiltrate

(b) Biopsy 2 weeks after steroid pulse therapy showing marked improvement with only minimal portal inflammation and mild residual bile duct damage

FIGURE 2: Histomicrograph of liver biopsy in December 2009.

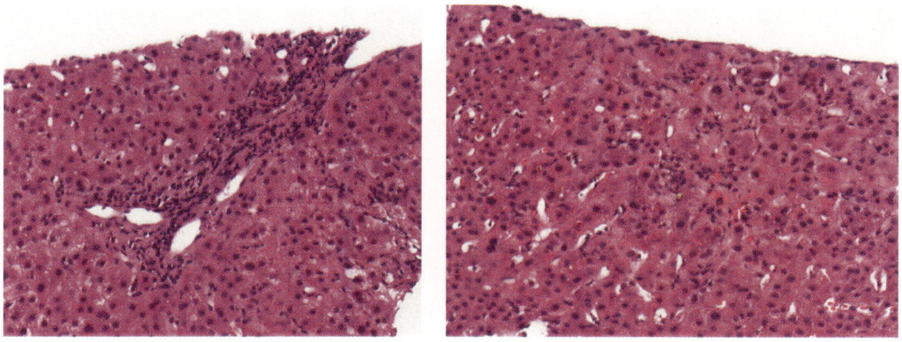

(a) Mild portal, periportal inflammation

(b) Lobular inflammation with cholestasis

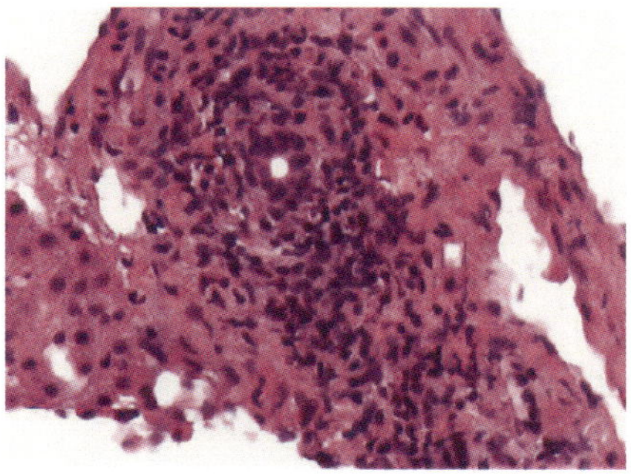

(c) Preserved bile duct within a portal tract; lymphocytic inflammation

FIGURE 3: Histomicrograph of liver biopsy in February 2010.

is the most prevalent and widespread. Genotype 2 has been reported in Mexico and West Africa. Genotype 3 has been isolated from nonendemic regions such as the United States, Europe, and Japan. Genotype 4 is less commonly isolated and has been found in specimens from China, Taiwan, Japan and Vietnam. HEV genotypes 1 and 2 primarily infect humans, whilst genotypes 3 and 4 have been isolated in swine and other animals in areas where human isolates have been found [9]. Reverse zoonotic transmission has also been reported [10].

Although previously assumed to manifest only as an acute hepatitis with spontaneous resolution, recent data and literature now suggest that HEV infection does have a chronic form, more commonly seen in the immunocompromised host. Most reports of chronic HEV have been in transplant recipients on immunosuppression. CD4+ IFNγ-secreting cells and natural killer T cells may be involved in the pathogenesis of HEV [11]. The greater severity of hepatitis E infection in pregnant women suggests a relation to the Th2 response [12]. Solid-organ transplant recipients with chronic hepatitis E have been found to have significantly lower total lymphocyte and CD2, CD3, and CD4 subset counts as opposed to recipients who had cleared the HEV [13]. Interestingly, HEV reactivation has also been reported in a patient after stem cell transplantation [14]. Hence, it is probably under these circumstances that nonpersistent viruses may result in chronic colonization and recurrent infection [15]. Chronic HEV infection may induce a rapid and severe liver disease, ranging from protracted HEV infection to chronic active hepatitis to progressive cirrhosis [16–18].

The diagnosis of HEV infection is usually made on the basis of positive serology in the immunocompetent host. However, in the context of immunosuppression, antibody testing has been reported to be repeatedly negative despite detectable HEV RNA in the blood [19]. Transplant clinicians should be mindful of this, and molecular testing should be performed if the index of suspicion is high, regardless of serological results.

Our case report is interesting for the following reasons.

Firstly, our patient returned from the overseas centre 3 weeks after transplant with a persistent, progressive liver dysfunction which did not improve despite successful biliary stenting and treatment for graft rejection. HEV serology was positive within 5 weeks post-LT. To our knowledge, our patient is one of the earliest to be diagnosed with HEV infection so soon after LT. As HEV genotype 3 is of the swine variety, it is possible that the patient had acquired it from ingestion of contaminated pork. However, it could also have been the result of implantation of an organ from a cadaveric donor who previously had HEV infection, resulting in reactivation with immunosuppression. HEV serology was not tested in our patient prior to LT as there had been no clinical indication to do so. How our patient would have acquired HEV and if transplant tourism increased the risk for this, we are unable to prove in this recipient. HEV is not endemic in our country. However, the implications of transplant tourism include having broad differentials for the cause of graft hepatitis. In light of the scarcity of available organs and the rising costs of healthcare, transplant clinicians should be mindful to consider unusual/uncommon infections from their patients returning from other centers.

Secondly, our patient also had concurrent EBV infection as demonstrated by serology and detectable DNA in the blood and liver tissue. EBV infections are commonly observed in patients after liver transplantation, and serologic evidence of active infection is demonstrable in close to 25% of cases [20]. This is usually asymptomatic disease. However, 1-2% of liver transplant recipients may have persistent or recurrent disease resulting in the development of posttransplant lymphoproliferative disorders (PTLDs) and lymphomas [21]. Although our patient did not demonstrate the classical features of infectious mononucleosis-like EBV infection, the decision was made to commence acyclovir treatment in view of persistent hepatitis and demonstrable EBV DNA in the blood and liver tissue. It is possible that this patient's EBV infection was a red herring, as graft function continued to deteriorate despite EBV treatment which had some documented response (one log drop in viral load). Furthermore, death or graft failure reported from EBV is commonly in the context of PTLD, rather than from viral infection per se. On the other hand, despite recent reports of HEV infection in solid-organ transplant recipients, most were not described to have concurrent EBV infection as well. Except for the report of a kidney-pancreas transplant recipient by Kamar et al., who developed acute hepatitis from HEV 6 months after transplant and who also had detectable EBV DNA in the blood, we are not aware of other reports of patients with concurrent EBV-HEV infection [18]. EBV was not demonstrable by immunohistochemistry in the liver tissue of Kamar et al.'s patient, and the EBV DNA level in the blood was relatively unchanged both before and after the acute hepatitis episode (4.3 $\log_{10}$ copies/mL). In their case report, a liver biopsy performed 16 months from the diagnosis of HEV infection demonstrated moderate hepatitis with a Metavir fibrosis score of F2.22 months from the diagnosis of HEV infection; their patient was cirrhotic and soon after succumbed to a bacterial infection. It is possible that EBV hepatitis or infection contributed to or aggravated the rapid progression of HEV in our patient. After all, both retrospective and prospective data from India and China suggest that superimposed HEV infection on patients with chronic liver hepatitis or liver disease has a poorer prognosis [22–24]. Whether EBV infection or reactivation contributes to hepatitis with a poor outcome in recipients with HEV infection should be explored in future studies, as positive EBV serology is not uncommon in solid organ transplant recipients.

Thirdly, as inferred from the pathogenesis of chronic HEV above, reducing immunosuppression that targets T cells may be a possible therapeutic option [18]. However, cellular rejection in our patient's graft necessitated steroid pulses and also made it difficult to tail immunosuppressants early. Recent reports suggest that pegylated interferon-α-2a/2b may have a role in the treatment of liver transplant recipients with chronic HEV in whom the lowering of immunosuppressant doses alone is insufficient [25, 26]. However, optimal treatment duration and the risk of associated graft rejection with interferon therapy are yet to be determined in this patient population. Kamar et al.'s case series of 3 liver transplant recipients treated with pegylated interferon-α-2a for chronic HEV infection reported acute humoral rejection in the liver biopsy of one of their patients after 12 weeks of therapy. Fortunately for that patient, HEV RNA was undetectable by then and remained so, despite steroid pulses required to treat graft rejection [26].

Transplant recipients should be cautioned against consuming meat from partially cooked animal sources which may harbor the HEV. Although a recent large, phase 3 study has demonstrated efficacy of an HEV recombinant vaccine [27], more studies would be required before formal recommendations can be made on whether HEV vaccination should be offered to all potential transplant candidates prior to transplantation, especially in endemic areas, or whether HEV serology testing should be performed pre-LT, assuming its positive implications for reactivation in a potential transplant candidate.

Transplant tourism may be an enticing option for the deteriorating LT candidate waiting at length for a suitable graft. Even some global medical insurance programs are promoting this option [28]. However, it is fraught with both clinical and public health implications. Apart from the standard of hygiene and quality of postoperative care in overseas centers, recipients have been reported to have contracted infections endemic to overseas centers (e.g., tuberculosis, aspergillus, and hepatitis B) or even donor malignancies [29–31]. Medical records from overseas centers are often incomplete, scant, in a foreign language, or unobtainable [29, 32, 33]. Fatal postoperative bleeding has also been reported, as have both under or over-immunosuppresion, and infection with the HIV virus [29, 30, 32, 34, 35]. Renal transplant tourists have been reported to have a more complex posttransplantation course with a higher incidence of graft rejection and severe infectious complications [36].

4. Conclusion

The transplant tourist presents a unique set of potential complications and problems not usually encountered in one's own center. The physician is required to consider a wide list of differentials and to think "out-of-the-box" when managing such recipients, especially in the first year after transplant.

Abbreviations

HEV: Hepatitis E virus
EBV: Epstein-Barr virus
LT: Liver transplantation
PCR: Polymerase chain reaction
PTLD: Post-transplant lymphoproliferative disorders

References

[1] K. Matsubayashi, J. H. Kang, H. Sakata et al., "A case of transfusion-transmitted hepatitis e caused by blood from a donor infected with hepatitis e virus via zoonotic food-borne route," *Transfusion*, vol. 48, no. 7, pp. 1368–1375, 2008.

[2] K. Matsubayashi, Y. Nagaoka, H. Sakata et al., "Transfusion-transmitted hepatitis E caused by apparently indigenous hepatitis E virus strain in Hokkaido, Japan," *Transfusion*, vol. 44, no. 6, pp. 934–940, 2004.

[3] J. M. Mansuy, A. Huynh, F. Abravanel, C. Recher, J. M. Peron, and J. Izopet, "Molecular evidence of patient-to-patient transmission of hepatitis E virus in a hematology ward," *Clinical Infectious Diseases*, vol. 48, no. 3, pp. 373–374, 2009.

[4] E. Boxall, A. Herborn, G. Kochethu et al., "Transfusion-transmitted hepatitis E in a 'nonhyperendemic' country," *Transfusion Medicine*, vol. 16, no. 2, pp. 79–83, 2006.

[5] P. Colson, C. Coze, P. Gallian, M. Henry, P. De Micco, and C. Tamalet, "Transfusion-associated hepatitis E, France," *Emerging Infectious Diseases*, vol. 13, no. 4, pp. 648–649, 2007.

[6] R. Aggarwal and K. Krawczynski, "Hepatitis E: an overview and recent advances in clinical and laboratory research," *Journal of Gastroenterology and Hepatology*, vol. 15, no. 1, pp. 9–20, 2000.

[7] G. G. Schlauder and I. K. Mushahwar, "Genetic heterogeneity of hepatitis E virus," *Journal of Medical Virology*, vol. 65, no. 2, pp. 282–292, 2001.

[8] H. Okamoto, "Genetic variability and evolution of hepatitis E virus," *Virus Research*, vol. 127, no. 2, pp. 216–228, 2007.

[9] R. H. Purcell and S. U. Emerson, "Hepatitis E: an emerging awareness of an old disease," *Journal of Hepatology*, vol. 48, no. 3, pp. 494–503, 2008.

[10] S. Pischke, P. V. Suneetha, C. Baechlein et al., "Hepatitis E virus infection as a cause of graft hepatitis in liver transplant recipients," *Liver Transplantation*, vol. 16, no. 1, pp. 74–82, 2010.

[11] R. Srivastava, R. Aggarwal, S. Jameel et al., "Cellular immune responses in acute hepatitis E virus infection to the viral open reading frame 2 protein," *Viral Immunology*, vol. 20, no. 1, pp. 56–65, 2007.

[12] R. Pal, R. Aggarwal, S. R. Naik, V. Das, S. Das, and S. Naik, "Immunological alterations in pregnant women with acute hepatitis E," *Journal of Gastroenterology and Hepatology*, vol. 20, no. 7, pp. 1094–1101, 2005.

[13] N. Kamar, J. Selves, J. M. Mansuy et al., "Hepatitis E virus and chronic hepatitis in organ-transplant recipients," *New England Journal of Medicine*, vol. 358, no. 8, pp. 811–817, 2008.

[14] P. Le Coutre, H. Meisel, J. Hofmann et al., "Reactivation of hepatitis E infection in a patient with acute lymphoblastic leukaemia after allogeneic stem cell transplantation," *Gut*, vol. 58, no. 5, pp. 699–702, 2009.

[15] O. Schildgen, A. Müller, and A. Simon, "Chronic hepatitis E and organ transplants," *New England Journal of Medicine*, vol. 358, no. 23, pp. 2521–2522, 2008.

[16] R. Gérolami, V. Moal, and P. Colson, "Chronic hepatitis E with cirrhosis in a kidney-transplant recipient," *New England Journal of Medicine*, vol. 358, no. 8, pp. 859–860, 2008.

[17] E. B. Haagsma, A. P. van den Berg, R. J. Porte et al., "Chronic hepatitis E virus infection in liver transplant recipients," *Liver Transplantation*, vol. 14, no. 4, pp. 547–553, 2008.

[18] N. Kamar, J. M. Mansuy, O. Cointault et al., "Hepatitis E virus-related cirrhosis in kidney-and kidney-pancreas- transplant recipients," *American Journal of Transplantation*, vol. 8, no. 8, pp. 1744–1748, 2008.

[19] A. Tamura, Y. K. Shimizu, T. Tanaka et al., "Persistent infection of hepatitis E virus transmitted by blood transfusion in a patient with T-cell lymphoma," *Hepatology Research*, vol. 37, no. 2, pp. 113–120, 2007.

[20] N. Singh, J. S. Dummer, S. Kusne et al., "Infections with cytomegalovirus and other herpesviruses in 121 liver transplant recipients: transmission by donated organ and the effect of OKT3 antibodies," *Journal of Infectious Diseases*, vol. 158, no. 1, pp. 124–131, 1988.

[21] M. A. Nalesnik, R. Jaffe, T. E. Starzl et al., "The pathology of posttransplant lymphoproliferative disorders occurring in the setting of cyclosporine A-prednisone immunosuppression," *American Journal of Pathology*, vol. 133, no. 1, pp. 173–192, 1988.

[22] A. Kumar, R. Aggarwal, S. R. Naik, V. Saraswat, U. C. Ghoshal, and S. Naik, "Hepatitis E virus is responsible for decompensation of chronic liver disease in an endemic region," *Indian Journal of Gastroenterology*, vol. 23, no. 2, pp. 59–62, 2004.

[23] S. Kumar Acharya, P. Kumar Sharma, R. Singh et al., "Hepatitis E virus (HEV) infection in patients with cirrhosis is associated with rapid decompensation and death," *Journal of Hepatology*, vol. 46, no. 3, pp. 387–394, 2007.

[24] W. M. Ke, X. J. Li, L. N. Yu et al., "Etiological investigation of fatal liver failure during the course of chronic hepatitis B in southeast China," *Journal of Gastroenterology*, vol. 41, no. 4, pp. 347–351, 2006.

[25] E. B. Haagsma, A. Riezebos-Brilman, A. P. van den Berg, R. J. Porte, and H. G. M. Niesters, "Treatment of chronic hepatitis E in liver transplant recipients with pegylated interferon alpha-2b," *Liver Transplantation*, vol. 16, no. 4, pp. 474–477, 2010.

[26] N. Kamar, L. Rostaing, F. Abravanel et al., "Pegylated interferon-α for treating chronic hepatitis e virus infection

after liver transplantation," *Clinical Infectious Diseases*, vol. 50, no. 5, pp. e30–e33, 2010.

[27] F. C. Zhu, J. Zhang, X. F. Zhang et al., "Efficacy and safety of a recombinant hepatitis e vaccine in healthy adults: a large-scale, randomised, double-blind placebo-controlled, phase 3 trial," *The Lancet*, vol. 376, no. 9744, pp. 895–902, 2010.

[28] K. A. Bramstedt and J. Xu, "Checklist: passport, plane ticket, organ transplant," *American Journal of Transplantation*, vol. 7, no. 7, pp. 1698–1701, 2007.

[29] S. E. Kennedy, Y. Shen, J. A. Charlesworth et al., "Outcome of overseas commercial kidney transplantation: an Australian perspective," *Medical Journal of Australia*, vol. 182, no. 5, pp. 224–227, 2005.

[30] M. T. Canales, B. L. Kasiske, and M. E. Rosenberg, "Transplant tourism: outcomes of United States residents who undergo kidney transplantation overseas," *Transplantation*, vol. 82, no. 12, pp. 1658–1661, 2006.

[31] G. V. Prasad, A. Shukla, M. Huang, R. J. D'A Honey, and J. S. Zaltzman, "Outcomes of commercial renal transplantation: a Canadian experience," *Transplantation*, vol. 82, no. 9, pp. 1130–1135, 2006.

[32] A. K. Salahudeen, H. F. Woods, A. Pingle et al., "High mortality among recipients of bought living-unrelated donor kidneys," *Lancet*, vol. 336, no. 8717, pp. 725–728, 1990.

[33] W. Qunibi, D. Abulrub, F. Shaheen, A. B. Shehab El-Din, O. Alfurayh, and K. Almeshari, "Attitudes of commercial renal transplant recipients toward renal transplantation in India," *Clinical Transplantation*, vol. 9, no. 4, pp. 317–321, 1995.

[34] H. Khalaf, S. Farag, and E. El-Hussainy, "Long-term follow-up after liver transplantation in Egyptians transplanted abroad," *Saudi Medical Journal*, vol. 25, no. 12, pp. 1931–1934, 2004.

[35] W. Qunibi, "Commercially motivated renal transplantation: results in 540 patients transplanted in India," *Clinical Transplantation*, vol. 11, no. 6, pp. 536–544, 1997.

[36] J. Gill, B. R. Madhira, D. Gjertson et al., "Transplant tourism in the United States: a single-center experience," *Clinical Journal of the American Society of Nephrology*, vol. 3, no. 6, pp. 1820–1828, 2008.

10

Isolated Aspergillosis Myocardial Abscesses in a Liver-Transplant Patient

Kim-Diêp Dang-Tran,[1] Valérie Chabbert,[1] Laure Esposito,[2] Céline Guilbeau-Frugier,[3,4] Fabrice Dédouit,[1,5] Lionel Rostaing,[2,4,6] Hervé Rousseau,[1,4] Phillippe Otal,[1,4] and Nassim Kamar[2,4,6]

[1] *Service de Radiologie Générale, Centre Hospitalier Universitaire Rangueil, 1 avenue du Professeur Jean Poulhès, TSA 50032, 31059 Toulouse Cedex 9, France*
[2] *Department of Nephrology and Organ Transplantation, CHU Rangueil, TSA 50032, 31059 Toulouse Cedex 9, France*
[3] *Service d'Anatomo-Pathologie, Centre Hospitalier Universitaire Rangueil, 1 avenue du Professeur Jean Poulhès, 31059 Toulouse Cedex 4, France*
[4] *Université Paul Sabatier, 31059 Toulouse, France*
[5] *Service de Médecine Légale, Centre Hospitalier Universitaire Rangueil, 1 avenue du Professeur Jean Poulhès, 31059 Toulouse Cedex 4, France*
[6] *INSERM U1043, IFR-BMT, CHU Purpan, 31059 Toulouse, France*

Correspondence should be addressed to Nassim Kamar; kamar.n@chu-toulouse.fr

Academic Editors: D. Capone, C. Costa, S. Faenza, and G. Forrest

Cardiac abscess is an uncommon and fatal complication after transplantation. We report a case of an initially isolated aspergillosis myocardial abscess diagnosed by cardiac magnetic resonance imaging (CMRI). At that time, there was no other biological evidence or other extracardiac manifestations. A three-month course of dual antifungal therapy followed by a single antifungal therapy was empirically given. Six month after admission, *Aspergillus fumigatus* was isolated for the first time and the patient deceased from a disseminated aspergillosis.

1. Introduction

Infections are commonly observed after solid-organ transplantation and generally require rapid and adequate therapy within this setting [1]. Although they seldom occur in cardiac locations, endocarditis is the main heart infection observed, whereas a cardiac abscess is rare. Concomitant clinical and/or biological abnormalities usually lead to etiologic diagnosis of a cardiac abscess. Herein, we report a case of an initially isolated cardiac abscess that occurred in a liver-transplant patient. Cardiac magnetic resonance imaging (CMRI) was found to be helpful in assessing the evolution of the abscess under empiric therapy.

2. Case Presentation

A 68-year-old man underwent a first cadaveric orthotopic liver transplantation for hepatitis B virus and alcohol-induced cirrhosis that was complicated by hepatocellular carcinoma. After an induction therapy using antithymocyte globulins (ATG), his initial immunosuppressive therapy was based on tacrolimus, mycophenolate mofetil, and steroids. At day 11, because *Aspergillus fumigatus* was found in a systematic tracheal aspiration, a 21-day course of voriconazole was given. By day 60, he experienced a steroid-resistant acute rejection, which required ATG antirejection therapy. By day 78, he presented with isolated fever. C-reactive protein

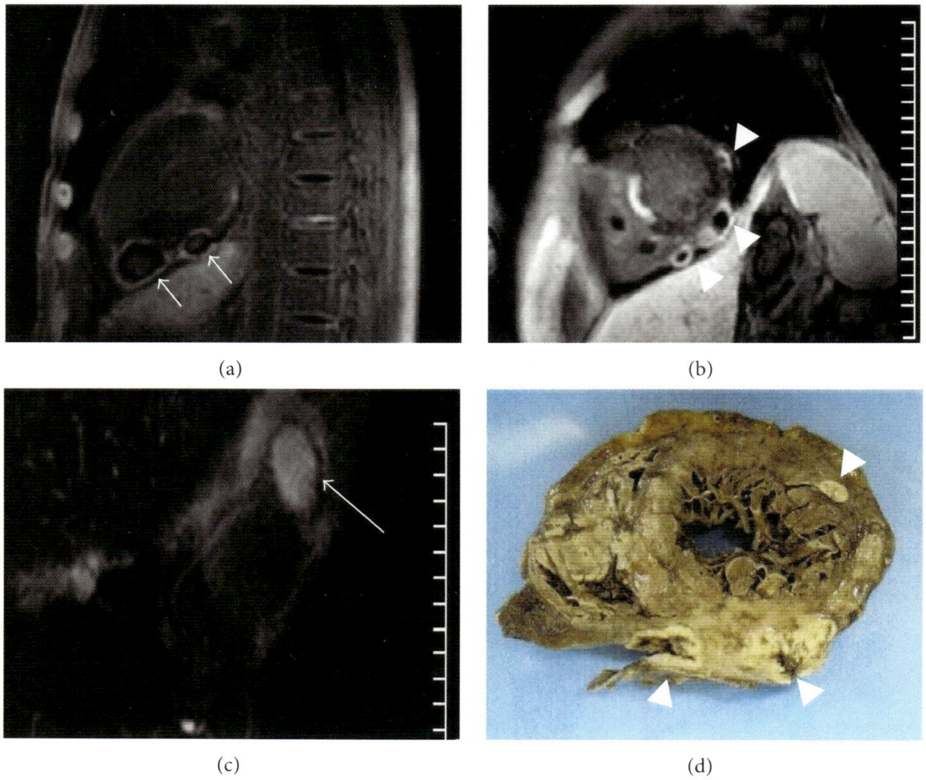

FIGURE 1: Cardiac MRI performed 6 months after diagnosis and autopsy study. (a) T1-weighted postgadolinium MRI—long axis view. Two collections (white arrows) with thick enhancing rim and hypointense core in the epicardium and myocardium of the left ventricle posterior wall. (b) T1-weighted postgadolinium MRI—short axis view. Lesions (arrow heads) in the left ventricle wall. A hyperintense calcified lesion located in the interventricular septum is also visualized. (c) T2-black blood MRI—axial view. Hyperintense core suggesting a cystic core (black arrow). (d) Autopsy study. Heart short axis view pointing out the three left ventricle abscesses observed on image (b) (arrow heads).

was 100 mg/L. Total lymphocyte count was 375/mm^3. CD4-positive cell count was 60/mm^3. Liver function tests were within the normal ranges. Blood-culture and urine-culture were negative for bacteria and fungi. *Aspergillus* antigenemia was negative. *Cytomegalovirus* DNAemia was negative. The bronchoalveolar lavage did not reveal the presence of any bacteria, virus, or fungi. In the absence of any identified cause of infection, he underwent a chest and abdominal CT scan, which showed an isolated rounded cardiac collection. Thus, a cardiac MRI was performed as soon as possible to enable diagnosis and close monitoring of the evolution of the cardiac lesion.

The CMRI pointed out a 3 cm diameter collection within the epicardium and myocardium, on the apex posterior wall, without any mass effect. On T1-weighted MRI, the lesion showed a thick rim and a hypointense core. The core was hyperintense on T2-weighted and T2-black blood SPIR MRI, suggesting a cystic core. Only the thick rim was enhanced on postgadolinium MRI. No ischemic lesion or heart-motion abnormality was found. Thus, we hypothesized an infectious cardiac abscess. Because the abscess was very close to the anterior interventricular artery, the radiologists and cardiac surgeons could not perform any abscess puncture for microbial diagnosis. Despite a negative *Aspergillus* antigenemia and because of the patient's recent history of aspergillosis, we initiated a dual antifungal therapy of caspofungin and liposomal Fungizone.

A second CMRI, performed one week later, showed the abscess had grown. Because of a history of tuberculosis in childhood, this prompted us to initiate an antituberculosis therapy (isoniazid, rifampicin, ethambutol, and pyrazinamide) though mainly pericardial abscess has been described [2]. A CMRI performed 3 months after diagnosis showed stability of the abscess, with the patient still receiving antituberculosis and double antifungal therapies. At that time, liposomal Fungizone was replaced by voriconazole. Because of increased liver-enzyme levels, voriconazole was stopped 1 month later, and the patient was continued on caspofungin alone. Antituberculosis therapy was also continued. By 6 months after diagnosis, a CMRI showed several new growing epi- and myocardial abscesses on both left and right atria and ventricles (Figure 1). Multiple small and confluent soft-contoured nodules were observed on CT examination and could definitively be attributed to *Aspergillus fumigatus* infection as, at that time point, the latter was found for the first time in serum, blood, urine, and lung. For the first time, *Aspergillus* antigens were also positive. Urgent heart surgery was discussed but was rejected due to the patient's altered physiological status and to the extent of the lesions. A few days later, the patient died from a septic shock and multiple organ failure caused by disseminated aspergillosis. Postmortem examination confirmed that multiple aspergillosis abscesses were located in the epicardium, myocardium, and endocardium and were associated with lung, liver, kidney, and skin aspergillosis abscesses.

3. Discussion

Pulmonary form of invasive aspergillosis is commonly observed after transplantation, but it is seldom located on the heart wall. Few aspergillosis cardiac locations have been described in severely immunocompromised AIDS patients with less than 200 CD4 T-lymphocytes/μL [3], but no cardiac abscess has been related after solid transplantation. To the best of our knowledge, this is the first reported case of cardiac aspergillosis abscess as first aspergillosis imaging abnormality in a transplanted patient. At admission there was no evidence of aspergillosis. *Aspergillus* antigenemia remained negative until 6 months after the diagnosis of the myocardial abscess. *Aspergillus* was also not found in the BAL. The antifungal therapy was initiated based on the patient's posttransplant history, that is, heavy immunosuppression and *Aspergillus fumigatus* detected in tracheal aspiration taken early after transplantation. Under dual antifungal therapy, the abscess size remained stable. Three months after the presentation, one of the two antifungal drugs was withdrawn: a disseminated aspergillosis was observed. However, the relationship between the number of antifungal drugs used and the outcome cannot be established.

Other organisms are known to cause a myocardial abscess: *Staphylococcus aureus, Streptococcus*, *Candida*, and *Salmonella* [4]. Those myocardial abscesses have been described with quite similar imaging characteristics but can be diagnosed with specific biological assessments (e.g., for *Staphylococcus aureus*, blood cultures) [5]. Our patient did not show any positive results from these assessments.

In the present case, CMRI was a valuable asset and permitted us to detect heart-wall lesions and to assess their extent and progression and enabled a definitive diagnosis: a collection with a thick enhancing rim. CMRI also allowed us to study the remaining heart-wall thickness and to evaluate the rupture prognosis and heart-wall motion, which is in contrast to results obtained using CT. With its precise images, CMRI could offer guidance to a surgical approach. The use of CMRI is an efficient, simple, accurate, and noninvasive technique but does lack etiology specificity. Other methods to detect a cardiac abscess have their shortfalls. Transthoracic echocardiography, performed a few days after the first CMRI, was only able to show an inferior pericardial thickening, due to reduced apex visibility. A transoesophageal echocardiography could not be planned because of the patient's altered clinical status. At admission, a puncutre of the abcess may have allow the early identification of the *Aspergillus*, and to adapt anti-fungal therapy consequently.

In conclusion, myocardial abscess can be observed as first imaging evidence of an invasive aspergillosis. Early diagnosis and treatment are required because of the high risk of mortality.

References

[1] J. A. Fishman, "Infection in solid-organ transplant recipients," *The New England Journal of Medicine*, vol. 357, no. 25, pp. 2601–2614, 2007.

[2] G. S. Gulati and S. Sharma, "Pericardial abscess occurring after tuberculous pericarditis: image morphology on computed tomography and magnetic resonance imaging," *Clinical Radiology*, vol. 59, no. 6, pp. 514–519, 2004.

[3] L. Xie, W. Gebre, K. Szabo, and J. H. Lin, "Cardiac aspergillosis in patients with acquired immunodeficiency syndrome: a case report and review of the literature," *Archives of Pathology and Laboratory Medicine*, vol. 129, no. 4, pp. 511–515, 2005.

[4] M.-J. Kim, J.-M. Song, and J.-K. Song, "Multiple myocardial abscesses successfully treated with medical management in an immunosuppressed patient," *European Heart Journal*, vol. 28, no. 9, article 1051, 2007.

[5] J. Iqbal, I. Ahmed, and W. Baig, "Metastatic myocardial abscess on the posterior wall of the left ventricle: a case report," *Journal of Medical Case Reports*, vol. 2, article 258, 2008.

11

Use of Methylene Blue for Treatment of Severe Sepsis in an Immunosuppressed Patient after Liver Transplantation

Saravanan Ramamoorthy,[1] Shachi Patel,[2] Eric Bradburn,[3] Zakiyah Kadry,[4] Tadahiro Uemura,[4] Piotr K. Janicki,[2] Riaz Ali Shah,[4] and Dmitri Bezinover[2]

[1] *Department of Anesthesiology, Penn State Hershey Medical Center, 500 University Drive, H187 Hershey, PA 17033-0850, USA*
[2] *Department of Anesthesiology, Penn State Hershey Medical Center, Hershey, PA-17033, USA*
[3] *Department of Surgery, Penn State Hershey Medical Center, Hershey, PA-17033, USA*
[4] *Department of Transplant Surgery, Penn State Hershey Medical Center, Hershey, PA-17033, USA*

Correspondence should be addressed to Dmitri Bezinover; dbezinover@hmc.psu.edu

Academic Editors: M. Ferraresso, J. Jazbec, J. A. Kari, and M. Klinger

Sepsis in the immunosuppressed patient is associated with very high mortality and morbidity. Treatment of sepsis in immunocompromised patients is especially challenging due to an unbalanced systemic inflammatory reaction with subsequent development of profound vasoplegia. Methylene blue (MB) has been successfully used for the treatment of refractory hypotension, but its use has not previously been reported for treatment of sepsis in immunosuppressed patients. The mechanism of MB's action is thought to be due to its inhibitory effect on cGMP-mediated vasodilatation. This case report describes the successful use of MB for treatment of severe septic shock in an immunosuppressed patient after liver transplantation. Hypotension in this patient was refractory to volume repletion and a combination of vasopressors. After MB administration, hemodynamic stability was rapidly reestablished. In the setting of severe sepsis in an immunosuppressed patient, MB should be considered early as a therapeutic option for treatment of refractory vasoplegia.

1. Introduction

Sepsis in the immunosuppressed patient is often resistant or unresponsive to conventional pharmacologic therapy and is associated with mortality significantly higher than in the immunocompetent patient. The fulminant course of sepsis in immunosuppressed patients is related to an unbalanced systemic inflammatory response with subsequent development of pharmacologically resistant hemodynamic depression. Severe septic shock with vasoplegia is a devastating complication of sepsis in the immunocompromised patient. Therapy resistant hypotension is thought to be the result of dysregulation of nitric oxide (NO) synthesis. A number of investigations performed in critically ill, although not pharmacologically immunosuppressed patients, have demonstrated the efficacy of methylene blue (MB) administration in reducing plasma NO and restoring hemodynamic stability [1–4].

2. Case Description

Before the preparation of this paper, written informed consent was obtained from the patient.

A 64-year-old male patient presented for a routine liver biopsy after orthotopic deceased donor liver transplantation (OLT). The original cause of the patient's liver failure was nonalcoholic steatohepatitis complicated by hepatocellular carcinoma. The patient's past medical history was otherwise not significant. Postoperative immunosuppressive medications included both mycophenolate and tacrolimus.

Two years after transplantation, the patient underwent a scheduled liver biopsy. A few hours after the procedure, he developed severe right upper quadrant pain which became diffuse and significantly worsened despite repeated administration of morphine sulfate boluses. A CT scan of the abdomen with contrast demonstrated the presence of fluid surrounding the liver as well as fluid accumulation in the lower abdomen and pelvis. There were no other pathological findings.

The patient's condition continued to rapidly deteriorate. He became febrile to 38.7°C and developed signs of respiratory distress with oxygen saturations below 90% despite 6 L/min oxygen via nasal cannula. On postprocedure day (PPD) 1, the patient became tachycardic to 129 bpm and hypotensive with a blood pressure of 96/68 mmHg. After further deterioration of the patient's cardiopulmonary status, he was intubated and transferred to the Medical Intensive Care Unit (MICU). Due to profound hypotension, intravenous administration of phenylephrine was initiated, first as boluses (100–200 mcg) and later as an infusion of 30 mcg/min. The patient also received an infusion of 0.9% normal saline solution at 200 mL/h. While in the MICU, the patient developed symptoms of peritonitis. CT-guided drainage of the peri-hepatic accumulation demonstrated fluid compatible with an infected biliary drainage. Blood cultures and peri-hepatic fluid cultures were positive for gram-negative *Escherichia coli*. Broad-spectrum antibiotic therapy was initiated with meropenem, ciprofloxacin, vancomycin, tobramycin, as well as caspofungin. Despite antibiotic administration and vasoactive support, arterial hypotension and tachycardia persisted (a low of 88/59 mmHg and heart rate of 135 bpm). Norepinephrine (NE) and vasopressin (VP) infusions were initiated. Infusion rates were titrated up to a maximum of 3 mcg/kg/min of NE and 0.08 units/min of VP without significant improvement in the patient's hemodynamic status. An exploratory laparotomy was performed which demonstrated a bile containing fluid accumulation and a laceration of the liver at the biopsy site. Repair of the laceration and an abdominal lavage were performed.

After surgery, the patient was admitted to the Surgical Intensive Care Unit (SICU) in critical condition. In the SICU, a pulmonary artery catheter was placed for hemodynamic monitoring. The patient displayed a pattern of circulation consistent with sepsis, with a cardiac output of 9.4 L/min, SVR of 298 dyne·s^{-1}·cm^{-5}, and mixed venous saturation of 78%. In addition to continued vasoactive agent administration, volume therapy was initiated. Overall, 8 liters of crystalloid was administered over the next 10 hours. The patient continued to be hemodynamically unstable. Subsequently, an epinephrine infusion, titrated up to 0.07 mcg/kg/min, was started. The patient's hemodynamics did not improve and deterioration of liver function was noted. Cholangitis from stricture formation was suspected and the patient underwent a bedside endoscopic retrograde cholangiopancreatography (ERCP) with stent placement in the common bile duct.

After ERCP, the patient's condition continued to deteriorate. He remained febrile and hemodynamically unstable, with a heart rate of 137 bpm and BP of 87/55 mmHg despite support of multiple pressors and inotropes. Urine output decreased and serum creatinine rose to over 3 mg/dL. Acute kidney failure developed requiring continuous renal replacement therapy (CRRT). In order to counteract a presumed suppression of the adrenal hypothalamic axis, intermittent boluses of hydrocortisone and a levothyroxine infusion (30 mcg/h) were started.

On PPD 2, after exhausting all therapeutic measures and with further deterioration of the patient's condition, MB therapy was initiated with two 100 mg doses (2 mg/kg) infused over a period of 2 hours. Three hours after administration of the first dose of MB, the patient's hemodynamic parameters markedly improved (BP of 117/62, HR of 117, SVR increased to 536 dyne·s^{-1}·cm^{-5}, and mixed venous saturation decreased to 60%). These changes reflect recovery of systemic microperfusion with subsequent increase in oxygen consumption and a reduction of arterio-venous shunting. The patient was subsequently weaned from vasoactive support (Figure 1) and mechanical ventilation was discontinued 3 days later. The patient's urine output markedly improved, CRRT was stopped, and he was transferred to the ward. The patient was discharged home on PPD 12.

3. Discussion

There are a number of publications demonstrating effectiveness of MB for treatment of sepsis-associated vasoplegia. This paper is the first known documentation of the therapeutic effects of MB for treatment of severe sepsis in an *immunocompromised* patient. The treatment of sepsis in immunosuppressed patients is one of most difficult challenges in modern critical care. The unbalanced inflammatory reaction, frequently seen in septic immunosuppressed patients, produces massive vasodilatation with subsequent severe injury to organ microperfusion.

Sepsis itself is associated with significant immune dysregulation. Defects in the function of leukocytes, alterations in antigen-presenting ability, and accelerated apoptosis contribute to the systemic inflammatory response which results in the release of cytokines and endotoxins [5, 6]. Endotoxins directly initiate production of inducible NO synthase (iNOS) [7–9]. In addition, they activate release of interleukin 1-b, tumor necrosis factor-α, and interferon-γ. These cytokines are responsible for increasing iNOS release in target cells, which leads to an elevation in NO production from L-arginine in vascular endothelium [10]. NO, in turn, activates guanyl-cyclase (GC) with subsequent increasing concentrations of cGMP in vascular smooth muscle. This results in systemic vasodilation.

There is a significant difference in the immune response to sepsis between the immunocompetent and immunocompromised patient. Immunocompetent patients usually demonstrate a specific *anti-inflammatory* reaction as an immediate response to sepsis in order to localize the inflammatory process and prevent diffuse vascular damage [11]. This reaction includes release of various cytokines including interleukin-1 and interleukin-10 receptor antagonists as well as soluble tumor necrosis factor receptor. These substances inhibit the T-cell network with subsequent downregulation of monocyte activation. In addition, the development of

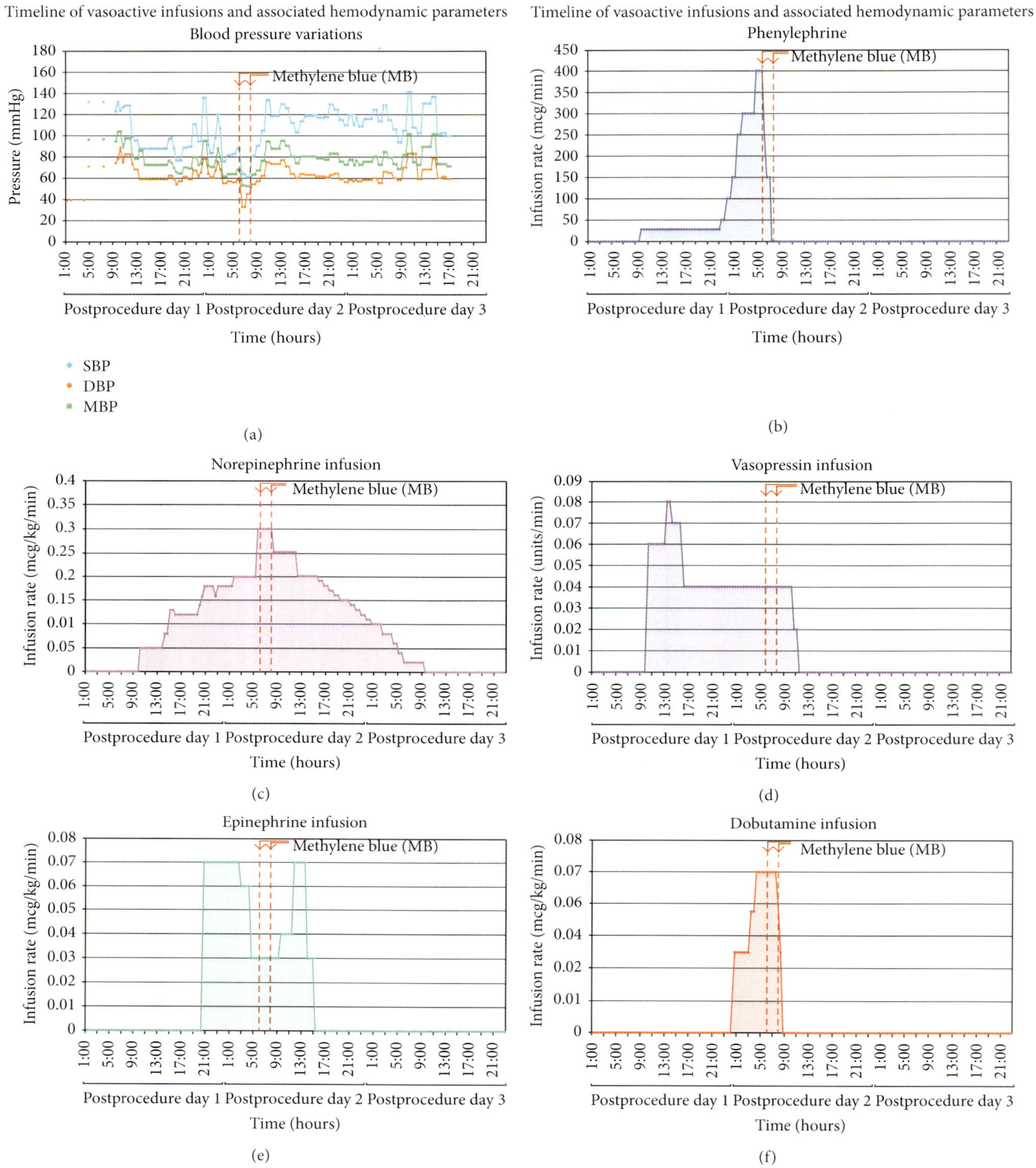

FIGURE 1: (a) Graph showing blood pressure variations across time period; blood pressure (Blue—SBP; brown—DBP; green—MAP) in *Y* axis and time elapsed in hours from postprocedure day 1 to post procedure 3 in *X* axis. (b) Graph showing phenylephrine infusion with infusion rate (mcg/min) in *Y* axis and time elapsed in hours from postprocedure day 1 to postprocedure 3 in *X* axis. (c) Graph showing norepinephrine infusion with infusion rate (mcg/kg/min) in *Y* axis and time elapsed in hours from postprocedure day 1 to postprocedure 3 in *X* axis. (d) Graph showing vasopressin infusion with infusion rate (Units/min) in *Y* axis and time elapsed in hours from postprocedure day 1 to postprocedure 3 in *X* axis. (e) Graph showing epinephrine infusion with infusion rate (mcg/kg/min) in *Y* axis and time elapsed in hours from postprocedure day 1 to postprocedure 3 in *X* axis. (f) Graph showing dobutamine infusion with infusion rate (mcg/kg/min) in *Y* axis and time elapsed in hours from postprocedure day 1 to postprocedure 3 in *X* axis. Double dash vertical lines across graphs (a, b, c, d, e and f) depict the period of methylene blue (MB) infusion.

tolerance to lipopolysaccharide (a major constituent of gram negative bacterial cell walls) as well as cellular deactivation of macrophages and monocytes is part of this protective process [12].

This anti-inflammatory mechanism is severely depressed in immunocompromised patients which results in an uncontrolled inflammatory response with subsequent hyper-resistant hemodynamic instability [13]. It has been demonstrated that immunosuppressed septic patients are prone to develop septic shock and demonstrate an even more refractory hypotension in comparison to patients without immunosuppression [14].

The main cause of this vasoplegia is the overpowering activation of the NO pathway due to an unbalanced systemic inflammatory reaction. Administration of MB has been demonstrated to reverse the course of hemodynamic deterioration and prevent development of severe septic shock.

MB acts on multiple sites in the cGMP pathway. Specifically, MB inhibits iNOS in vascular endothelium which effectively reduces NO production [15]. MB also binds soluble GC which results in a reduction in cGMP levels [16, 17]. Additionally, it has been demonstrated that MB contributes to increasing cardiac contractility depressed by cGMP [18].

Severe sepsis is associated with a mortality rate over 40% [18]. Sepsis-associated mortality in immunosuppressed patients is even higher. Poutsiaka et al. [14] reviewed the outcome of immunosuppressed patients with severe sepsis. They demonstrated significantly higher 28-day mortality in patients with preexisting immunosuppression in comparison with immunocompetent septic patients.

The main cause of sepsis associated mortality is multiorgan failure related to breakdown of tissue microcirculation. Considering that organ perfusion in the immunosuppressed septic patient is more severely affected than in the immunocompetent septic patient due to the uncontained inflammatory response, early administration of MB can be beneficial.

References

[1] R. L. Levin, M. A. Degrange, G. F. Bruno et al., "Methylene blue reduces mortality and morbidity in vasoplegic patients after cardiac surgery," *Annals of Thoracic Surgery*, vol. 77, no. 2, pp. 496–499, 2004.

[2] G. W. Fischer, Y. Bengtsson, S. Scarola, and E. Cohen, "Methylene blue for vasopressor-resistant vasoplegia syndrome during liver transplantation," *Journal of Cardiothoracic and Vascular Anesthesia*, vol. 24, no. 3, pp. 463–466, 2010.

[3] G. Brown, D. Frankl, and T. Phang, "Continuous infusion of methylene blue for septic shock," *Postgraduate Medical Journal*, vol. 72, no. 852, pp. 612–614, 1996.

[4] E. S. H. Kwok and D. W. Howes, "Use of methylene blue in sepsis: a systematic review," *Journal of Intensive Care Medicine*, vol. 21, no. 6, pp. 359–363, 2006.

[5] K. Lyn-Kew and T. J. Standiford, "Immunosuppression in sepsis," *Current Pharmaceutical Design*, vol. 14, no. 19, pp. 1870–1881, 2008.

[6] J. S. Boomer, K. To, K. C. Chang et al., "Immunosuppression in patients who die of sepsis and multiple organ failure," *The Journal of the American Medical Association*, vol. 306, no. 23, pp. 2594–2605, 2011.

[7] G. Laffi, M. Foschi, E. Masini et al., "Increased production of nitric oxide by neutrophils and monocytes from cirrhotic patients with ascites and hyperdynamic circulation," *Hepatology*, vol. 22, no. 6, pp. 1666–1673, 1995.

[8] H. F. Galley, D. Coomansingh, N. R. Webster, and P. W. Brunt, "Nitric oxide synthase activity is increased in relation to the severity of liver dysfunction," *Clinical Science*, vol. 95, no. 3, pp. 355–359, 1998.

[9] C. Nathan and Q. W. Xie, "Nitric oxide synthases: roles, tolls, and controls," *Cell*, vol. 78, no. 6, pp. 915–918, 1994.

[10] H. Tilg, A. Wilmer, W. Vogel et al., "Serum levels of cytokines in chronic liver diseases," *Gastroenterology*, vol. 103, no. 1, pp. 264–274, 1992.

[11] R. S. Munford and J. Pugin, "Normal responses to injury prevent systemic inflammation andcan be immunosuppressive," *The American Journal of Respiratory and Critical Care Medicine*, vol. 163, no. 2, pp. 316–321, 2001.

[12] J. C. Gea-Banacloche, S. M. Opal, J. Jorgensen, J. A. Carcillo, K. A. Sepkowitz, and C. Cordonnier, "Sepsis associated with immunosuppressive medications: an evidence-based review," *Critical Care Medicine*, vol. 32, no. 11, pp. S578–S590, 2004.

[13] J. Cohen, "The immunopathogenesis of sepsis," *Nature*, vol. 420, no. 6917, pp. 885–891, 2002.

[14] D. D. Poutsiaka, L. E. Davidson, K. L. Kahn, D. W. Bates, D. R. Snydman, and P. L. Hibberd, "Risk factors for death after sepsis in patients immunosuppressed before the onset of sepsis," *Scandinavian Journal of Infectious Diseases*, vol. 41, no. 6-7, pp. 469–479, 2009.

[15] G. W. Fischer and M. A. Levin, "Vasoplegia during cardiac surgery: current concepts and management," *Seminars in Thoracic and Cardiovascular Surgery*, vol. 22, no. 2, pp. 140–144, 2010.

[16] R. M. J. Palmer, "The discovery of nitric oxide in the vessel wall: a unifying concept in the pathogenesis of sepsis," *Archives of Surgery*, vol. 128, no. 4, pp. 396–401, 1993.

[17] B. Mayer, F. Brunner, and K. Schmidt, "Novel actions of methylene blue," *European Heart Journal*, vol. 14, no. 1, pp. 22–26, 1993.

[18] G. S. Martin, D. M. Mannino, S. Eaton, and M. Moss, "The epidemiology of sepsis in the United States from 1979 through 2000," *New England Journal of Medicine*, vol. 348, no. 16, pp. 1546–1554, 2003.

12

Diffuse Hepatic Epithelioid Hemangioendothelioma Developed in a Patient with Hepatitis C Cirrhosis

Pedro W. Baron,[1] Thomas Amankonah,[1] Robert F. Cubas,[2] Arputharaj H. Kore,[1] Arvand Elihu,[1] Michael E. de Vera,[1] and Mia C. N. Perez[3]

[1] *Transplantation Institute, Loma Linda University Medical Center, 25865 Barton Road, Suite 101, Loma Linda, CA 92354, USA*
[2] *Department of Surgery, Loma Linda University Medical Center, 25865 Barton Road, Suite 101, Loma Linda, CA 92354, USA*
[3] *Departments of Pathology and Laboratory Medicine, Loma Linda University Medical Center, 25865 Barton Road, Suite 101, Loma Linda, CA 92354, USA*

Correspondence should be addressed to Pedro W. Baron; pbaron@llu.edu

Academic Editor: Piero Boraschi

Hepatic epithelioid hemangioendothelioma (HEHE) is an infrequent vascular tumor of endothelial origin that primarily occurs in women in the mid-fifth decade of life without underlying chronic liver disease or cirrhosis. Liver transplant should be the first-line of therapy in patients with large or diffuse unresectable tumors even in the presence of metastatic disease due to the favorable long-term outcome. We report the case of a 48-year-old female who complained of abdominal pain and weight loss. She has a history of cirrhosis secondary to chronic hepatitis C (HCV) and was treated with interferon and ribavirin with sustained virological response. Her work-up revealed multiple confluent infiltrating bilobar liver masses diagnosed as HEHE. She underwent a successful liver transplant without evidence of recurrent HCV infection. She developed cervical spine (C4-C6) HEHE metastases 4 years after transplant. She underwent surgical resection and local radiotherapy after resection with good clinical response. To the best of our knowledge, this is the first report of HEHE that developed in a patient with HCV cirrhosis successfully treated with antiviral therapy before transplant and liver transplant with good allograft function without evidence of recurrent liver tumor or HCV infection but developed metastases to the cervical spine 4 years after transplant.

1. Introduction

Hepatic epithelioid hemangioendothelioma (HEHE) is an infrequent vascular tumor of endothelial origin, not associated with cirrhosis, with a histological appearance intermediate between hemangioma and angiosarcoma [1].

HEHE has an incidence of less than 0.1 per 100,000 population [2], accounts for less than 1% of all hepatic malignancies, and shows a 3 : 2 female preponderance [3]. HEHE was first described in 1982 by Weiss and Enzinger [4]. Ishak et al. reported the first series of 32 primary hepatic hemangioendotheliomas in 1984 [5]. There are no clearly established risk factors for its development; however, association with oral contraceptive pill intake, vinyl chloride exposure, major hepatic trauma, and viral hepatitis has been implicated [1, 3]. Generally, HEHE behaves as a low-grade malignant tumor with a slowly progressive phenotype [6]. Its clinical presentation is nonspecific and can vary from no symptoms to overt hepatic failure and death [7].

Patients with HEHE are often candidates for liver transplant (LT) as the disease is usually multifocal at diagnosis and it is also resistant to both chemotherapy and radiotherapy.

2. Case Report

We report the case of a 48-year-old Caucasian female who complained of abdominal pain and 30-pound-weight loss over a three-month period. She had a history of chronic hepatitis C (HCV), genotype 3a, that was treated with peginterferon alpha and ribavirin with HCV RNA negative after 8 weeks of treatment. She continued HCV therapy for about 24 weeks until transplant. On initial physical examination, patient was anicteric but with increased liver span of 14 cm by dull percussion which is consistent with hepatomegaly. Additional pretransplant work-up showed normal hemoglobin and serum alpha-fetoprotein (AFP), low platelet count, and mildly elevated serum aminotransferase levels. Abdominal and pelvic computerized tomography (CT) scan showed multiple confluent infiltrating bilobar low density liver masses and cirrhosis (Figure 1). A percutaneous liver core biopsy was performed. The initial histopathologic interpretation was inconclusive. Following an additional positive factor VIII-related antigen stain, the diagnosis of HEHE was rendered. She was listed for LT following a Liver Regional Review Board approval with a model for end-stage liver disease score exception of 22 and gained additional points corresponding to 10% waiting-list mortality every 3 months. Patient underwent a successful LT 13 months later.

The explanted liver showed hepatomegaly (2,480 grams in weight) and a micronodular capsular surface. Cut sections revealed cirrhosis and multiple, firm, tan-white nodules measuring up to 2.2 cm in greatest diameter. Histopathologic examination confirmed multifocal HEHE in the background of cirrhosis and steatosis (Figure 2). The typical HEHE features, consisting of anastomosing cords of epithelioid cells, mostly with intracytoplasmic lumina, in a hyalinized and myxoid stroma, were seen (Figure 2 inset). There were also atypical features with a solid growth pattern and spindle cell cytology. A positive CD31 stain again confirmed the vascular endothelial nature. The tumor additionally showed extracapsular spread with direct extension to perihilar lymph nodes and hilar vessels. Proliferation marker Ki-67 showed differential staining with less than 5% positivity in the typical areas and 10–15% positivity in the atypical areas.

Her immunosuppressive therapy consisted of methylprednisolone IV bolus after hepatectomy was completed and then tacrolimus and prednisone as maintenance therapy. The patient was discharged home with excellent allograft function on postoperative day 8. She has not had an episode of acute rejection. Prednisone was discontinued 6 months after transplant. She underwent total right shoulder replacement due to severe degenerative arthritis and chronic pain without complications 15 months after transplant. She developed cervical spine (C4-C6) HEHE metastases 4 years after transplant. She underwent surgical resection and local radiotherapy after resection. Her allograft function is normal and she has no evidence of recurrent HCV infection. This report was completed after obtaining written authorization from the patient, as per our standard Institutional Review Board policy.

3. Discussion

To the best of our knowledge, this is the first report in English literature of a case of HEHE that developed in a patient with HCV cirrhosis, RNA-negative following pretransplant therapy and treated with LT, without HCV recurrence for more than 48 months after transplant. However, she developed metastatic cervical spine disease 4 years after transplant treated with resection and radiotherapy with good clinical response.

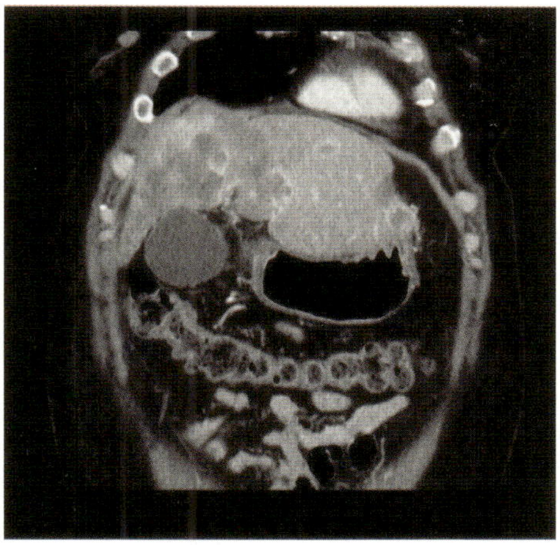

FIGURE 1: CT scan of the abdomen and pelvis.

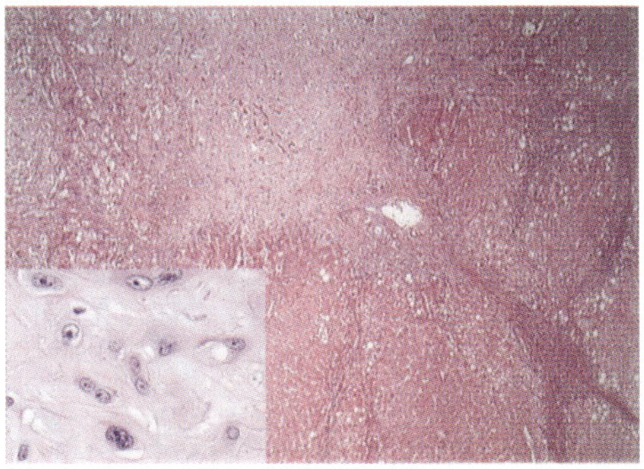

FIGURE 2: Photomicrograph of explanted liver. Transition zone between HEHE (upper-left corner) and cirrhosis. Inset is high-power view of HEHE showing epithelioid cells with intracytoplasmic lumina.

Several factors, including viral hepatitis, have been implicated in the pathogenesis of HEHE. Makhlouf et al. reported three HEHE patients who tested positive for hepatitis B virus and another three HEHE patients who tested positive for hepatitis C virus. None of the six patients had cirrhosis at the time of the HEHE diagnosis [8]. Grotz et al. reported 30 patients with HEHE, none of whom had underlying chronic liver disease or cirrhosis [1]. Mehrabi et al. stated that HEHE, in contrast to many other types of primary liver tumor, does not arise in a background of chronic liver disease [9–12]. No clear association was found between HEHE and HCV cirrhosis in patients who underwent LT between 1990 and 2010 after reviewing the Organ Procurement and Transplantation Network (OPTN) database*. Two LTs were done for a vascular tumor of the liver as a diagnosis group that includes HEHE, hemangiosarcoma, and angiosarcoma with a secondary diagnosis of HCV cirrhosis. It was not possible to determine whether these two patients had HEHE and HCV cirrhosis.

Most patients with HEHE seek medical attention after the tumor burden has become large enough to cause symptoms [13]. Upper abdominal pain or discomfort appears to be the most frequent symptom. Although CT scan may detect the lesions, no imaging features of HEHE are pathognomonic [1].

Histopathologic examination is the only way to confirm the diagnosis of HEHE. Distinguishing HEHE from other liver tumors is vital, because the 5-year survival rate of HEHE has been reported to be greater than 55%, which is favorable compared to other primary liver malignant neoplasms [14].

There is no standard treatment for HEHE due to its infrequent incidence. Either surgical resection or LT has been generally recommended as curative treatment for this disease [1, 15]. HEHE is usually multifocal and therefore not suitable for partial hepatectomy in about 87% of the cases [12]. It also seems to be resistant to both chemotherapy and radiotherapy.

Mehrabi et al. reviewed 434 patients treated for HEHE since 1984 and concluded that LT is the treatment of choice because of the hepatic multicentricity with 96% and 54% patient survival rates at 1 and 5 years, respectively [12]. Lerut et al. reported that the outcome of LT as a treatment for HEHE was excellent with 83% and 72% patient survival rates at 1 and 5 years, respectively [16]. Rodriguez et al. analyzed 110 patients from the UNOS database who underwent LT between 1987 and 2005. These data indicated that survival after LT was favorable for all patients, including patients with diffuse intrahepatic tumor, with 1-year and 5-year patient survival rates of 80% and 64%, respectively [13]. Preexisting extrahepatic disease spread and lymph node involvement are not contraindications to LT. However, microscopic and/or macroscopic vascular invasion significantly influence post-LT survival [16–18].

Although these patients achieve excellent post-LT outcomes, there is very little data regarding tumor markers that can further direct chemotherapy in HEHE to prevent disease recurrence [18]. Tumor markers (i.e., AFP, carcinoembryonic antigen/CEA, and cancer antigen/CA 19-9) are usually in the normal range; however, vascular endothelial growth factor expression was identified in all specimens from a cohort of six patients with HEHE at a single center (100%) [13, 18].

If radiologic characteristic of hepatocellular carcinoma (HCC) is not present, high index of suspicion is necessary to rule in this very rare liver tumor in the background of hepatitis C cirrhosis, granting that HCC is the most common malignancy by far.

In conclusion, to the best of our knowledge, this is the first report of HEHE that developed in a patient with HCV cirrhosis successfully treated with antiviral therapy before transplant and liver transplant with good liver allograft function without evidence of recurrent liver tumor or HCV infection but developed metastases to the cervical spine 4 years after transplant.

Abbreviations

HEHE: Hepatic epithelioid hemangioendothelioma
LT: Liver transplant
HCV: Hepatitis C virus
AFP: Alpha-fetoprotein
CT: Computerized tomography
HCC: Hepatocellular carcinoma.

Disclosure

These data were presented as a Poster at the 24th International Congress of the Transplantation Society in Berlin, Germany, July 16–19, 2012.

Acknowledgments

*OPTN data as of June 21, 2013. This work was supported in part by Health Resources and Services Administration contract 234-2005-371011C. The content is the responsibility of the authors alone and does not necessarily reflect the views or policies of the Department of Health and Human Services nor does the mention of trade names, commercial products, or organizations imply endorsement by the US Government.

References

[1] T. E. Grotz, D. Nagorney, J. Donohue et al., "Hepatic epithelioid haemangioendothelioma: is transplantation the only treatment option?" *HPB*, vol. 12, no. 8, pp. 546–553, 2010.

[2] M. Hertl and A. B. Cosimi, "Liver transplantation for malignancy," *Oncologist*, vol. 10, no. 4, pp. 269–281, 2005.

[3] N. Agrawal, S. Parajuli, P. Zhao et al., "Liver transplantation in the management of hepatic epithelioid hemangioendothelioma: a single-center experience and review of the literature," *Transplantation Proceedings*, vol. 43, no. 7, pp. 2647–2650, 2011.

[4] S. W. Weiss and F. M. Enzinger, "Epitheloid hemangioendothelioma: a vascular tumor often mistaken for a carcinoma," *Cancer*, vol. 50, no. 5, pp. 970–981, 1982.

[5] K. G. Ishak, I. A. Sesterhenn, M. Z. Goodman, L. Rabin, and F. W. Stromeyer, "Epithelioid hemangioendothelioma of the liver: a clinicopathologic and follow-up study of 32 cases," *Human Pathology*, vol. 15, no. 9, pp. 839–852, 1984.

[6] K. Mucha, B. Foroncewicz, K. Zieniewicz et al., "Patient with liver epithelioid hemangioendothelioma treated by transplantation: 3 years' observation," *Transplantation Proceedings*, vol. 38, no. 1, pp. 231–233, 2006.

[7] G. H. Kim, Y. S. Kim, H. O. Kim et al., "A case of primary hepatic epithelioid hemangioendothelioma with spontaneous rupture," *The Korean journal of hepatology*, vol. 15, no. 4, pp. 510–516, 2009.

[8] H. R. Makhlouf, K. G. Ishak, and Z. D. Goodman, "Epithelioid hemangioendothelioma of the liver: a clinicopathologic study of 137 cases," *Cancer*, vol. 85, pp. 562–582, 1999.

[9] M. D'Annibale, P. Piovanello, P. Carlini et al., "Epithelioid hemangioendothelioma of the liver: case report and review of the literature," *Transplantation Proceedings*, vol. 34, no. 4, pp. 1248–1251, 2002.

[10] Y. Hayashi, K. Inagaki, S. Hirota, T. Yoshikawa, H. Ikawa, and H. Itoh, "Epithelioid hemangioendothelioma with marked liver deformity and secondary Budd-Chiari syndrome: pathological and radiological correlation," *Pathology International*, vol. 49, no. 6, pp. 547–552, 1999.

[11] J. M. Lauffer, A. Zimmermann, L. Krahenbuhl, J. Triller, and H. U. Baer, "Epithelioid hemangioendothelioma of the liver. A rare hepatic tumor," *Cancer*, vol. 78, no. 11, pp. 2318–2327, 1996.

[12] A. Mehrabi, A. Kashfi, H. Fonouni et al., "Primary malignant hepatic epithelioid hemangioendothelioma: a comprehensive review of the literature with emphasis on the surgical therapy," *Cancer*, vol. 107, no. 9, pp. 2108–2121, 2006.

[13] J. A. Rodriguez, N. S. Becker, C. A. O'Mahony, J. A. Goss, and T. A. Aloia, "Long-term outcomes following liver transplantation for hepatic hemangioendothelioma: the UNOS experience from 1987 to 2005," *Journal of Gastrointestinal Surgery*, vol. 12, no. 1, pp. 110–116, 2008.

[14] J. Cardinal, M. E. de Vera, J. W. Marsh et al., "Treatment of hepatic epithelioid hemangioendothelioma: a single-institution experience with 25 cases," *Archives of Surgery*, vol. 144, no. 11, pp. 1035–1039, 2009.

[15] N. Oshima, H. Terajima, and R. Hosotani, "Surgical therapy for a solitary form of hepatic epithelioid hemangioendothelioma: a long-term survival case," *Case Reports in Gastroenterology*, vol. 3, pp. 214–221, 2009.

[16] J. P. Lerut, G. Orlando, R. Adam et al., "The place of liver transplantation in the treatment of hepatic epitheloid hemangioendothelioma: report of the European liver transplant registry," *Annals of Surgery*, vol. 246, no. 6, pp. 949–957, 2007.

[17] S. Bufton, G. Haydon, and D. Neil, "Liver transplantation for hepatic epithelioid hemangioendothelioma: a case series," *Progress in Transplantation*, vol. 17, no. 1, pp. 70–72, 2007.

[18] J. A. Emamaullee, R. Edgar, C. Toso et al., "Vascular endothelial growth factor expression in hepatic epithelioid hemangioendothelioma: implications for treatment and surgical management," *Liver Transplantation*, vol. 16, no. 2, pp. 191–197, 2010.

13

Liver Transplantation for Acute Liver Failure at 11-Week Gestation with Successful Maternal and Fetal Outcome

Vinaya C. Maddukuri,[1] Courtney D. Stephenson,[2] Lon Eskind,[3] William A. Ahrens,[4] Preston Purdum,[5] and Mark W. Russo[1,6]

[1] *Division of Hepatology, Carolinas Medical Center, 1000 Blythe Boulevard, Charlotte, NC 28203, USA*
[2] *Department of Obstetrics and Gynecology, Carolinas Medical Center, 1000 Blythe Boulevard, Charlotte, NC 28203, USA*
[3] *Department of Surgery, Carolinas Medical Center, 1000 Blythe Boulevard, Charlotte, NC 28203, USA*
[4] *Department of Pathology, Carolinas Medical Center, 1000 Blythe Boulevard, Charlotte, NC 28203, USA*
[5] *Carolinas Digestive Health Associates, Charlotte, NC 28211, USA*
[6] *Transplant Center, Carolinas Medical Center, 3rd Floor Annex building, Charlotte, NC 28203, USA*

Correspondence should be addressed to Mark W. Russo, mark.russo@carolinashealthcare.org

Academic Editors: J. Kaneko and G. Schlaf

Acute liver failure (ALF) during pregnancy is very uncommon. Pregnancy-specific liver conditions like hemolysis, elevated liver enzymes, and low platelets (HELLP) syndrome and acute fatty liver of pregnancy can cause ALF at term or postpartum, but, typically occur during the third trimester. Most of these patients recover spontaneously after delivery, but, on occasion, they require liver transplantation in the postpartum period. However, ALF during the first and second trimester of pregnancy requiring antepartum liver transplantation is rare. Only fifteen cases of liver transplantation during pregnancy have been reported, and very few occurred during the first trimester. We report a Woman who developed acute liver failure during the first trimester of pregnancy and underwent successful liver transplantation at 11-week gestation, followed by successful delivery of the fetus at 30 weeks. To our knowledge, this is the earliest case of successful liver transplantation during pregnancy followed by successful fetal outcome. We discuss management of the patient and fetus before, during, and after liver transplantation and review the literature on antepartum liver transplant in pregnancy.

1. Introduction

Abnormal liver tests can be seen in 3% to 5% of pregnant women and are usually due to pregnancy related conditions [1]. Pregnancy related conditions, such as intrahepatic cholestasis of pregnancy (ICP), pre-eclampsia, HELLP (hemolysis, elevated liver enzymes, and low platelets) syndrome, and acute fatty liver of pregnancy (AFLP) [1], almost always occur during the third trimester. Conditions unrelated to pregnancy, such as viral hepatitis, gallstones, and drug-induced liver injury can occur at any time during pregnancy, including the first and second trimesters, and cause significant liver dysfunction. However, acute liver failure (ALF) during pregnancy is very rare, and the exact incidence is unknown. HELLP syndrome and AFLP can cause ALF late in pregnancy or postpartum, and most patients recover spontaneously after delivery [2]. On occasion, these patients may require orthotopic liver transplantation (OLT) in the immediate postpartum period [2]. According to the European Liver Transplantation Registry (ELTR), ten of 75,530 liver transplants performed between 1968 and 2008 were performed for acute liver failure due to AFLP and HELLP syndrome [3].

Liver transplant during pregnancy (antepartum or before delivery) has been previously reported (Table 2). However, OLT during the first trimester has been reported in only two previous cases, of which, only one case resulted in successful delivery of the fetus. We report a 29 year-old woman who suffered cryptogenic ALF in the 11th week of her pregnancy requiring emergent antepartum OLT. She continued her

TABLE 1: Selected laboratory values.

Day →	Day 1 (presentation)	2	3	4	5	6	7	8 transplant	9	10	16 discharge	Week 24	Week 26
Lab↓													
Creatinine (mg/dL)	0.6	0.7	0.6	0.7	0.7	0.7	0.6	0.7	0.7	1.0	0.6	1.0	1.1
Albumin (g/dL)	2.2	2.6	2.2	2.4	2.4	2.3	2.3	2.5	2.6	2.9	2.5	3.1	3.1
Total bilirubin (mg/dL)	16.4	16.2	16.0	19.0	21.2	22.1	22.3	24.0	13	4.4	2.6	0.8	0.5
Alkaline phosphatase (IU/L)	105	116	112	143	152	176	166	172	98	63	56	152	152
AST (IU/L)	1001	757	684	729	733	637	580	567	808	370	38	29	30
ALT (IU/L)	1269	883	818	842	834	726	633	607	582	357	117	53	50
INR (s)	3.3	1.7*	2.6	2.9	3.2	3.5	4	5	1.4	1.2			
GGT (IU/L)	66								37	24	50	119	131
Bile acids (μmol/L)												44	

pregnancy after transplant and delivered at 30 weeks, with a successful maternal and fetal outcome. Both mother and child are healthy 4 years after liver transplantation and delivery.

2. Case

A 29 year-old woman, G1 P0, at week 10 of her pregnancy, was admitted with five days of jaundice, nausea, diarrhea, and right upper quadrant pain. She otherwise had no significant past medical history and was not taking any medications, including over the counter medications, except for prenatal vitamins. There was no family history of liver disease. On admission, she was jaundiced, and her abdomen was appropriate for her gestational age with no evidence of ascites. She had no asterixis or encephalopathy on presentation. Admission laboratory tests revealed acute hepatitis and were as follows (Table 1): total bilirubin 16.4 mg/dL, aspartate aminotransferase (AST) 1001 IU/L, alanine aminotransferase (ALT) 1269 IU/L, alkaline phosphatase 105 IU/L, gamma glutamyl transferase (GGT) 66 IU/L, serum albumin 2.2 gm/dL, serum creatinin 0.6 mg/dL, white blood cell count (WBC) 12.6 K/μL, platelets 161 K/μL, and hemoglobin 12.6 gm/dL.

A thorough evaluation for the etiology of acute hepatitis was unrevealed. The following tests were negative: hepatitis A IgM, hepatitis B surface antigen, hepatitis B core antibody [total & IgM], hepatitis C antibody, hepatitis E antibody, cytomegalovirus (CMV) IgM, Epstein-Barr virus IgM, human immunodeficiency virus antibodies, herpes simplex virus (HSV) IgM, varicella IgM, antinuclear antibodies, antimitochondrial antibodies, and antismooth muscle antibodies. The serum ceruloplasmin and immunoglobulin levels [IgG, IgM, and IgA] and plasma alpha −1 antitrypsin level were within the normal range. The serum acetaminophen level was <10 mcg/mL, and urine drug screen was negative. An abdominal ultrasound with Dopplers showed heterogeneous appearing liver with patent hepatic vasculature, without intra- or extrahepatic biliary dilatation. An MRI of the abdomen showed heterogeneous enhancement of the liver with periportal edema, patent portal, and hepatic veins but no cirrhosis.

On the third hospital day, a transjugular liver biopsy was performed that showed intense, active, interface hepatitis (Figures 1(a) and 1(b)) with lymphocytes, neutrophils, and scant plasma cells, bile ductular proliferation, and massive hepatocyte dropout. A Masson's trichrome stain showed bridging fibrosis (stage 3) with lobular architectural collapse. Liver biopsy HSV stains were negative. She received intravenous methylprednisolone for presumed autoimmune hepatitis (AIH), but her condition continued to worsen. She underwent emergent evaluation for liver transplantation and was listed for liver transplant.

On day five of admission, she developed intermittent vaginal bleeding because of coagulopathy. Her Factor V and Factor VII activity levels on day seven of admission were very low at 6% and 4%, respectively. On the morning of the eighth day, she was lethargic and developed asterixis, but was arousable, consistent with stage 3 hepatic encephalopathy. On the eight hospital day, she underwent orthotopic liver transplantation from a 25 year-old donor who died from a self-inflicted gunshot wound to the head. The donor was CMV positive, and the patient was CMV negative.

Abdominal transplant surgery, hepatology, high-risk obstetrics, and anesthesiology teams were involved in her care throughout the hospitalization. Pretransplant obstetric ultrasound was performed by high-risk obstetrics team to confirm fetal viability and to accurately date the pregnancy. The potential complications of posttransplant immunosuppression on the pregnancy were discussed with the patient, by the obstetrics team, before transplant. Medical termination of pregnancy was not recommended as there was no evidence to suggest that pregnancy caused or worsened the patient's liver disease.

Liver transplantation was performed with venovenous bypass. A suprahepatic caval anastomosis was created between the donor liver and the hepatic vein confluence of the recipient. A common cuff of gastroduodenal artery and proper hepatic artery was fashioned on the recipient's side and using the celiac axis of the donor, an end-to-end hepatic arterial anastomosis was created. An end-to-end portal venous anastomosis and an end-to-end choledochochledochostomy were performed. There was excellent perfusion of the liver, and it synthesized bile within 5 minutes of

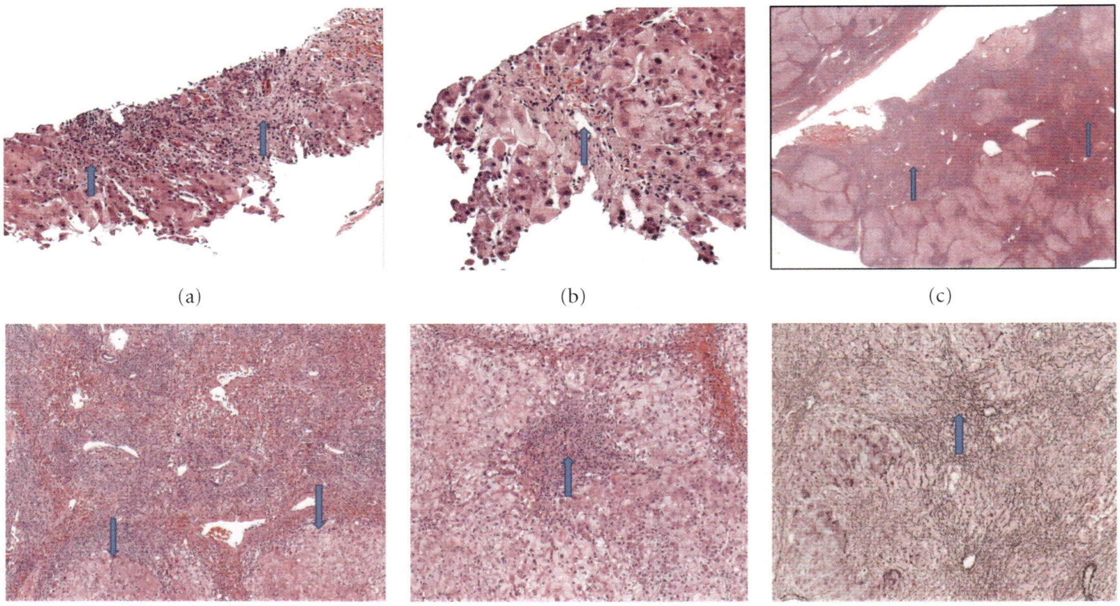

(a) (b) (c) (d) (e) (f)

Figure 1: (a) Transjugular biopsy-portal tract showing inflammation with bile ductular proliferation and interface hepatitis (arrows) (H&E 200x). (b) Transjugular biopsy-central vein (arrow) with pericentral hepatocyte dropout, ballooning degeneration, and hemorrhage (H&E 200x). (c) Explant showing architectural collapse (arrows) (H&E 40x). (d) Explant with interface between area of collapse and residual viable parenchyma (arrows) (H&E 100x). (e) Explant with portal/interface hepatitis (arrow). Periportal hepatocytes showing ballooning/cytoplasmic clearing (H&E 100x). (f) Reticulin stain highlights areas of collapse (arrow) adjacent to viable parenchyma.

recirculation. She remained hemodynamically stable during the procedure without any vasopressor requirement. She received one unit of packed red blood cells, nine units of fresh frozen plasma and ten units of platelets during surgery. A posttransplant X-ray was not obtained due to her pregnancy. Intraoperative fetal monitoring was not performed during the liver transplant since the fetus was less than 24 weeks and not viable. Postoperatively, an obstetric ultrasound was performed which confirmed fetal cardiac activity and normal amniotic fluid volume.

Pathology from her explanted liver revealed a small organ (total weight 509 grams), prominent interface hepatitis, extensive hepatocyte necrosis, and confluent collapse (Figures 1(c)–1(f)), but there was focal preservation of some lobules (Figure 1(d)). Interestingly, Masson's trichrome stain of the explanted liver showed very little fibrosis. The findings from explant were different from the transjugular liver biopsy which showed stage 3 fibrosis.

Tacrolimus was administered with goal plasma trough levels of 10–12 ng/mL, and our center's standard steroid protocol were administered for immunosuppression (Table 2) after liver transplantation. Although mycophenolate mofetil is part of our center's immunosuppression protocol for patients transplanted for ALF, it was avoided due to its potential teratogenic effects. CMV prophylaxis was initiated with intravenous ganciclovir in the immediate postoperative period, and it was changed to oral valganciclovir at the time of discharge. Trimethoprim-sulfamethoxazole for pneumocystis prophylaxis was started after the first trimester. She did not have any immediate posttransplant complications and was discharged on hospital day 16, seven days after surgery, with a viable intrauterine pregnancy.

She was closely followed by abdominal transplant surgery, hepatology and high-risk obstetrics teams after discharge. Outpatient laboratory testing and imaging studies were performed per respective team protocols. Specifically, obstetric ultrasounds were performed every 2-3 weeks to monitor fetal well-being. The graft function remained stable, and her pregnancy progressed without any complications until 24 weeks. At 24 weeks, she developed severe, diffuse pruritus due to intrahepatic cholestasis of pregnancy (ICP). Blood work revealed elevated alkaline phosphatase and gamma glutamyl transferase (Table 1). Her serum bile acid levels were also elevated at 44 μmol/L, but total bilirubin and aminotransferases were normal. There was no evidence of liver graft rejection or posttransplant biliary stricture. She was treated with ursodeoxycholic acid (UDCA) and cholestyramine for the relief of pruritus. She also developed gestational diabetes at 24 weeks and was treated appropriately with insulin. After the diagnosis of ICP, she was evaluated weekly for fetal well-being by ultrasound biophysical profile studies. At 30 weeks gestation, fetal growth began to slow, and the amniotic fluid volume started decreasing. At that point, she received betamethasone for fetal lung maturation. During the same week, she experienced spontaneous rupture of membranes and delivered by normal vaginal delivery. She had no postpartum complications. The newborn was a healthy female weighing 3 lbs, 12 ounces

Table 2: Review of cases of liver transplantation during pregnancy.

Reference	Diagnosis	Gestational age at transplant	Immunosuppression	Outcome
Morris et al. [20]	Acute liver failure from drug induced liver injury	27 weeks	Prednisone and cyclosporine	Successful deceased donor liver transplant and neonatal death
Laifer et al. [6, 17]	Fulminant Hepatitis B	26 weeks	Prednisone and cyclosporine	Delivery by c section at 28 weeks and neonatal death
Fair et al. [18]	21 y/o woman with acute liver failure from Hepatitis B	22 weeks gestation	Steroids, OKT3, and cyclosporine	Deceased donor liver transplant with primary malfunction, followed by successful retransplantation on postop day 2. C section at 30 weeks. Fetus survived and healthy. Fetus had IUGR and severe oligohydramnios
Moreno et al. [14]	32 y/o female with cryptogenic acute liver failure	27 weeks	Methylprednisolone, cyclosporine, and azathioprine	Successful deceased donor liver transplantation Fetus survived. C-section at 39 weeks. Infant healthy at 11 months
Hamilton et al. [19]	20 y/o woman with acute liver failure from Hepatitis B	18 weeks	n/a	Successful deceased donor liver transplantation. Fetal death on posttransplant day 5
Finlay et al. [22]	Acute liver failure	17 weeks	n/a	Successful deceased donor liver transplantation. Fetal death at 22 weeks
Lo et al. [15]	25 y/o with cryptogenic acute liver failure	26 weeks	n/a	Successful left lobe living donor liver transplantation. Spontaneous abortion posttransplant day 2
Catnach et al. [21]	27 y/o woman with end stage autoimmune hepatitis	20 weeks	Cyclosporine, prednisolone, and azathioprine	Successful deceased donor liver transplantation. Successful delivery at 28 weeks. Recipient developed CMV infection
Laifer et al. [6, 17]	30 y/o female decompensated cirrhosis from autoimmune liver disease	23 weeks	Tacrolimus and prednisone	Fetal death posttransplant day 6
Eguchi et al. [7]	28 y/o woman with cryptogenic acute liver failure	15 weeks	Prednisone and tacrolimus	Successful adult living donor liver transplant. Artificial abortion posttransplant day 31. Recipient developed CMV infection
Kato et al. [8]	31 y/o female with cryptogenic acute liver failure	14 weeks	Methylprednisolone, tacrolimus, and 2 days of mycophenolate mofetil	Left lateral segment adult to adult living donor liver transplantation. Spontaneous abortion immediately after transplant
Jarufe et al. [9]	35 y/o female with cryptogenic acute liver failure	22 weeks	Prednisone and tacrolimus	Successful deceased donor liver transplantation. Delivery at 27 weeks of gestation. Normal psychomotor development at 1-year followup
Jankovic et al. [10]	26 y/o female with cryptogenic familial biliary cirrhosis	13.5 weeks	Tacrolimus, azathioprine, and prednisolone	Successful liver transplantation. Vaginal delivery at 36 weeks
Anders et al. [16]	18 y/o female with cryptogenic acute liver failure	20 weeks	n/a	Successful liver transplantation. Fetal death 48 hours after transplantation
Sequeira et al. [11]	36 y/o female with drug induced acute liver failure due to propylthiouracil	18 weeks	Tacrolimus, cyclosporine, and prednisolone	Successful liver transplantation. Elective cesarean section at 37 weeks. Child had IUGR, oligohydramnios, decreased cerebral volume, ventriculomegaly, microcephaly, seizures, and delayed developmental milestones

Table 2: Continued.

Reference	Diagnosis	Gestational age at transplant	Immunosuppression	Outcome
Current case	29 y/o female with cryptogenic acute liver failure	11 weeks	Tacrolimus and prednisone	Successful deceased donor liver transplantation. Healthy female fetus delivered at 30 weeks. Normal psychomotor development at 4-year followup

(1700 grams) with an Apgar score of 9 and 9 at one and five minutes, respectively. The child did not breast feed. She is now four years old, healthy, and reaching her age with appropriate developmental milestones.

3. Discussion

Although planned pregnancy after liver transplantation is relatively common, acute liver failure requiring liver transplantation during pregnancy is rare. Liver transplantation during the first trimester of pregnancy is an exceptionally uncommon event. A search in the literature found only fifteen cases of antepartum liver transplantation, and only six (40%) of those cases resulted in successful delivery of the fetus (Table 2). Among those six cases, first trimester (14 weeks or less) liver transplantation was performed only in two patients. Spontaneous abortion occurred in one of those two, and the other pregnancy resulted in a successful fetal outcome. Thus, our case represents only the second case of successful liver transplantation during the first trimester, followed by a successful pregnancy outcome, reported in the literature. To our knowledge, our case is the earliest successful liver transplant during pregnancy with successful fetal outcome. Furthermore, we provide long term followup of the child who has met developmental milestones.

Management of ALF in pregnancy is complicated as both maternal and fetal well-being need to be considered, although maternal outcome takes precedent. An algorithm proposed by Greenberg et al. in 2009 is a useful tool in the management of ALF in pregnancy [4].

We used a combination of corticosteroids and tacrolimus for posttransplant immunosuppression. Corticosteroids and tacrolimus are categorized by Food and Drug Administration (FDA) as pregnancy category B and C medications, respectively [5]. We choose tacrolimus instead of cyclosporine as it is a more potent calcineurin inhibitor, with lower rates of maternal complications like renal dysfunction, pre-eclampsia, and hypertension [5]. We avoided mycophenolate mofetil because it is teratogenic, and (FDA category D) and is associated with very high rates of first trimester pregnancy loss and birth defects [5]. In one report on 33 pregnancies exposed to mycophenolate mofetil, (from National Transplant Pregnancy Registry (NTPR)), 15 (45%) pregnancies resulted in spontaneous abortions and 4 among 18 live births (22%) had congenital malformations [5]. Azathioprine is also FDA category D medication [3] and should be avoided. Other immunosuppressive agents such as muromonab, antithymocyte globulin, and sirolimus belong to FDA category C, and available data on safety in pregnancy is insufficient [3]. Among the fifteen case reports that we reviewed, information about immunosuppression was provided in eleven reports (Table 2). In six of these eleven patients (54%), similar to our case, a combination of corticosteroids and tacrolimus was used [6–11]. Our patient received trimethoprim-sulfamethoxazole for pneumocystis prophylaxis. It was started after the first trimester as the medication is a folate antagonist (pregnancy category C), with potential for teratogenicity [12]. We initiated intravenous ganciclovir (Cytovene) immediately after transplant for CMV prophylaxis and later changed to oral valganciclovir (Valcyte) at the time of discharge. Both ganciclovir and valganciclovir are pregnancy category C medications (Cytovene and Valcyte prescribing information. Roche Laboratories, Inc., 2010), but the benefits of treatment outweighed the risks in our patient.

Etiologies of acute liver failure during pregnancy include causes that occur in the general population or pregnancy specific conditions, such as HELLP syndrome and AFLP [2]. In many cases a cause is not determined. In a study from India, a workup for an etiology of ALF was negative in 68 of 249 (27.9%) of pregnant patients with ALF [13]. In the fifteen cases that we reviewed, six (40%) were cryptogenic [7–9, 14–16], three (20%) were due to hepatitis B [17–19], two (13%) were due to drug induced liver injury [11, 20], two (13%) were due to AIH [6, 21], one (6%) patient had PBC [10], and a cause was not reported in one case [22] (Table 2). It is interesting that none of the fifteen patients that we reviewed developed ALF due to HELLP syndrome, pre-eclampsia or AFLP. In our patient, a thorough evaluation for a cause of ALF, including the histology of explanted liver, did not reveal a definitive cause. Autoimmune hepatitis was suspected based upon both transjugular liver biopsy and explant histology; however, her autoimmune serologies were negative, and she did not respond to corticosteroids.

Unfavorable fetal outcomes were noted in nine of the fifteen cases (60%) that we reviewed (Table 2). Four fetal deaths (26%) [6, 16, 19, 22], two neonatal deaths (13%) [17, 20], two spontaneous abortions (13%) [8, 15], and one artificial abortion (6%) [7] were reported. Favorable fetal outcomes were noted in six of the fifteen cases (40%). Three neonates were born prematurely [9, 18, 21], and the remaining three [10, 11, 14] were born at term. Fetal malformation rate in pregnant women treated with corticosteroids is 4%, and tacrolimus is 6% which is slightly higher than the malformation rate of 2-3% in general population [5]. Fortunately, no congenital malformations were present in our case. Corticosteroids are associated with premature rupture of membranes [5]. Our patient developed premature rupture of membranes at 30 weeks and delivered a premature, low-birth weight (1700 grams) baby. Neonatal adrenal insufficiency and infections may occur in corticosteroid-treated pregnancies [5], but those complications were not seen in our case. The baby survived without any complications in spite of prematurity. The child is now 4 years old, and she has met all her developmental milestones with no cognitive or physical deficits.

Other lessons that can be learned from our case include preoperative management of the pregnant patient with acute liver failure. Preoperatively, we did not routinely give fresh frozen plasma to prevent uterine bleeding for her coagulopathy but managed her similar to nonpregnant patients. She was transfused with fresh frozen plasma, as needed, in an attempt to control her intermittent vaginal bleeding that occurred three days before her liver transplantation. She received fresh frozen plasma for procedures, such as transjugular liver biopsy. Since the fetus had not reached viability (24 weeks) at the time of transplant, pre- and intraoperative fetal monitoring were not conducted as that would not have altered the management.

An interesting and particularly concerning event was the development of intrahepatic cholestasis of pregnancy (ICP) at 24-week gestation. In general, ICP is a self-limited condition which resolves after delivery of the fetus and usually occurs in the second half of pregnancy [1]. Fetal and perinatal mortality associated with ICP is 0.4%−1.4%, but there is no increased maternal mortality [1]. The goal of the treatment is to control maternal pruritus and prevent fetal mortality. Our patient was treated with UDCA and cholestyramine for symptom relief, and ultrasound biophysical profile studies were performed weekly to document fetal well-being.

In conclusion, acute liver failure during pregnancy requiring liver transplantation can be performed with successful fetal outcome, even during the first trimester of pregnancy. Intraoperative management did not include fetal monitoring, but high-risk obstetrics was present in the operating room at the time of transplant. Hemodynamic monitoring and volume management were performed similar to nonpregnant patients undergoing liver transplantation. A multidisciplinary approach with hepatology, transplant surgery, high-risk obstetrics, and anesthesiology may result in a healthy mother and child.

Acknowledgment

This work was carried out with informed consent of the patient.

References

[1] J. E. Hay, "Liver disease in pregnancy," *Hepatology*, vol. 47, no. 3, pp. 1067–1076, 2008.

[2] W. M. Lee, "Etiologies of acute liver failure," *Seminars in Liver Disease*, vol. 28, no. 2, pp. 142–152, 2008.

[3] M. A. Heneghan, M. Selzner, E. M. Yoshida, and B. Mullhaupt, "Pregnancy and sexual function in liver transplantation," *Journal of Hepatology*, vol. 49, no. 4, pp. 507–519, 2008.

[4] M. Greenberg, T. J. Daugherty, A. Elihu et al., "Acute liver failure at 26 weeks' gestation in a patient with sickle cell disease," *Liver Transplantation*, vol. 15, no. 10, pp. 1236–1241, 2009.

[5] B. Surti, J. Tan, and S. Saab, "Pregnancy and liver transplantation," *Liver International*, vol. 28, no. 9, pp. 1200–1206, 2008.

[6] S. A. Laifer, K. Abu-Elmagd, and J. J. Fung, "Hepatic transplantation during pregnancy and the puerperium," *Journal of Maternal-Fetal and Neonatal Medicine*, vol. 6, no. 1, pp. 40–44, 1997.

[7] S. Eguchi, K. Yanaga, F. Fujita et al., "Living-related right lobe liver transplantation for a patient with fulminant hepatic failure during the second trimester of pregnancy: report of a case," *Transplantation*, vol. 73, no. 12, pp. 1970–1971, 2002.

[8] T. Kato, J. R. Nery, J. J. Morcos et al., "Successful living related liver transplantation in an adult with fulminant hepatic failure," *Transplantation*, vol. 64, no. 3, pp. 415–417, 1997.

[9] N. Jarufe, A. Soza, R. M. Pérez-Ayuso et al., "Successful liver transplantation and delivery in a woman with fulminant hepatic failure occurring during the second trimester of pregnancy," *Liver International*, vol. 26, no. 4, pp. 494–497, 2006.

[10] Z. Jankovic, D. Stamenkovic, B. Duncan, R. Prasad, and M. Davies, "Successful outcome after a technically challenging liver transplant during pregnancy," *Transplantation Proceedings*, vol. 39, no. 5, pp. 1704–1706, 2007.

[11] E. Sequeira, S. Wanyonyi, and R. Dodia, "Severe propylthiouracil-induced hepatotoxicity in pregnancy managed successfully by liver transplantation: a case report," *Journal of Medical Case Reports*, vol. 5, no. 1, article 461, 2011.

[12] F. Forna, M. McConnell, F. N. Kitabire et al., "Systematic review of the safety of trimethoprim-sulfamethoxazole for prophylaxis in HIV-infected pregnant women: implications for resource-limited settings," *AIDS Reviews*, vol. 8, no. 1, pp. 24–36, 2006.

[13] V. Bhatia, A. Singhal, S. K. Panda, and S. K. Acharya, "A 20-year single-center experience with acute liver failure during pregnancy: is the prognosis really worse?" *Hepatology*, vol. 48, no. 5, pp. 1577–1585, 2008.

[14] E. G. Moreno, G. I. Garcia, S. R. Gomez et al., "Fulminant hepatic failure during pregnancy successfully treated by orthotopic liver transplantation," *Transplantation*, vol. 52, no. 5, pp. 923–926, 1991.

[15] C. M. Lo, P. Gertsch, and S. T. Fan, "Living unrelated liver transplantation between spouses for fulminant hepatic failure," *British Journal of Surgery*, vol. 82, no. 8, p. 1037, 1995.

[16] M. Anders, E. Quiñonez, N. Goldaracena et al., "Liver transplantation during pregnancy in a patient with acute liver failure," *Acta Gastroenterologica Latinoamericana*, vol. 40, no. 3, pp. 268–270, 2010.

[17] S. A. Laifer, M. J. Darby, V. P. Scantlebury, J. H. Harger, and S. N. Caritis, "Pregnancy and liver transplantation," *Obstetrics and Gynecology*, vol. 76, no. 6, pp. 1083–1088, 1990.

[18] J. Fair, A. S. Klein, T. Feng, W. T. Merritt, and J. F. Burdick, "Intrapartum orthotopic liver transplantation with successful outcome of pregnancy," *Transplantation*, vol. 50, no. 3, pp. 534–535, 1990.

[19] M. I. R. Hamilton, R. Alcock, L. Magos, S. Mallett, K. Rolles, and A. K. Burroughs, "Liver transplantation during

pregnancy," *Transplantation Proceedings*, vol. 25, no. 5, pp. 2967–2968, 1993.

[20] C. V. Morris, R. M. Goldstein, J. B. Cofer, H. Solomon, and G. B. Klintmalm, "An unusual presentation of fulminant hepatic failure secondary to propylthiouracil therapy," *Clinical Transplants*, p. 311, 1989.

[21] S. M. Catnach, M. McCarthy, E. Jauniaux et al., "Liver transplantation during pregnancy complicated by cytomegalovirus infection," *Transplantation*, vol. 60, no. 5, pp. 510–511, 1995.

[22] D. E. Finlay, M. C. Foshager, D. G. Longley, and J. G. Letourneau, "Ischemic injury to the fetus after maternal liver transplantation," *Journal of Ultrasound in Medicine*, vol. 13, no. 2, pp. 145–148, 1994.

14

Acute Liver Failure Occurring during the First Trimester of Pregnancy Successfully Treated with Living Donor Liver Transplantation

Naoya Kanogawa,[1] Tatsuo Kanda,[1] Masayuki Ohtsuka,[2] Masato Nakamura,[1] Tatsuo Miyamura,[1] Shin Yasui,[1] Makoto Arai,[1] Hitoshi Maruyama,[1] Keiichi Fujiwara,[1] Makio Shozu,[3] Shigeto Oda,[4] Masaru Miyazaki,[2] and Osamu Yokosuka[1]

[1] *Department of Gastroenterology and Nephrology, Chiba University, Graduate School of Medicine, 1-8-1 Inohana, Chuo-ku, Chiba 260-8677, Japan*
[2] *Department of General Surgery, Chiba University, Graduate School of Medicine, Chuo-ku, Chiba 260-8677, Japan*
[3] *Department of Reproductive Medicine, Chiba University, Graduate School of Medicine, Chuo-ku, Chiba 260-8677, Japan*
[4] *Department of Emergency and Critical Care Medicine, Chiba University, Graduate School of Medicine, Chuo-ku, Chiba 260-8677, Japan*

Correspondence should be addressed to Tatsuo Kanda; kandat-cib@umin.ac.jp

Academic Editors: D. Capone, C. F. Classen, C. Costa, and F. Keller

Acute liver failure (ALF) during pregnancy remains difficult to treat, and despite advances in treatment, liver transplantation must be selected as treatment option in certain cases. We report a 30-year-old woman with ALF of unknown etiology, occurring during the first trimester of pregnancy. Her condition was complicated by consciousness disturbance and coagulopathy due to ALF, but she was successfully treated with living donor liver transplantation 7 days after dilatation and curettage. At 9-month followup, she was in good medical condition. Liver transplantation has been reported as one of the treatment options for ALF during pregnancy with the prognosis varying depending on the trimester, from living donor or deceased donor liver transplantation. Of importance is that clinicians always think of emergent liver transplantation as a therapeutic option in ALF even in the first trimester of pregnancy.

1. Introduction

Liver disease during pregnancy is classified into three categories as follows: (1) specific to pregnancy, (2) coincidental with pregnancy, and (3) preexisting liver disease [1, 2]. In the first trimester of a normal pregnancy, hyperemesis gravidarum occurs in 1–20 per 1000 pregnancies [3, 4]. On the other hand, fatty liver of pregnancy, preeclampsia or eclampsia, and HELLP (haemolysis, elevated liver enzymes, and low platelets) syndrome are three representative pregnancy-related diseases whose onset is usually between the 34th and the 36th weeks [1].

Treatment decisions for acute liver failure (ALF) are complicated by the diversity of its clinical presentations especially in pregnant women. Although liver transplantation supersedes empirical drug therapy in decompensated patients, pregnant patients warrant treatment modifications, and it is difficult to plan their therapies in certain cases because the lives of mother and baby should be rescued.

Although there have been several reports about liver transplantation from deceased donors for ALF occurring during pregnancy [5–26], it is relatively rare in the first trimester of pregnancy [13, 15]. We experienced a case of acute liver failure, successfully treated with liver transplantation from a living related donor, which we report here.

2. Case Report

A 30-year-old woman at week 12 of pregnancy was referred and transferred to Chiba University School of Medicine

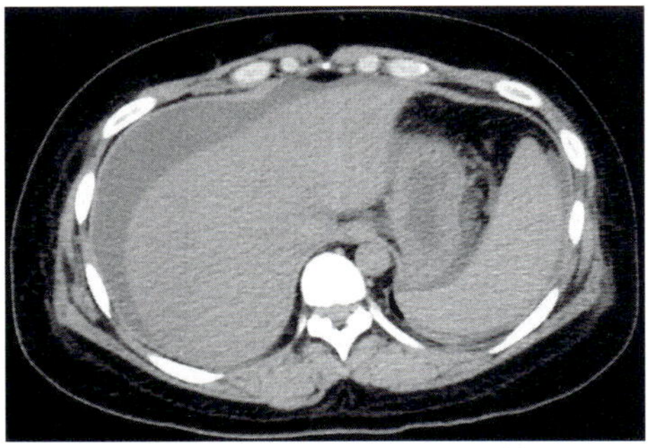

Figure 1: Computed tomography on admission showed atrophic liver and mild splenomegaly. There was moderate ascites but no evidence of cirrhosis.

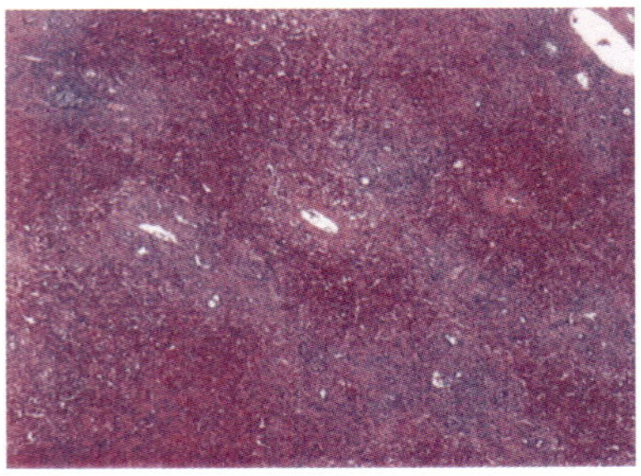

(a)

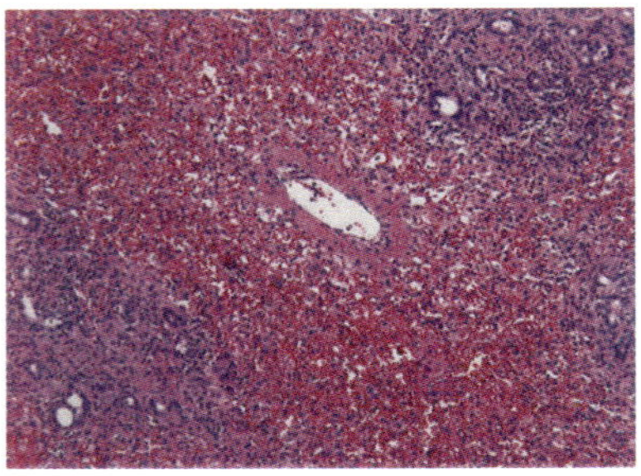

(b)

Figure 2: The recipient's explanted liver showed no cirrhosis, and the hepatic architecture was preserved (hematoxylin and eosin; original magnification 40x) (a). Massive hemorrhagic hepatic necrosis was also seen (hematoxylin and eosin; original magnification 200x) (b).

Hospital from another hospital with 10 days of liver test abnormalities and jaundice, for consciousness disturbance and coagulopathy. On the first admission into another hospital, two days after her first symptom of jaundice, her laboratory findings were total bilirubin, 15.6 mg/dL; AST, 2286 IU/L; ALT, 1818 IU/L; and prothrombin time, 37%. She had been healthy, apart from suffering from a left wrist fracture three years earlier and occasionally taking loxoprofen for lower back pain. There was no history of liver disease, alcohol consumption, or transfusion. She had 5 children, who were born via normal vaginal delivery, and she did not show liver test abnormalities at the time of their births. Her family had no history of liver disease. On physical examination, she was obese (her weight, 95 kg; body length, 1.70 m; and body mass index, 32.5 kg/m^2) and found to be deeply jaundiced. Flapping tremor, disorientation, and hepatic encephalopathy grade III were noted. On admission to our hospital, her laboratory findings had deteriorated as follows: total bilirubin, 20.5 mg/dL; AST, 281 IU/L; ALT, 495 IU/L; prothrombin time, 12%; international normalized ratio (INR), 3.25; NH_3, 131 μg/dL; AFP, 10 ng/mL; and hepatocyte growth factor, 4.43 ng/mL (normal < 0.4 ng/mL). Serum IgG, IgM, ceruloplasmin and copper were at normal levels, but IgA (418 mg/dL) and urine copper (471.6 μg/day) were slightly elevated. Viral serology was negative for HBsAg, anti-HBc IgM, anti-HAV IgM, anti-HCV, anti-HEV IgA, anti-HSV IgM, anti-VZV IgM, anti-EBV VCA, and anti-HIV. Serum HBV DNA, HCV RNA, and HEV RNA were all negative. Anti-CMV IgM was weakly positive but CMV-antigen was negative. Serum antinuclear antibody was slightly positive, but antimitochondrial and antismooth muscle antibodies were negative. Abdominal ultrasound and computed tomography (CT) demonstrated moderate ascites, atrophic liver, and slight splenomegaly but no collateral vessels (Figure 1). On admission, MELD score was 31. We started to perform online hemodiafiltration concomitant with slow plasma exchange twice as artificial liver supports, and performed dilatation and curettage one day after admission to improve consciousness disturbance and coagulopathy. Seven days later, as her general hepatic status and MELD score did not improve, urgent transplant of a liver from a living related donor, her healthy father, was performed. The patient was discharged with nearly normal liver function at 3 months after surgery, and she and her father were at home in good health at 9 months.

The explanted liver weighed 720 g; there was no sign of cirrhosis, and the hepatic architecture was preserved (Figure 2(a)). Liver histology of the affected liver was consistent with massive necrosis and extensive coagulative necrosis (Figure 2(b)).

3. Discussion

Severe hepatic injury and hepatotoxicity including ALF are also occasionally seen in the first trimester of pregnancy [2], although representative pregnancy-related diseases, such as pregnancy-related fatty liver diseases, often causing ALF, occur more often in the late stage of pregnancy [1]. The present case occurred during the first trimester of pregnancy. After dilatation and curettage, the patient's liver function did not improve and living donor liver transplantation from her father was performed for her rescue.

There have been several reports about liver transplantation for ALF, occurring during pregnancy, either from deceased donors [5–15] or living donors [16–20]. The causes of ALF during pregnancy requiring liver transplantation were various as follows: hepatitis viral infection [6, 8, 14, 20, 21], drug-associated [5, 21, 24, 25], autoimmune hepatitis [10], acute fatty liver of pregnancy (AFLP) [11, 22], and unknown etiology [7, 9, 12, 13, 15–19, 26]. Thus, the majority of causes of ALF during pregnancy requiring liver transplantation are reported to be unknown, as was the cause of the present case, although drug-associated hepatitis induced by loxoprofen could not be completely ruled out. We did not expect our case as AFLP, which is one of the diseases of late pregnancy [1].

Gestational age of expectant mothers with ALF requiring liver transplantation was also related to various etiologies for their ALF. Only three cases of ALF with unknown etiology, including the present case, and occurring during the first trimester of pregnancy, required liver transplantation [13, 15].

Horikoshi et al. [19] reported that successful living donor liver transplantation for ALF of unknown etiology with onset immediately after cesarean delivery was performed at 33 weeks and 3 days of gestation and that this patient and her baby were in good medical condition. Living donor liver transplantation for ALF during the earlier trimester of pregnancy looked to relieve not the mother but her baby [17, 18, 20]. In the present case, living donor liver transplantation was also performed 7 days after her dilatation and curettage. In some cases of deceased donor liver transplantation, both mother and baby were alive [13, 15]. Further studies about the differences between living donor and deceased donor transplantation will be needed.

In conclusion, liver transplantation for ALF during pregnancy was not rare and living donor related transplantation should be available on demand. Even if the ALF patient was in the first trimester of pregnancy, we should consider liver transplantation as a treatment option.

References

[1] A. K. Burroughs and E. J. Heathcote, "The liver in pregnancy," in *Sherlock's Diseases of the Liver and Biliary System*, J. S. Dooly, A. S. F. Lok, A. K. Burroughs, and E. J. Heathcoate, Eds., pp. 602–614, John Wiley & Sons, West Sussex, UK, 12th edition, 2011.

[2] T. Miyamura, T. Kanda, S. Minemura et al., "Acute liver failure associated with propylthiouracil in a pregnant 26-year-old woman," *Case Reports in Gastroenterology*, vol. 7, no. 2, pp. 240–244, 2013.

[3] N. K. Kuşcu and F. Koyuncu, "Hyperemesis gravidarum: current concepts and management," *Postgraduate Medical Journal*, vol. 78, no. 916, pp. 76–79, 2002.

[4] D. B. Fell, L. Dodds, K. S. Joseph, V. M. Allen, and B. Butler, "Risk factors for hyperemesis gravidarum requiring hospital admission during pregnancy," *Obstetrics and Gynecology*, vol. 107, no. 2, part 1, pp. 277–284, 2006.

[5] C. V. Morris, R. M. Goldstein, J. B. Cofer, H. Solomon, and G. B. Klintmalm, "An unusual presentation of fulminant hepatic failure secondary to propylthiouracil therapy," *Clinical transplants*, p. 311, 1989.

[6] J. Fair, A. S. Klein, T. Feng, W. T. Merritt, and J. F. Burdick, "Intrapartum orthotopic liver transplantation with successful outcome of pregnancy," *Transplantation*, vol. 50, no. 3, pp. 534–535, 1990.

[7] E. G. Moreno, G. I. Garcia, S. R. Gomez et al., "Fulminant hepatic failure during pregnancy successfully treated by orthotopic liver transplantation," *Transplantation*, vol. 52, no. 5, pp. 923–926, 1991.

[8] M. I. R. Hamilton, R. Alcock, L. Magos, S. Mallett, K. Rolles, and A. K. Burroughs, "Liver transplantation during pregnancy," *Transplantation Proceedings*, vol. 25, no. 5, pp. 2967–2968, 1993.

[9] D. E. Finlay, M. C. Foshager, D. G. Longley, and J. G. Letourneau, "Ischemic injury to the fetus after maternal liver transplantation," *Journal of Ultrasound in Medicine*, vol. 13, no. 2, pp. 145–148, 1994.

[10] S. M. Catnach, M. McCarthy, E. Jauniaux et al., "Liver transplantation during pregnancy complicated by cytomegalovirus infection," *Transplantation*, vol. 60, no. 5, pp. 510–511, 1995.

[11] P. Remiszewski, J. Pawlak, A. Skwarek et al., "Orthotopic liver transplantation for acute liver failure resulting from 'acute fatty liver of pregnancy'," *Annals of Transplantation*, vol. 8, no. 3, pp. 8–11, 2003.

[12] N. Jarufe, A. Soza, R. M. Pérez-Ayuso et al., "Successful liver transplantation and delivery in a woman with fulminant hepatic failure occurring during the second trimester of pregnancy," *Liver International*, vol. 26, no. 4, pp. 494–497, 2006.

[13] Z. Jankovic, D. Stamenkovic, B. Duncan, R. Prasad, and M. Davies, "Successful outcome after a technically challenging liver transplant during pregnancy," *Transplantation Proceedings*, vol. 39, no. 5, pp. 1704–1706, 2007.

[14] L. Toti, T. M. Manzia, P. Romano et al., "Successful management of a same-day emergency delivery and liver transplant in a 27 weeks pregnant woman with fulminant hepatic failure," *Transplant International*, vol. 23, no. 1, pp. 114–115, 2010.

[15] V. C. Muddukuri, C. D. Stephenson, L. Eskind, W. A. Ahrens, P. Purdum, and M. W. Russo, "Liver transplantation for acute liver failure at 11-week gestation with successful maternal and fetal outcome," *Case Reports in Transplantation*, vol. 2012, Article ID 484080, 7 pages, 2012.

[16] C. M. Lo, P. Gertsch, and S. T. Fan, "Living unrelated liver transplantation between spouses for fulminant hepatic failure," *British Journal of Surgery*, vol. 82, no. 8, p. 1037, 1995.

[17] T. Kato, J. R. Nery, J. J. Morcos et al., "Successful living related liver transplantation in an adult with fulminant hepatic failure," *Transplantation*, vol. 64, no. 3, pp. 415–417, 1997.

[18] S. Eguchi, K. Yanaga, F. Fujita et al., "Living-related right lobe liver transplantation for a patient with fulminant hepatic failure during the second trimester of pregnancy: report of a case," *Transplantation*, vol. 73, no. 12, pp. 1970–1971, 2002.

[19] Y. Horikoshi, H. Itoh, S. Kikuchi et al., "Successful living donor liver transplantation for fulminant hepatic failure that manifested immediately after cesarean delivery," *ASAIO Journal*, vol. 58, no. 2, pp. 174–176, 2012.

[20] Y. Simsek, B. Isik, A. Karaer et al., "Fulminant hepatitis A infection in second trimester of pregnancy requiring living-donor liver transplantation," *Journal of Obstetrics and Gynaecology*, vol. 38, no. 4, pp. 745–748, 2012.

[21] S. A. Laifer, M. J. Darby, V. P. Scantlebury, J. H. Harger, and S. N. Caritis, "Pregnancy and liver transplantation," *Obstetrics and Gynecology*, vol. 76, no. 6, pp. 1083–1088, 1990.

[22] S. A. Ockner, E. M. Brunt, S. M. Cohn, E. S. Krul, D. W. Hanto, and M. G. Peters, "Fulminant hepatic failure caused by acute fatty liver of pregnancy treated by orthotopic liver transplantation," *Hepatology*, vol. 11, no. 1, pp. 59–64, 1990.

[23] M. Bourliere, Y. P. Le Treut, J. C. Manelli et al., "Chlormezanone-induced fulminant hepatitis in a pregnant woman: successful delivery and liver transplantation," *Journal of Gastroenterology and Hepatology*, vol. 7, no. 3, pp. 339–341, 1992.

[24] E. J. Gill, M. J. Contos, and T. C. C. Peng, "Acute fatty liver of pregnancy and acetaminophen toxicity leading to liver failure and postpartum liver transplantation: A case report," *Journal of Reproductive Medicine for the Obstetrician and Gynecologist*, vol. 47, no. 7, pp. 584–586, 2002.

[25] E. Sequeira, S. Wanyonyi, and R. Dodia, "Severe propylthiouracil-induced hepatotoxicity in pregnancy managed successfully by liver transplantation: a case report," *Journal of Medical Case Reports*, vol. 5, article 461, 2011.

[26] M. Anders, E. Quiñonez, N. Goldaracena et al., "Liver transplantation during pregnancy in a patient with acute liver failure," *Acta Gastroenterologica Latinoamericana*, vol. 40, no. 3, pp. 268–270, 2010.

15

Liver Transplantation Using a Graft from a Donor with Situs Inversus Totalis

Xu-Yong Sun, Ke Qin, Jian-Hui Dong, Hai-Bin Li, Liu-Gen Lan, Ying Huang, Song Cao, and Zhuang-Jiang Li

Guangxi Key Laboratory of Transplant Medicine, Institute of Transplant Medicine, 303 Hospital of People's Liberation Army, Nanning 530021, China

Correspondence should be addressed to Xu-Yong Sun; xuyongsun303@gmail.com

Academic Editors: I. Engelmann and M. R. Moosa

It is critical to effectively use every available organ to meet the increasing demands for liver transplantation. Situs inversus is a rare congenital anomaly caused by obstruction of viscus rotation during embryonic development. Situs inversus was once regarded as a contraindication to liver transplantation because of the technical difficulties associated with the unique vascular anatomy and concern about achieving accurate graft positioning. Here, we present a successful case of liver transplantation using a graft from a donor with situs inversus totalis. The related experience will contribute to opening up new realms for the use of such rare organ resources.

1. Introduction

Situs inversus is a rare congenital anomaly caused by obstruction of viscus rotation during embryonic development. Its incidence is about 0.01% worldwide. The viscus distribution in the situs inversus individuals is opposite to ordinary people. All thoracoabdominal organs and retroperitoneal organs (i.e., kidneys and adrenal glands) are symmetrically positioned to the midline, which is often called mirror-image reversal [1]. Situs inversus was once regarded as a contraindication to liver transplantation because of the technical difficulties associated with the unique vascular anatomy and concern about achieving accurate graft positioning [2, 3]. For a number of patients with situs inversus, liver transplantation has been successfully performed during the last two decades [4–8]. However, few cases of deceased donor organs with situs inversus used for liver transplantation have been reported [3, 9–11]. Here, we present a case of liver transplantation using a graft from a donor with situs inversus totalis.

2. Case Report

A 23-year-old male was referred to our hospital in May 2008 due to severe traumatic brain injury caused by a traffic accident and was diagnosed as brain dead shortly after admission. Dextrocardia was found during physical examination and situs inversus totalis was verified by further X-ray and ultrasonic inspection. During the retrieval of donor organs, it was found that the liver, pancreas, and stomach were located in the opposite positions. The descending aorta was located directly in front of the spine and the inferior vena cava was found in the front left of the spine. Organ procurement was smoothly performed without great difficulty even though the procedure took a little longer due to the operator's habitual thinking about the anatomy. During preparation of the donated liver, the anatomical relations were clearly identified, that is, liver artery locating in right side and common bile duct in the left, and portal vein still being behind common bile duct and liver artery. The hepatic superior and inferior vena cava was cut to angle well in preparation for vascular anastomosis.

A 58-year-old female recipient was diagnosed with end-stage liver disease caused by type B hepatitis. Preoperative condition was evaluated with Child-Pugh (class A) and MELD (4.3). The liver transplantation was performed in May 2008. The incision was made double subcostally. Following isolation of porta hepatis and hepatic ligament, the retrohepatic inferior vena cava was partially clamped and then the diseased liver was removed preserving the inferior vena cava. The right hepatic vein was suture ligated while preserving the left and middle hepatic veins. At the point of left hepatic vein entering the hepatic superior and inferior vena cava, a transection was taken on an anterior wall of the interval between the left and middle hepatic veins, and meanwhile, the anterior wall of inferior vena cava was cut downward 2 cm, thereby forming a "T" type anastomotic rim in preparation for hepatic venous outflow reconstruction.

Liver transplantation was performed with a modified piggyback technique. The donor liver was directly placed into the recipient's right upper quadrant without rotating adjustment, that is, the right hepatic lobe was positioned in the recipient's left side and the smaller lobe was positioned in the recipient's liver fossa. The hepatic superior and inferior vena cava was directly anastomosed to recipient's inferior vena cava with 3-0 vascular suture. Portal veins were end-to-end anastomosed with 6-0 vascular suture followed by albumin solution perfusion. The residual UW solution (University of Wisconsin solution) in the donated liver was flushed away with albumin solution. Then, the intrahepatic vena cava was completely ligated and the clamps were removed from portal vein and vena cava, thereby ending an hepatic phase. Cold and warm ischemia times were 7 hr and 2 min, respectively. For artery reconstruction, the cut off at the junction of the proper hepatic artery and gastroduodenal artery (recipient) was anastomosed with the cut off at the junction of common hepatic artery and splenic artery (donor) with 7-0 vascular suture. Biliary reconstruction was performed by duct-to-duct anastomosis between recipient's common hepatic duct and donor's common bile duct with 6-0 vascular suture without placing a "T" type drainage tube. The total operation time was 6.5 hr and life support was withdrawn at 6 hr after operation. Figure 1 illustrates the status of the transplanted liver after reconstruction of the portal vein. The immunosuppression was induced with anti CD25 antibody and maintained with FK506/MMF. The patient recovered well postoperatively with normal hepatic function in 2 weeks and discharged from hospital at day 20 after transplantation. By now, the patient has been followed up for 36 months. The liver function remains normal without biliary complication and rejection reactions.

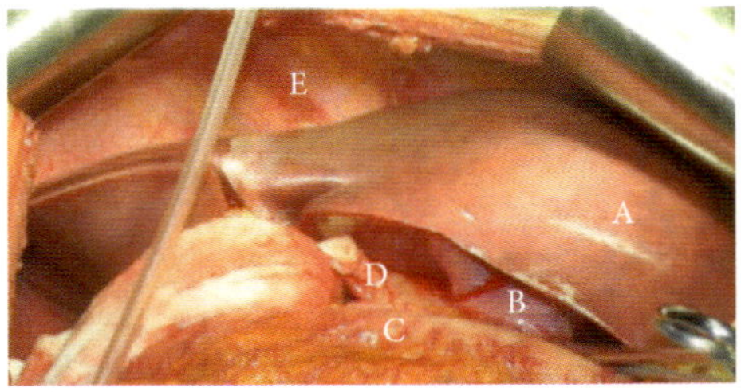

Figure 1: The status of transplanted liver. Orthotopic liver transplantation was performed with a graft from a donor with situs inversus totalis. Piggyback technique was used for the transplantation. The photograph was taken prior to the reconstruction of hepatic artery and postreconstruction of portal vein. (A) Liver; (B) gallbladder; (C) colon; (D) hepatic artery; (E) diaphragm.

3. Discussion

The shortage of donated organs has been a critical issue with regard to the increasing demand. In order to enhance usable organ sources, people try to expand the criteria for donor evaluation and attempt the maximum possible use of every donor resources. Situs inversus totalis is a very rare anatomical abnormality, which is characterized by dextrocardia and "mirror-image" distribution of abdominal organs. It may coexist with other malformations such as underdevelopment of portal vein and inferior vena cava, polysplenia syndrome, and congenital biliary atresia [12]. Situs inversus totalis was considered as an absolute contraindication in organ transplantation mainly due to the anatomic deformities of viscera and blood vessels. Along with the extensive implementation and technological advance of liver transplantation, a number of ELD patients with situs inversus totalis had successful liver transplants, and few patients received liver implantation from donors with situs inversus totalis. However, a standard operation procedure has not been established in terms of this type of liver transplantation.

In 1995, Asfar et al. [9] reported a case of liver transplantation using a graft from a donor with situs inversus totalis. A 23-year-old female DBD (donation after brain death) donor was identified with situs inversus totalis and dextrocardia. The recipient was a 63-year-old male who suffered from alcoholic cirrhosis. During the operation, the liver was counterclockwise rotated at 90°, that is, left side of the liver was located in recipient's right subphrenic space and the right side of the liver was placed in paracolic sulci. The hepatic inferior vena cava was ligated followed by an end-to-side anastomose between the intrahepatic vena cava and recipient's inferior vena cava and end-to-end anastomoses between portal veins and hepatic arteries. Youx-en-Y biliary anastomosis was performed for biliary reconstruction. Liver function was restored in 1 week following liver implantation. The patient died from ARDS and septicemia at day 20 after the operation. This case indicated the feasibility of liver transplantation using a graft from a donor with situs inversus totalis even though long-term survival was not achieved on this recipient. In another two cases using liver grafts from donors with situs inversus totalis, orthotopic liver transplantation was performed with piggyback technique [10, 13]. The liver was implanted in the original orientation without adjustment and recipients achieved long-term survival. In Pomposelli et al.'s report, piggyback technique was also used for orthotopic liver transplantation, but the donor liver was backward rotated at 180° along the axis of inferior vena cava allowing a big part of the left side of the liver to be located in the right upper abdominal cavity. After the directional adjustment, the common bile duct of the graft was toward the up front, and Roux-en-Y biliary intestinal anastomosis was carried out for biliary reconstruction. The long-term survival of the patient was achieved following liver transplantation. In 2011, a modified piggyback technique was used in orthotopic liver transplantation with a situs inversus liver [14]. Recipient's right hepatic vein was suture ligated and a "T" type anastomotic rim composed of left and middle hepatic veins and inferior vena cava was created for hepatic venous outflow of the transplanted liver. Recently, Dou et al. [15] successfully performed a classical orthotopic liver transplantation from a donor with situs inversus totalis. The liver graft was placed in the recipient's right upper abdominal cavity with a slightly rightward rotation. After finishing the conjunctions of suprahepatic and intrahepatic inferior vena cava, the interspace was filled with omentum majus. The implanted liver was fixed to the diaphragm with falciform ligament.

In the present report, the donor with situs inversus totalis died from severe traumatic brain injury caused by-traffic accident. The distribution of viscera was confirmed with X-ray and type-B ultrasonic checks, and a planned procedure was laid out before the organ retrieval. In consideration of the recipient being at the end-stage of liver disease without cancerization, a modified piggyback technique was used for the orthotopic liver transplantation. During operation, the liver graft was slightly rightward rotated and a water bag was temporarily placed in the liver fossa supporting the graft in order to avoid its self rotating. After the removal of the diseased liver, there was enough space in right upper quadrant to hold the liver graft, and vascular bypass was not required. The inferior vena cava involved a "T" type anastomotic rim which ensured the hepatic venous outflow to be unobstructed. The hepatic artery was closely related to bile duct, which was adjusted by slightly changing liver position during anastomosis of vascular and biliary systems. End-to-end anastomosis was applied for the reconstruction of hepatic artery and biliary duct. Since the left hepatic lobe was relatively large, the liver graft was laid up in situ placement. The remaining space in the right upper quadrant was filled with omentum majus and the liver was mounted to the diaphragm with falciform ligament. This manipulation could protect the liver from graft self-rotation without repressing the stomach and the surrounding intestinal tract. The achievement of long-term survival proved the rationality of the planned procedure in this particular case.

In the face of critical shortage of donor livers, we treasured every valuable donor resource to save as many lives as possible. All donors received routine auxiliary examinations and the condition of the anticipated organ was predetermined prior to organ procurement. Especially to liver graft with situs inversus, timely awareness of the exceptional situation and a detailed procedure in advance are prerequisites to the success of transplantation. During donor liver retrieval, the location and relationship among various vessels need to be carefully distinguished to prevent operation damage to the organ. During implantation of the liver graft, the following two aspects should be seriously considered, the reconstruction of hepatic venous outflow which is not to be obstructed and fixation of liver graft to prevent self-rotation. Thus to our experience, the success of transplantation using such infrequently donated organs could be achieved through careful preoperative examination and an elaborately planned operation procedure.

Acknowledgments

We are grateful to the Ministry of Education (985 program of China) and Guangxi Science and Technology Projects (0719006-2-7, 0993003A-17, 10169-05) for funding and supporting this project.

References

[1] A. S. Aylsworth, "Clinical aspects of defects in the determination of laterality," *American Journal of Medical Genetics*, vol. 101, no. 4, pp. 345–355, 2001.

[2] S. C. Raynor, R. P. Wood, A. D. Spanta, and B. W. Shaw Jr., "Liver transplantation in a patient with abdomimal situs inversus," *Transplantation*, vol. 45, no. 3, pp. 661–663, 1988.

[3] J. M. Chun, G. O. Jung, G. S. Choi et al., "Living donor liver transplantation using a graft from a donor with situs inversus totalis," *Liver Transplantation*, vol. 15, no. 6, pp. 666–669, 2009.

[4] G. B. Klintmalm, M. S. Bell, B. S. Husberg et al., "Liver transplant in complete situs inversus: a case report," *Surgery*, vol. 114, no. 1, pp. 102–106, 1993.

[5] C. J. E. Watson, A. Rasmussen, N. V. Jamieson et al., "Liver transplantation in patients with situs inversus," *British Journal of Surgery*, vol. 82, no. 2, pp. 242–245, 1995.

[6] H. Kamei, M. Kasahara, K. Uryuhara et al., "Living-donor liver transplantation for situs inversus: 2 case reports," *Journal of Pediatric Surgery*, vol. 40, no. 3, pp. E35–E37, 2005.

[7] J. K. Heimbach, K. V. N. Menon, M. B. Ishitani et al., "Living donor liver transplantation using a right lobe graft in an adult with situs inversus," *Liver Transplantation*, vol. 11, no. 1, pp. 111–113, 2005.

[8] C. J. Qiao, Y. N. Liu, and J. M. Wei, "Liver transplantation with situs inversus totalis: a case report," *Chinese Journal of General Surgery*, vol. 20, no. 8, pp. 518–519, 2005.

[9] S. Asfar, N. Ozcay, D. Grant, and W. Wall, "Transplantation of the liver from a donor with complete situs inversus and dextrocardia," *Transplantation*, vol. 59, no. 3, pp. 442–444, 1995.

[10] L. A. Herrera, J. Castillo, E. Martino, J. M. Rabanal, and M. G. Fleitas, "Orthotopic liver transplantation from a donor with abdominal situs inversus," *Transplantation*, vol. 62, no. 1, pp. 133–135, 1996.

[11] J. J. Pomposelli, M. A. DaCosta, K. McPartland, and R. L. Jenkins, "Retroversus implantation of a liver graft: a novel approach to the deceased donor with situs inversus totalis," *American Journal of Transplantation*, vol. 7, no. 7, pp. 1869–1871, 2007.

[12] J. Vazquez, J. C. Lopez Gutierrez, M. Gamez et al., "Biliary atresia and the polysplenia syndrome: its impact on final outcome," *Journal of Pediatric Surgery*, vol. 30, no. 3, pp. 485–487, 1995.

[13] F. Braun, B. Rodeck, T. Lorf et al., "Situs inversus of donor or recipient in liver transplantation," *Transplant International*, vol. 11, no. 3, pp. 212–215, 1998.

[14] B. Liu, F. J. Zeng, L. Lan et al., "A case report of liver transplantation withsitus inversus totalis," *Chinese Journal of Organ Transplantation*, vol. 32, no. 12, pp. 759–760, 2011.

[15] J. Dou, T. Yang, J.-L. Cao, Q.-J. Gao, Y.-L. Su, and Z.-J. Zhu, "Classical orthotopic liver transplantation from a donor with situs inversus totalis using slight rotation of the liver graft," *Chinese Medical Journal*, vol. 123, no. 10, pp. 1353–1355, 2010.

16

Successful Treatment of Recurrent Primary Sclerosing Cholangitis after Orthotopic Liver Transplantation with Oral Vancomycin

Yinka K. Davies,[1] Cynthia J. Tsay,[2] Dario V. Caccamo,[3] Kathleen M. Cox,[1,4] Ricardo O. Castillo,[1,4] and Kenneth L. Cox[1,4]

[1] *Division of Gastroenterology, Hepatology, and Nutrition, Department of Pediatrics, School of Medicine, Stanford University, Stanford, CA 95762, USA*
[2] *Yale University, New Haven, CT 06510, USA*
[3] *Department of Pathology, Sutter Medical Center, Sacramento, CA 95816, USA*
[4] *Department of Pediatrics, Lucile Packard Children's Hospital, Stanford University, Palo Alto, CA 94304, USA*

Correspondence should be addressed to Yinka K. Davies; ydavies@aol.com

Academic Editors: A. Beiras-Fernandez and J. Kaneko

Primary sclerosing cholangitis (PSC) is a progressive, cholestatic disease of the liver that is marked by inflammation of the bile ducts and damage to the hepatic biliary tree. Approximately 60–70% of patients also have inflammatory bowel disease and progression of PSC can lead to ulcerative colitis and cirrhosis of the liver. Due to limited understanding of the etiology and mechanism of PSC, the only existing treatment option is orthotopic liver transplantation (OLT); however, recurrence of PSC, after OLT is estimated to be between 5% and 35%. We discuss the successful treatment of a pediatric patient, with recurrent PSC, after OLT with oral Vancomycin.

1. Introduction

Primary sclerosing cholangitis (PSC) is a progressive inflammatory disease, of unknown etiology and with significant morbidity and mortality, which damages the intra- and/or extrahepatic biliary tree leading to portal hypertension and cirrhosis of the liver. The clinical course is variable including hepatobiliary carcinoma, especially cholangiocarcinoma in 6–20% of patients [1–6]. Additionally, it is estimated that 60–70% of people with PSC have inflammatory bowel disease [7, 8]. Orthotopic liver transplantation (OLT) is the only treatment option for patients with end-stage liver disease due to the progressive damage caused from PSC [9, 10]. The recurrence of PSC in the new graft is estimated to be between 5–35% [11–13]. We report the successful treatment of a patient after OLT, who had shown recurrence of disease, with oral Vancomycin.

2. Case Report

A 12-year-old girl presented with a three-week history of jaundice and lethargy, with periumbilical pain every other day. There had been no recent travel or sick contacts. Screening tests revealed platelet level was low (89 K/uL; normal range 150 to 400). Antinuclear Antibody (ANCA) was positive with a homogeneous pattern, and Antinuclear Antibody Titer was elevated (640; normal range <40). Serum copper was normal at 1065 ug/L and ceruloplasmin was normal at 24 mg/dL. γ-Glutamyl transpeptidase (GGT) level was elevated (139 U/L; reference range from 5 to 36). C-Reactive Protein (CRP) was elevated at 2.80 mg/dL; reference range was from 0.0 to 0.5. PTT was elevated at 48.6 sec; normal range was from 23.3 to 33.8. Prothrombin Time was elevated at 21.0 sec; normal range was from 11.8 to 14.2. INR was increased to 1.9 sec; normal range was from

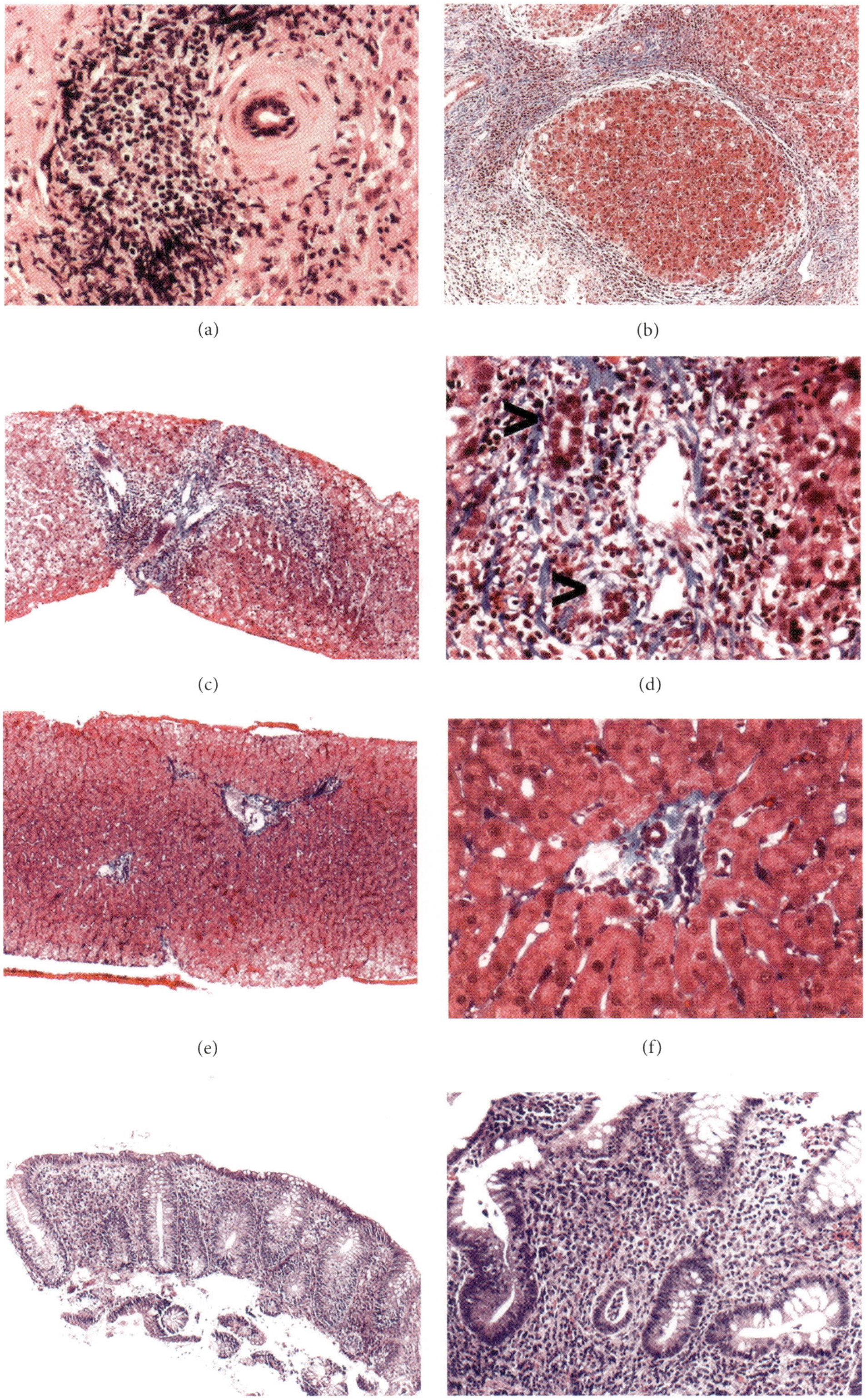

(a) (b) (c) (d) (e) (f) (g) (h)

FIGURE 1: Liver and colon biopsies (stained with trichomere): *thoracic liver before OLT*: (a) onion skin fibrosis and periductular inflammation; (b) cirrhosis nodules surrounded by normal tissue; *after OLT with recurrence of PSC* (c) periductular fibrosis and inflammation; (d) damaged bile ductules noted with arrows; *after Vancomycin treatment with no immune suppression* (e) normal bile ducts; (f) resolution of portal space ductile damage. Biopsies from (g) descending colon (100x) and (h) sigmoidal colon (200x) show mild irregularities in the contours of the crypts, mild loss of mucin, and evidence of cryptitis with neutrophilic infiltrate within the crypt epithelium.

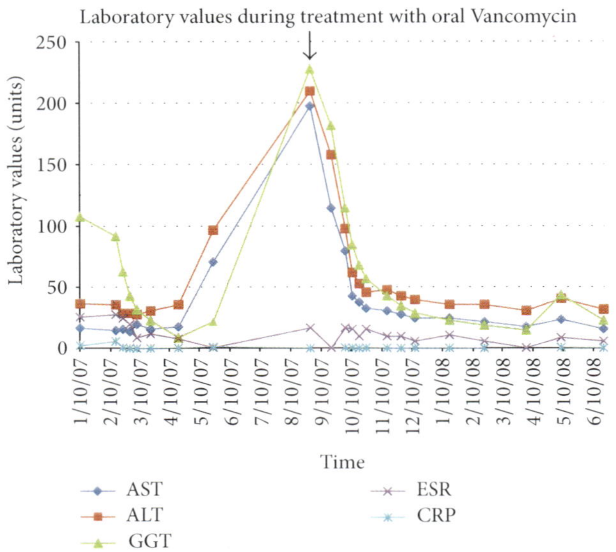

Figure 2: Blood liver markers (AST, ALT, GGT, ESR, CRP) returned to normal values after treatment with oral Vancomycin was started in August 2007 (see arrow). To this date, she remains on oral Vancomycin with normal laboratory values (AST: 15–37 U/L, ALT: 30–65 U/L, GGT: 5–36 U/L, ESR: 0–20 mm/hr, CRP: 0.0–0.5 mg/dl).

0.9 to 1.1. Erythrocyte sedimentation rate (ESR) was elevated at 107 mm/hr; bilirubin was elevated at 3.5 mg/dL, and ammonia was elevated at 55 umol/L. Patient underwent an open liver biopsy, which demonstrated the hepatic parenchyma being completely replaced by extensive compartmentalizing fibrosis and regenerative nodules. There was marked bile duct proliferation in the fibrotic areas. The fibrous septae showed a dense inflammatory infiltrate that consisted predominantly of small lymphocytes admixed with plasma cells and neutrophils. There was prominent interface hepatitis at the periphery of the inflamed septae. There was also a component of acute cholangitis showing focal bile duct infiltration and destruction by inflammatory cells, but most of the bile ducts were intact. There was minimal intrahepatocytic cholestasis, but no significant cholestasis was present in the large bile ducts (Figures 1(a) and 1(b)). She underwent colonoscopy and colonic biopsies which demonstrated focal cryptitis, occasional crypt abscesses, and some crypt distortion, mainly in the descending and sigmoid colon, correlating with her serologic marker ANCA, elevated at 640 (Figures 1(g) and 1(h)) consistent with ulcerative colitis. The patient was diagnosed with primary sclerosing cholangitis with inflammatory bowel disease (ulcerative colitis).

She underwent an orthotopic liver transplant three months later with postoperative complications consisting of hypertension. She was discharged home on postoperative day ten. Her postoperative medications included Prograf (Tacrolimus), CellCept (Mycophenolate), Prednisone, Actigall (Ursodiol), Magnesium, Septra (Trimethoprim and Sulfamethoxazole), and Valcyte (Valganciclovir). Over the next three years she did well weaning off everything except Prograf and CellCept. On routine labs (three years after transplant) she was found to have an elevated alkaline phosphatase level (204 U/L; normal range from 50 to 136). Her aspartate aminotransferase (AST) was elevated (267 U/L; normal range from 15 to 37). Her alanine aminotransferase (ALT) was elevated (290 U/L; normal range from 30 to 65). Her GGT was also elevated (309 U/L; normal range from 5 to 55). Her sedimentation rate was elevated (25 mm/hr; normal range from 0 to 20). EBV and CMV titers were negative and she had a therapeutic Prograf level of 7.9.

The patient underwent liver biopsy to distinguish between liver rejection or recurrence of primary sclerosing cholangitis. The transplanted liver biopsy demonstrated prominent portal inflammation consisting of large numbers of plasma cells and lymphocytes and rare neutrophils and eosinophils. There was prominent interface inflammation with occasional acidophil bodies near the limiting plate. There was mild to moderate bile ductular proliferation with very prominent lymphocytic infiltration of the bile ducts. Some of the bile ductules showed branching and there was concentric inflammation and "onion skin" fibrosis around bile ductules. Overall, the lobular parenchyma was unremarkable. There was lymphocytic endothelialitis. Trichrome stain demonstrated little periportal fibrosis and no evidence of bridging fibrosis. Iron stain was unremarkable. The biopsy was compatible with recurrent primary sclerosing cholangitis (Figures 1(c) and 1(d)). The lack of eosinophils in the portal infiltrate was more consistent with recurrent disease rather than acute rejection.

She was treated for recurrent primary sclerosing cholangitis. Her immunosuppressant medication remained the same and oral Vancomycin was added to the regimen. She received 500 mg orally three times a day of Vancomycin. During the course of her treatment with oral Vancomycin, liver enzymes (AST, ALT, GGT, ESR, and CRP) returned to normal values (Figure 2). The patient is currently on Vancomycin and remains well, to date, with normal laboratory values. Her repeat liver biopsy after three years from the recurrence of her primary sclerosing cholangitis showed no evidence of onion skin around the large bile duct and no inflammation of the bile ducts (Figures 1(e) and 1(f)). Comparison of biopsy photos before and after Vancomycin reveals a return to normal liver structure and anatomy (Figure 3).

3. Discussion

In this paper, we describe the successful use of oral Vancomycin in the treatment of recurrent PSC, after OLT. Currently, there is no universally accepted treatment for PSC; progressive cirrhosis of the liver inevitably leads to the need for liver transplantation in most patients. The majority of available therapeutic options, such as immunosuppressants, corticoid steroids, and ursodeoxycholic acid (UDCA), deal with complications resulting from PSC and do not inhibit

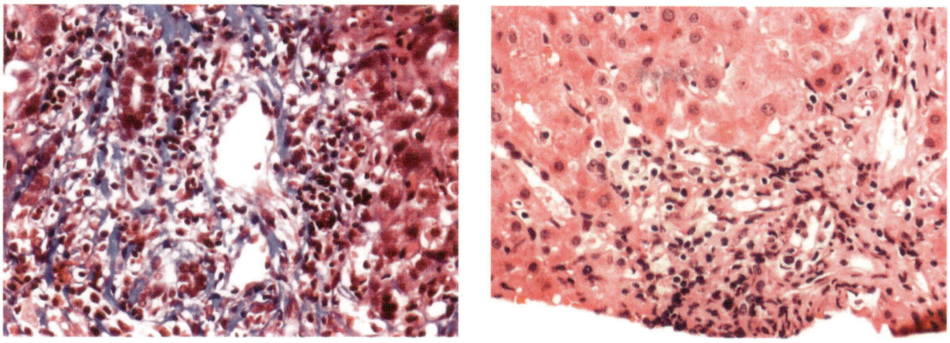

(a) (b)

Figure 3: Comparative liver biopsy of bile ductules (a) before Vancomycin (recurrent PSC) and (b) after Vancomycin. Resolution of inflammation and cirrhosis is visible.

progressive damage from the disease itself [14]. Studies have demonstrated that while UDCA can lead to improvements in biochemical markers, the potential for PSC recurrence requiring OLT is relatively high [15, 16]. Therefore, liver transplantation is the only life-extending option for individuals with advanced stage liver disease. Most data regarding PSC deals with adult cases, and some evidence has shown that the course of the disease in adolescents may follow a unique clinical course, notably an elevation in autoimmune features such as elevated antinuclear antibodies [17]. While juvenile PSC is rare, it contributes to around 2% of pediatric LT annually. The limited number of effective treatment options is primarily due to the unknown pathogenesis of PSC, although some speculate that the primary disease agent is from an enteric bacterial infection.

Previous studies have demonstrated that oral Vancomycin is a viable treatment for early stage PSC, before extensive cirrhosis of the liver is present [18, 19]. An extended clinical study demonstrated that long-term treatment with oral Vancomycin in fourteen juvenile PSC with IBD cases led to the normalization of liver blood markers and reversal of histological abnormalities. However, relapse in GGT and ALT occurred after treatment was suspended [19]. Oral Vancomycin is an immunomodulating bacteria glycopeptide antibiotic that is used to treat gram-positive infections with staphylococcal and has been shown to be poorly absorbed systemically [20, 21]. Vancomycin could also be acting as an anti-inflammatory agent, suggesting that PSC could be an autoimmune disease.

The successful use of oral Vancomycin in reversing the effects of early stage PSC can help develop current understanding regarding the mechanism of the disease. Ongoing clinical trials can potentially lead to new information in regard to the etiology and pathology of the disease. Specifically, this case demonstrates that oral Vancomycin was effective in a case of recurrent PSC after OLT, suggesting that the disease mechanism is not confined within the liver and has external causes—potentially from the backflow of gut bacteria or the spread of gut bacteria through the blood. However, larger cohorts of children with PSC are needed for a more thorough, longitudinal investigation regarding the mechanism, pathogenesis, and treatment of juvenile PSC.

References

[1] A. Wee, J. Ludwig, and R. J. Coffey, "Hepatobiliary carcinoma associated with primary sclerosing cholangitis and chronic ulcerative colitis," *Human Pathology*, vol. 16, no. 7, pp. 719–726, 1985.

[2] C. B. Rosen, D. M. Nagorney, R. H. Wiesner, R. J. Coffey, and N. F. LaRusso, "Cholangiocarcinoma complicating primary sclerosing cholangitis," *Annals of Surgery*, vol. 213, no. 1, pp. 21–25, 2001.

[3] J. M. Farrant, K. M. Hayllar, M. L. Wilkinson et al., "Natural history and prognostic variables in primary sclerosing cholangitis," *Gastroenterology*, vol. 100, no. 6, pp. 1710–1717, 1991.

[4] U. Broomé, R. Olsson, L. Lööf et al., "Natural history and prognostic factors in 305 Swedish patients with primary sclerosing cholangitis," *Gut*, vol. 38, no. 4, pp. 610–615, 1996.

[5] C. Y. Ponsioen, S. M. E. Vrouenraets, W. Prawirodirdjo et al., "Natural history of primary sclerosing cholangitis and prognostic value of cholangiography in a Dutch population," *Gut*, vol. 51, no. 4, pp. 562–566, 2002.

[6] J. J. W. Tischendorf, P. N. Meier, C. Stabburg et al., "Characterization and clinical course of hepatobiliary carcinoma in patients with primary sclerosing cholangitis," *Scandinavian Journal of Gastroenterology*, vol. 41, pp. 1227–1234, 2000.

[7] J. J. W. Tischendorf, H. Hecker, M. Kruger, M. P. Manns, and P. N. Meier, "Characterization, outcome and prognosis in 273 patients with primary sclerosing cholangitis," *The New England Journal of Medicine*, vol. 310, pp. 899–903, 1984.

[8] R. H. Wiesner, P. M. Grambsch, E. R. Dickson et al., "Primary sclerosing cholangitis: natural history, prognostic factors and survival analysis," *Hepatology*, vol. 10, no. 4, pp. 430–436, 1989.

[9] R. Olsson, A. Danielsson, G. Jarnerot et al., "Prevalence of primary sclerosing cholangitis in patients with ulcerative colitis," *Gastroenterology*, vol. 100, no. 5, pp. 1319–1323, 1991.

[10] K. M. Abu-Elmagd, M. Malinchoc, E. R. Dickson et al., "Efficacy of hepatic transplantation in patients with primary sclerosing cholangitis," *Surgery Gynecology and Obstetrics*, vol. 177, no. 4, pp. 335–344, 1993.

[11] K. M. Abu-Elmagd, R. Selby, S. Iwatsuki et al., "Cholangiocarcinoma and sclerosing cholangitis: clinical characteristics and effect on survival after liver transplantation," *Transplantation Proceedings*, vol. 25, no. 1, pp. 1124–1125, 1993.

[12] B. Nashan, H. J. Schlitt, G. Tusch et al., "Biliary malignancies in primary sclerosing cholangitis: timing for liver transplantation," *Hepatology*, vol. 23, no. 5, pp. 1105–1111, 1996.

[13] B. Brandsaeter, H. Isoneimi, U. Broome et al., "Liver transplantation for primary sclerosing cholangitis, predictors and consequences of hepatobiliary malignancy," *Journal of Hepatology*, vol. 40, pp. 815–822, 2004.

[14] R. Chapman, J. Fevery, A. Kalloo et al., "Diagnosis and management of primary sclerosing cholangitis," *Hepatology*, vol. 51, no. 2, pp. 660–678, 2010.

[15] N. L. Nikolaidis, O. I. Giouleme, K. A. Tziomalos et al., "Small-duct primary sclerosing cholangitis: a single-center seven-year experience," *Digestive Diseases and Sciences*, vol. 50, no. 2, pp. 324–326, 2005.

[16] A. E. Feldstein, J. Perrault, M. El-Youssif, K. D. Lindor, D. K. Freese, and P. Angulo, "Primary sclerosing cholangitis in children: a long-term follow-up study," *Hepatology*, vol. 38, no. 1, pp. 210–217, 2003.

[17] G. Mieli-Vergani and D. Vergani, "Unique features of primary sclerosing cholangitis in children," *Current Opinion in Gastroenterology*, vol. 26, no. 3, pp. 265–268, 2010.

[18] K. L. Cox and K. M. Cox, "Oral vancomycin: treatment of primary sclerosing cholangitis in children with inflammatory bowel disease," *Journal of Pediatric Gastroenterology and Nutrition*, vol. 27, no. 5, pp. 580–583, 1998.

[19] Y. K. Davies, K. M. Cox, B. A. Abdullah, A. Safta, A. B. Terry, and K. L. Cox, "Long-term treatment of primary sclerosing cholangitis in children with oral vancomycin: an immunomodulating antibiotic," *Journal of Pediatric Gastroenterology and Nutrition*, vol. 47, no. 1, pp. 61–67, 2008.

[20] M. Siedlar, A. Szczepanik, J. Więckiewicz, A. Pituch-Noworolska, and M. Zembala, "Vancomycin down-regulates lipopolysaccharide-induced tumour necrosis factor alpha (TNFα) production and TNFα-mRNA accumulation in human blood monocytes," *Immunopharmacology*, vol. 35, no. 3, pp. 265–271, 1997.

[21] G. Di Febo, C. Calabrese, and F. Matassoni, "New trends in non-absorbable antibiotics in gastrointestinal disease," *Italian Journal of Gastroenterology*, vol. 24, no. 9, pp. 10–13, 1992.

Salvage with a Secondary Infrahepatic Cavocavostomy of the Occluded Modified Piggyback Anastomosis during Split Liver Transplantation

Erdem Kinaci,[1,2] Cuneyt Kayaalp,[1] Sezai Yilmaz,[1] and Emrah Otan[1]

[1] *Inonu University, Liver Transplantation Institute, 44280 Malatya, Turkey*
[2] *Istanbul Training and Research Hospital, Department of General Surgery, 34098 Istanbul, Turkey*

Correspondence should be addressed to Erdem Kinaci; erdemkinaci@gmail.com

Academic Editor: Yasuhiko Sugawara

Hepatic venous outflow obstruction following liver transplantation is rare but disastrous. Here we described a 14-year-old boy who underwent a split right lobe liver transplantation with modified (side-to-side) piggyback technique which resulted in hepatic venous outflow obstruction. When the liver graft was lifted up, the outflow drainage returned to normal but when it was placed back into the abdomen, the outflow obstruction recurred. Because reanastomosis would have resulted in hepatic reischemia, alternatively, a second infrahepatic cavocavostomy was planned without requiring hepatic reischemia. During this procedure, the first assistant hung the liver up to provide sufficient outflow and the portal inflow of the graft continued as well. We only clamped the recipient's infrahepatic vena cava and the caudal cuff of the graft cava. After the second end-to-side cavocaval anastomosis, the graft was placed in its orthotopic position and there was no outflow problem anymore. The patient tolerated the procedure well and there were no problems after three months of follow-up. A second cavocavostomy can provide an extra bypass for some hepatic venous outflow problems after piggyback anastomosis by avoiding hepatic reischemia.

1. Introduction

There are several vascular complications of liver transplantation diagnosed intraoperatively. Venous outflow obstruction during liver transplantation is a serious problem which may lead to loss of the graft. It can be corrected with a reanastomosis; however, this is potentially harmful due to the necessity of reclamping of hepatic inflow that prolongs the warm ischemia time. Here, a case of hepatic outflow obstruction during a split right lobe liver transplantation with a modified piggyback cavocaval anastomosis technique was described. The problem was solved by an infrahepatic second cavocaval anastomosis without occlusion of the hepatic inflow or outflow.

2. Case Presentation

A 14-year-old boy, weighing 24 kg, with hepatic failure secondary to Wilson's disease was admitted for liver transplantation. Physical examination revealed decreased skin tonus, jaundice, malnutrition, oliguria, and depression of mental status. Among laboratory test results, aspartate aminotransferase was 251 IU/L, alanine aminotransferase was 121 IU/L, alkaline phosphatase was 267 IU/L, gamma glutamyl transpeptidase was 56 IU/L, creatinine was 0.7 mg/dL, albumin was 4.1 g/dL, total bilirubin was 31.8 mg/dL, and INR was 1.6. Child-Pugh score was 8 and Model for End-Stage Liver Disease (MELD) score was 25.

During the transplant waiting period, a deceased liver was accepted from the National Organ Sharing System for a small baby who had acute liver failure. The full-size liver was divided into two parts as the left lobe was for this small baby and the remaining right lobe with the caudate lobe and retrohepatic inferior vena cava was used for the 14-year-old patient. The graft belonged to a 31-year-old male, weighing 60 kg. The right lobe graft weighed 695 g and the graft to recipient weight ratio (GRWR) was 2.89%.

At the back table, the graft was prepared for the modified piggyback cavocaval anastomosis. Supra- and infrahepatic

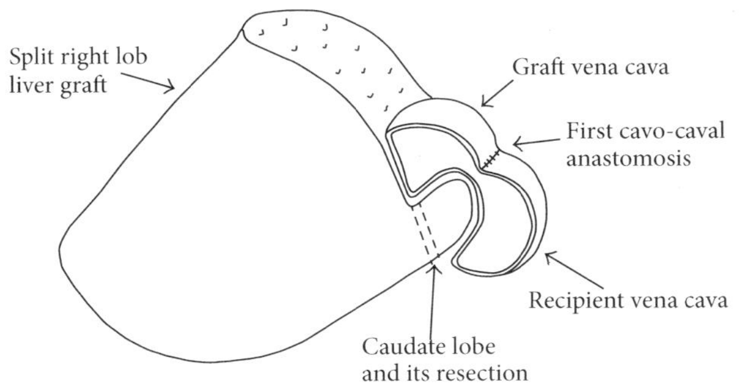

FIGURE 1: The caudate lobe was resected.

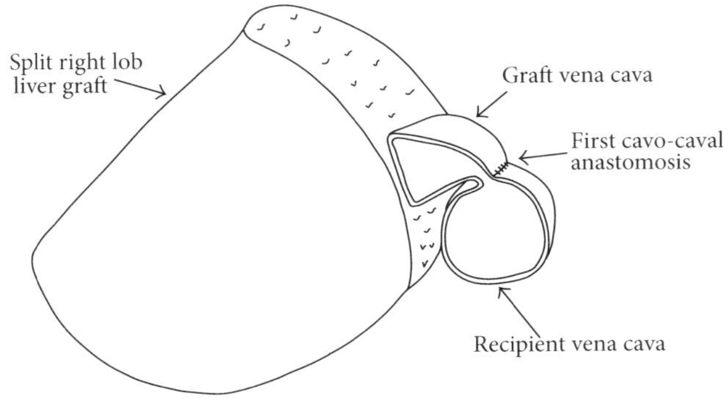

FIGURE 2: Rotational effect on the cavocaval anastomosis.

orifices of the graft vena cava were closed with 5/0 polypropylene sutures. It was anastomosed to the recipient's vena cava by side-to-side, under total caval clamping. A 4 cm length anastomosis was performed to the most cranial parts of the recipient's and the donor's vena cava. Anastomosis was accomplished to the anterior wall of the recipient vena cava without removing any slit from the cava. Before the portal anastomosis, preservation solution in the liver was washed out through a small orifice at the corner of the donor's infrahepatic vena cava and this orifice was closed by sutures after wash-out. Portal vein anastomosis was completed and reperfusion was accomplished.

The systolic arterial blood pressure was between 70 and 90 mmHg before the implantation and it dropped to 40 mm/Hg following reperfusion and did not recover. The liver became hard and dark, and venous bleeding came out from the cut surface. When we lifted the graft up, blood pressure increased to normal level, the tonus/color of the liver returned to normal, and cut surface bleeding ceased. When we left the graft to the right subphrenic space back, the same bad scenario repeated. At first, to eliminate the possibility of positional occlusion, we filled the right subphrenic space with a compress; however, the liver was not released. Secondly, to exclude the external pressure on the inferior vena cava, we resected the caudate lobe of the graft, but it did not provide any benefit (Figure 1). During all those maneuvers, the liver was always hung up by the first assistant. Afterwards, we checked the anastomosis externally by a finger through the recipient vena cava. There was no mechanical occlusion at the anastomosis, when the liver was hung up. However, we believed that a positional kinking of the cavocaval anastomosis could be the reason due to the anterior caval wall anastomosis without removing any caval slit (Figure 2). A reconstruction of the caval anastomosis was planned, but it would be risky because of the necessity of reclamping of the hepatic inflow and outflow that would result in a second ischemia/reperfusion injury of the split graft. Instead, a second anastomosis between both cavae without the risk of an additional second hepatic ischemia/reperfusion injury was preferred.

Caudal stump of the donor's vena cava clamped and the sutured end was released. The infrahepatic vena cava of the recipient was totally cross-clamped. The graft was lifted up for good drainage during the anastomosis. We performed

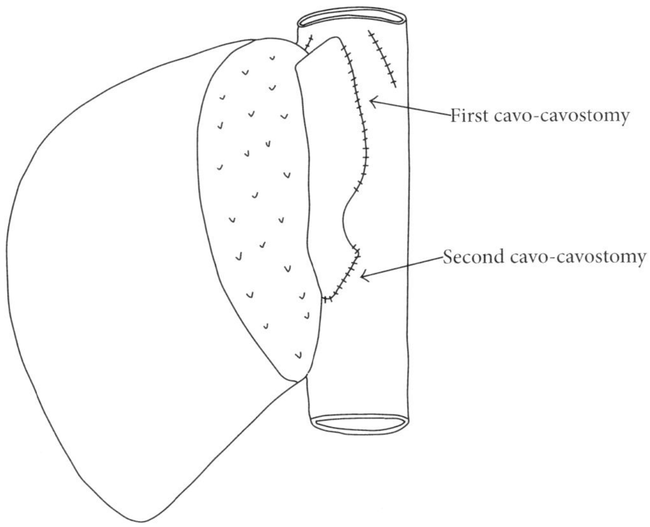

FIGURE 3: The second cavocaval anastomosis.

an infrahepatic anastomosis between the end of the graft's vena cava and the anterolateral wall of the recipient's vena cava. During the procedure, the venous inflow and outflow of the graft were not interrupted. After the new cavocavostomy, the caval clamps were released and the graft was left in the right subphrenic space (Figure 3). Systolic arterial pressure was normal and the graft seemed soft, normal in color, and without bleeding. Finally, the reconstruction of the hepatic artery and bile duct was completed. The postoperative course was uneventful and the patient was alive on the 3rd month of the transplantation.

3. Discussion

Several mechanisms can cause hepatic venous obstruction after liver transplantation. Positional problems can be a reason and placement of tissue expanders behind the graft is an option for correction [1] and compression of the native infrahepatic caval vein has also been described before [2]. External compression of the caudate lobe could be another defined mechanism for caval flow obstruction [3]. Risaliti [4] reported that venous outflow obstruction can be the result of the size discrepancy between the donor's suprahepatic vena cava and the stump of the recipient's hepatic veins. In this case, the GRWR was 2.89% and we checked the piggyback anastomosis but the obstruction was not related to size discrepancy. Outflow problems during and after liver transplantation are more common with reduced-size livers and the reason is usually the kinking of the venous anastomosis due to the rotation effect of a relatively small graft [5]. Large grafts also can be a reason of positional outflow obstruction [6]. In our case, a positional obstruction (rotational effect) at the anastomosis was thought to be the reason for the outflow problem. The patient's primary diagnosis was Wilson's disease and the removed liver was bulky with a deep subphrenic space. Despite the large volume of the graft, there should be a rotation effect. Possibly, anterior located side-to-side anastomosis without slit removal aggravated the obstructive problem. The second anastomosis (cavocavostomy) was located anterolaterally to the recipient's cava and in an end-to-side manner. At the end, the hepatic outflow was provided successfully.

A similar secondary caval anastomosis during liver transplantation was described in the literature by partial side clamping of the recipient's cava [4, 7]. In those cases, the piggyback techniques included the right and left hepatic vein orifices. Therefore, they had enough caval length for the secondary anastomosis. In our case, partial side clamping was not easy for the upper long anastomosis. Therefore, a total infrahepatic caval clamping and end-to-side anastomosis were preferred. It took almost 15 minutes without any serious hemodynamic instability. Quintini and coworkers [8] described a side-to-side cavocavostomy with an endovascular stapler to rescue the obstructed hepatic outflows in two deceased full-size liver grafts. Their cases were done under total hepatic vascular clamping; in other words, they clamped the hepatic artery and portal vein as well. We believe that performing an extra anastomosis without any additional hepatic ischemia is one of the major advantages of our technique.

Regardless of the reason, hepatic venous outflow occlusion and its treatment by an additional anastomosis after piggyback liver transplantation have been described in a limited number of studies [4, 6–8]. This paper presented the first case of a second anastomosis for outflow occlusion after a split liver transplantation. Moreover, this was the first case of a pediatric patient related to this topic.

As a conclusion, an infrahepatic second cavocavostomy is a good option for the intraoperative management of some hepatic venous outflow obstruction without resulting in any additional graft ischemia.

Acknowledgment

This case was presented as a poster presentation in the 11th Congress of Turkish Hepatopancreatobiliary Surgery, in November 2013 in Antalya, Turkey. Erdem Kinaci works in fellowship program.

References

[1] C.-C. Wang, A. M. Concejero, C.-C. Yong et al., "Improving hepatic and portal venous flows using tissue expander and Foley catheter in liver transplantation," *Clinical Transplantation*, vol. 20, no. 1, pp. 81–84, 2006.

[2] F. Zamboni and R. Sampietro, "Conversion to termino-terminal cavo-cavostomy as a rescue technique for infrahepatic obstruction after piggyback liver transplantation," *Transplant International*, vol. 21, no. 10, pp. 1008–1010, 2008.

[3] K. Takeda, K. Tanaka, T. Kumamoto et al., "Severe outflow block syndrome caused by compression by the swollen caudate lobe after living donor liver transplantation: report of a case," *Surgery Today*, vol. 42, no. 2, pp. 177–180, 2012.

[4] A. Risaliti, "Infrahepatic cavo-cavostomy as a rescue technique for complicated piggyback liver transplantation," *Transplantation Proceedings*, vol. 33, no. 1-2, pp. 1388–1389, 2001.

[5] J. C. Emond, T. G. Heffron, P. F. Whitington, and C. E. Broelsch, "Reconstruction of the hepatic vein in reduced size hepatic transplantation," *Surgery Gynecology and Obstetrics*, vol. 176, no. 1, pp. 11–17, 1993.

[6] F. Z. Eldeen, C. F. Lee, C. S. Lee, K. M. Chan, and W. C. Lee, "Passing Loop' technique: a new modification of the piggyback technique tailored to voluminous liver grafts: case report," *Transplantation Proceedings*, vol. 45, pp. 831–832, 2013.

[7] R. Merenda, G. E. Gerunda, D. Neri et al., "Infrahepatic terminolateral cavo-cavostomy as a rescue technique in complicated "modified" piggyback liver transplantation," *Journal of the American College of Surgeons*, vol. 185, pp. 576–579, 1997.

[8] C. Quintini, C. M. Miller, K. Hashimoto et al., "Side-to-side cavocavostomy with an endovascular stapler: rescue technique for severe hepatic vein and/or inferior vena cava outflow obstruction after liver transplantation using the piggyback technique," *Liver Transplantation*, vol. 15, no. 1, pp. 49–53, 2009.

18

Scedosporiosis in a Combined Kidney and Liver Transplant Recipient: A Case Report of Possible Transmission from a Near-Drowning Donor

Rachael Leek,[1] Erika Aldag,[1] Iram Nadeem,[1] Vikraman Gunabushanam,[1] Ajay Sahajpal,[1,2] David J. Kramer,[2,3] and Thomas J. Walsh[4]

[1]*Department of Abdominal Transplant, Aurora St. Luke's Medical Center, Milwaukee, WI, USA*
[2]*University of Wisconsin School of Medicine and Public Health, Madison, WI 53726, USA*
[3]*Department of Critical Care, Aurora St. Luke's Medical Center, Milwaukee, WI, USA*
[4]*Weill Cornell Medicine, Cornell University and New York Presbyterian Hospital, New York, NY, USA*

Correspondence should be addressed to Erika Aldag; erika.aldag@aurora.org

Academic Editor: Graeme Forrest

Scedosporium spp. are saprobic fungi that cause serious infections in immunocompromised hosts and in near-drowning victims. Solid organ transplant recipients are at increased risk of scedosporiosis as they require aggressive immunosuppression to prevent allograft rejection. We present a case of disseminated *Scedosporium apiospermum* infection occurring in the recipient of a combined kidney and liver transplantation whose organs were donated by a near-drowning victim and review the literature of scedosporiosis in solid organ transplantation.

1. Introduction

Scedosporium is a saprobic fungus that naturally occurs in soil, manure, sewage, and water bodies polluted by environmental contaminants. Cases of infections with *Scedosporium* spp. are reported worldwide and can range in severity from colonization or local infection to disseminated disease [1–5]. *S. apiospermum* most commonly infects the lungs as inhalation is often the suspected mode of organism acquisition [6].

The genus *Scedosporium* includes, but is not limited to, three species that cause life-threatening infections in humans: *Scedosporium apiospermum*, *Scedosporium prolificans* (recently renamed *Lomentospora prolificans*), and *Scedosporium aurantiacum* [7]. *Scedosporium* spp. appear as branching septate hyphae when isolated on standard culture media.

Scedosporium spp. have been implicated in near-drowning accidents [8–10]. Indeed *Scedosporium* spp. are the most common cause of fungal pneumonia, infection of the central nervous system, and disseminated disease following near-drowning events. There are few cases of donor to recipient transmission of infection of *Scedosporium* spp. and even fewer reports of near-drowning donor transmission of diseases [11, 12]. We report the clinical course and management of disseminated *S. apiospermum* infection in a combined kidney and liver transplantation case receiving organs from a brain-dead donor who suffered a near-drowning accident; we further review the literature on scedosporiosis in solid organ transplant recipients.

2. Case Presentation: Donor

A 41-year-old male fell into a freshwater lake. Emergency responders pulled him from the lake and return of spontaneous circulation was achieved after twenty minutes of resuscitation. Subsequent chest radiographs showed development and worsening of bilateral opacities suspicious for pneumonia. Brain death was declared three days after hospital admission.

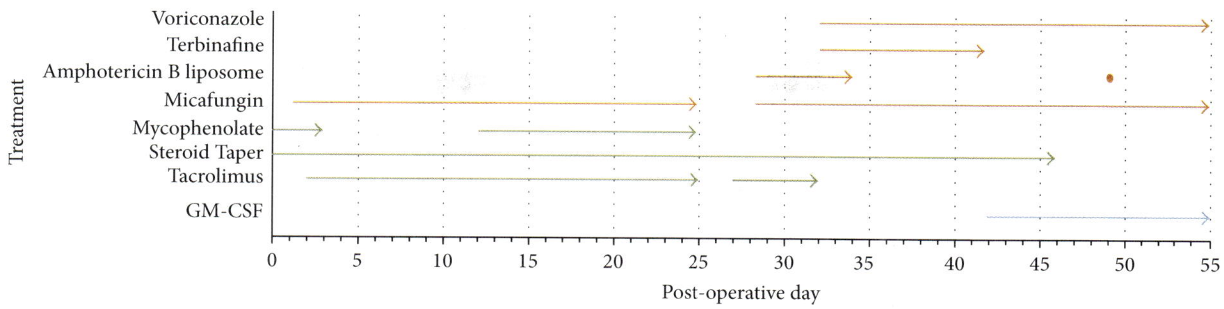

FIGURE 1: Antifungal agents and immunosuppression management.

3. Case Presentation: Recipient

A 66-year-old male actively listed for a kidney and liver transplant presented to the surgical intensive care unit with sepsis and an oxacillin-sensitive *Staphylococcus aureus* bacteremia. He was treated with appropriate antibiotic therapy. He then developed acute tubular necrosis requiring continuous venovenous hemofiltration (CVVH). The patient had a chest X-ray showing mild pulmonary congestion and bronchoscopy was not performed as the patient did not show signs of pneumonia. After two weeks within his admission, the patient was treated for *Escherichia coli* bacteremia with piperacillin-tazobactam. Repeat blood cultures were negative after two days of therapy.

While the patient was hospitalized, a donor became available. The donor kidney and liver were grossly normal. The patient underwent a combined kidney and liver transplant for chronic kidney failure with associated liver cirrhosis caused by the hepatitis C virus and alcoholism. The explanted liver was cirrhotic without any malignancy. At the time of transplantation, the patient's Model for End Stage Liver Disease (MELD) score was 40, having been decompensated in the surgical intensive care unit for the previous month. A summary of the patient's immunosuppression and antifungal management after transplant is provided in Figure 1.

The patient was given methylprednisolone 500 mg and mycophenolate mofetil 1,000 mg intraoperatively as induction immunosuppression. Maintenance immunosuppression protocols were followed after transplant. CVVH was performed intraoperatively and was discontinued on postoperative day (POD) 1 when renal graft function improved. The patient's hospital stay was complicated by a contained urine leak from the ureteroureterostomy which was managed nonoperatively with drains and ureteral stents. On POD 8, the patient was transferred out of the intensive care unit and on POD 14, to the inpatient rehab care unit as graft function continued to improve. The hepatic transaminases fluctuated and, on POD 25, he was transferred back to the surgical intensive care unit with peritonitis. As infection was suspected, immunosuppression was restricted to the use of corticosteroids tapered down to prednisone 5 mg daily. The patient was taken back to the operating room on POD 28 for a peritoneal washout. Cultures obtained during the procedure are presented in Tables 1 and 2. Of most concern was the *S. apiospermum* isolated from the perihepatic, perinephric, and biloma fluid. Endoscopic Retrograde Cholangiopancreatography (ERCP) was performed the following day, which did not reveal any extravasation. Discovery of *S. apiospermum* prompted contact with the Centers for Disease Control and Prevention (CDC), the Disease Transmission Advisory Committee (DTAC) of the United Network for Organ Sharing (UNOS), and the transplant centers treating recipients of allografts from the same donor. Other recipients had no evidence of infection.

On POD 28, due to worsening hemodynamics and peritonitis, another laparotomy and another washout were performed to evacuate an infected hematoma. The entire peritoneal surface was lined with mold. On POD 32, a mold suggestive of *Scedosporium* spp. grew from surgical cultures. Expert opinion for the management of our patient's suspected *S. apiospermum* infection was to use voriconazole targeting a trough of 2–4 mcg/mL, which we started on POD 32. Additionally, terbinafine was started for suspected synergy with voriconazole. A sample of the *S. apiospermum* was sent out for synergy studies which were expected to take a week or more to be conclusive. On POD 41 *S. apiospermum* was identified. Laboratory results suggested terbinafine was not synergistic with voriconazole. Additionally, terbinafine is distributed rapidly to skin and bone and as such is not distributed well into visceral tissue and accumulation of terbinafine may cause hepatotoxicity. In response, terbinafine was discontinued and granulocyte macrophage colony-stimulating factor (GM-CSF) initiated on POD 42. The patient developed neurologic deficits with decreased vision to the right side and blurred vision bilaterally on POD 46. Magnetic resonance imaging (MRI) of the brain, shown in Figure 2, revealed multiple ring-enhancing lesions in the supratentorial compartment consistent with hematogenous central nervous system (CNS) scedosporiosis. We continued treatment with antifungal therapy. He developed septic shock and expired on POD 55.

4. Discussion

Differential diagnoses for opportunistic pathogens causing pneumonia related to near-drowning events include several key pathogenic bacteria and fungi. Gram negative bacteria are most often the causative agents in near-drowning cases [13]. *Aeromonas spp.* have been described most often in near-drowning pneumonia cases. *Aeromonas* spp. naturally thrive in fresh and brackish waters and have been isolated

TABLE 1: Culture results.

Date	Culture site	Source	Result
POD 28	Abdominal fluid	Surgical specimen	*C. tropicalis* *E. faecalis* *E. coli* *M. morganii*
POD 28	Biloma fluid	Surgical specimen	*E. faecium* *E. faecalis* *S. apiospermum* *C. tropicalis*
POD 28	Perihepatic fluid	Surgical specimen	*S. apiospermum* *E. faecium* *C. tropicalis*
POD 28	Perinephric hematoma tissue	Surgical specimen	*S. apiospermum*
POD 32	Abdominal clot	Surgical specimen	*S. apiospermum*
POD 32	Intestinal serosal tissue	Surgical specimen	*S. apiospermum* *E. faecium*
POD 50	LUQ abdominal fluid	Surgical specimen	*C. glabrata* *C. tropicalis*
POD 50	Cerebrospinal fluid	Lumbar puncture	Negative

TABLE 2: Susceptibility testing of fungal isolates.

Isolate	Resistant (MIC)	Intermediate (MIC)	Susceptible (MIC)
Scedosporium apiospermum	5-Fluorocytosine (>64), amphotericin B (>16), caspofungin (>8), micafungin (>8), terbinafine (>2)	None	Voriconazole (1)
Candida tropicalis	None	None	Caspofungin (≤0.25), fluconazole (≤1), voriconazole (≤0.12)
Candida glabrata	None	None	Caspofungin (2), fluconazole (≤1), voriconazole (≤0.12)

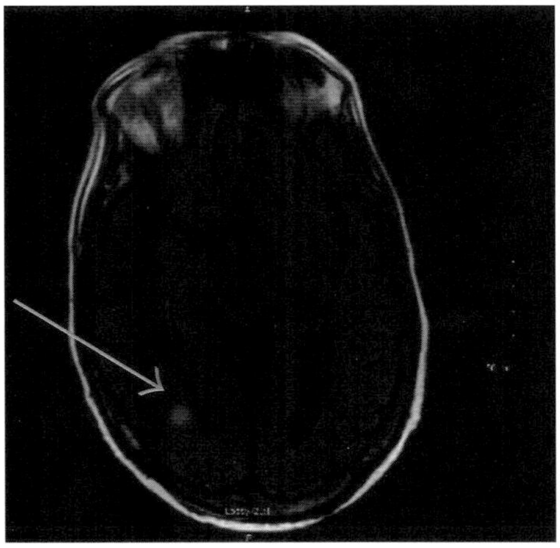

FIGURE 2: MRI of the brain. Multiple ring-enhancing lesions with associated diffusion restriction and T2/FLAIR hyperintensity are present throughout the supratentorial white matter.

in humans in wound and gastrointestinal infections after exposure to contaminated water. Other potential bacterial pathogens include *Pseudomonas aeruginosa*, *Legionella* spp., *Klebsiella* spp., and other Enterobacteriaceae [13]. *Scedosporium* spp. are the most common cause of invasive fungal infection, including pneumonia, CNS disease, and dissemination following near-drowning.

We identified 60 published cases of scedosporiosis after solid organ transplantation between the year 2000 and the present. Few were cases of scedosporiosis after solitary liver transplantation (5/60); most were reported following solitary lung (18/60) or kidney (18/60) transplantation. Table 3 [2, 12, 14–42] provides a summary of the comprehensive literature review performed. *S. apiospermum* was isolated in the majority of cases, though *S. prolificans* and *S. aurantiacum* were also isolated. In four cases, both *S. apiospermum* and *S. prolificans* were identified in the same patient. In patients who had infections with a single isolate of *Scedosporium* spp., the observed mortality rates of *S. apiospermum, S. prolificans*, and *S. aurantiacum* were 54.5% (24/44), 70% (7/10), and 100% (3/3), respectively (excluding four cases with combined infections). Observed mortality of all *Scedosporium* spp. infections was 59% (36/61) including our patient case.

Kim et al. reported three fatal and two nonfatal cases of scedosporiosis following solid organ transplantation from

TABLE 3: Review of solid organ transplant-associated *Scedosporium* infection.

Ref #	Year	Recipient information Age (years)	Gender	Recipient organ(s)	Species of *Scedosporium*	Treatment approach	Outcome
[14]	2000	67	Male	Heart	*apiospermum*	Voriconazole	Deceased
[15]	2001	42	Female	Heart/lung	*apiospermum*	Fluconazole, itraconazole	Deceased
		22	Female	Heart/lung	*prolificans + apiospermum*	Fluconazole, itraconazole	Deceased
		42	Male	Heart/lung	*prolificans + apiospermum*	Fluconazole, itraconazole	Alive
		49	Male	Lung	*prolificans + apiospermum*	Fluconazole, itraconazole	Deceased
		39	Male	Lung	*prolificans + apiospermum*	Fluconazole, itraconazole	Alive
		52	Female	Lung	*apiospermum*	Fluconazole, itraconazole	Alive
		38	Female	Heart/lung	*apiospermum*	Fluconazole, itraconazole	Deceased
[16]	2002	58	Female	Liver	*apiospermum*	Itraconazole, miconazole	Alive
		37	Male	Lung	*apiospermum*	Itraconazole	Deceased
		30	Male	Lung	*apiospermum*	Amphotericin B, miconazole	Deceased
		37	Female	Heart/lung	*apiospermum*	Miconazole	Deceased
		39	Male	Liver	*apiospermum*	5-Flucytosine, amphotericin B	Deceased
		67	Male	Heart	*apiospermum*	Itraconazole, voriconazole	Deceased
		36	Male	Kidney	*apiospermum*	Itraconazole, miconazole	Deceased
[17]	2002	49	Male	Kidney	*apiospermum*	Voriconazole	Deceased
[18]	2002	62	Female	Kidney	*apiospermum*	None	Deceased
		58	Male	Kidney	*apiospermum*	Itraconazole, voriconazole	Alive
[19]	2002	64	Female	Lung	*apiospermum*	Amphotericin B, itraconazole	Deceased
[20]	2002	71	Male	Heart	*apiospermum*	Itraconazole	Alive
[21]	2003	24	Male	Lung	*apiospermum*	Voriconazole	Alive
		59	Male	Kidney	*apiospermum*	Voriconazole	Alive
[22]	2004	50	Male	Kidney	*apiospermum*	Voriconazole	Alive
[23]	2004	58	Male	Kidney	*apiospermum*	Amphotericin B, fluconazole, itraconazole, miconazole	Alive
[24]	2004	56	Female	Lung	*prolificans*	Voriconazole	Deceased
[25]	2005	55	Male	Small bowel	*prolificans*	Amphotericin B	Deceased
		40	Male	Kidney/pancreas	*prolificans*	Voriconazole	Alive
		67	Male	Kidney	*apiospermum*	Amphotericin B	Alive
		51	Female	Small bowel	*prolificans*	Amphotericin B, Voriconazole, caspofungin	Deceased
		67	Male	Heart	*apiospermum*	Voriconazole	Deceased
		17	Male	Liver	*prolificans*	Voriconazole	Deceased
		64	Male	Liver	*apiospermum*	None	Deceased
		45	Male	Heart	*apiospermum*	Itraconazole	Deceased
		56	Male	Liver	*apiospermum*	Voriconazole	Deceased
		44	Female	Heart	*prolificans*	Amphotericin B	Deceased
		68	Male	Kidney	*prolificans*	Voriconazole	Alive
		52	Male	Small bowel	*apiospermum*	Amphotericin B, Voriconazole, caspofungin	Alive
		62	Male	Kidney/pancreas	*apiospermum*	Voriconazole	Alive
[26]	2005	26	Female	Lung	*apiospermum*	Miconazole, voriconazole	Deceased
[27]	2006	58	Male	Kidney	*apiospermum*	Miconazole, voriconazole	Alive
[28]	2006	57	Male	Lung	*apiospermum*	Terbinafine, voriconazole	Alive
		63	Male	Lung	*apiospermum*	Liposomal amphotericin B, terbinafine, voriconazole	Alive

Table 3: Continued.

Ref #	Year	Recipient information Age (years)	Gender	Recipient organ(s)	Species of *Scedosporium*	Treatment approach	Outcome
[29]	2007	59	Female	Kidney	*apiospermum*	Voriconazole	Alive
[30]	2007	43	Male	Lung	*apiospermum*	Caspofungin, itraconazole, liposomal amphotericin B	Deceased
[31]	2008	70	Male	Kidney	*prolificans*	Terbinafine, voriconazole	Alive
[32]	2009	65	Female	Kidney	*apiospermum*	Voriconazole	Alive
[33]	2010	37	Female	Lung	*apiospermum*	Caspofungin, terbinafine, voriconazole	Deceased
[34]	2011	16	Female	Lung	*apiospermum*	Voriconazole	Alive
[35]	2012	35	Male	Lung/liver	*apiospermum*	Caspofungin, voriconazole	Deceased
[36]	2012	37	Female	Lung	*apiospermum*	Aerosolized amphotericin B, caspofungin, itraconazole, voriconazole	Deceased
[37]	2013	17	Female	Lung	*apiospermum*	Caspofungin, posaconazole, voriconazole	Alive
[38]	2013	70	Female	Lung	*prolificans*	Caspofungin, terbinafine, voriconazole	Deceased
[39]	2014	50	Female	Kidney	*apiospermum*	Voriconazole	Alive
[40]	2014	35	Male	Kidney	*prolificans*	Itraconazole, liposomal amphotericin B, micafungin, voriconazole	Deceased
[41]	2015	70	Male	Heart	*apiospermum*	Posaconazole, terbinafine	Deceased
[12]	2015	19	Male	Heart	*aurantiacum*	Amphotericin B prophylaxis	Deceased
		56	Male	Kidney	*aurantiacum*	Itraconazole, liposomal amphotericin B	Deceased
		57	Female	Kidney	*aurantiacum*	Caspofungin, voriconazole	Deceased
[2]	2015	40	Male	Kidney	*apiospermum*	Voriconazole	Deceased
[42]	2015	18	Female	Lung	*apiospermum*	Terbinafine, voriconazole	Alive

the same donor who was victim to a near-drowning accident [12]. Additionally, they reviewed national Korean data on transplants and found that, among 2600 deceased-donor transplants over thirteen years, 27 (1%) of donors were victims of drowning. We accessed data from the United States Organ Procurement and Transplantation Network and found a similar rate: in 2015, 102/7586 (approximately 1.3%) of solid organ donors died of near-drowning events [43]. While this is a low percentage of all donors, the significance of our case is enhanced by the 58.3% mortality rate of infections involving *Scedosporium* spp. after solid organ transplantation.

At our center, liver transplant recipients are given antifungal prophylaxis based on their risk level. We stratify higher risk patients as those with MELD scores greater than 35, renal failure, requiring hemodialysis or CVVH prior to transplantation, recurrent spontaneous bacterial peritonitis, or preoperative prealbumin less than 10. High risk liver transplant recipients receive micafungin intravenously unless resistant *Candida glabrata*, *Aspergillus* spp., or *Cryptococcus* spp. are suspected; in such cases, amphotericin B lipid complex or voriconazole would be used. Our patient was classified as high risk and given micafungin prophylaxis.

All cases of suspected donor-derived infections should be reported to the DTAC. Communications with the CDC, DTAC, and the centers treating the recipients of the other organs provided by this donor revealed the recipient of the heart was receiving voriconazole prophylaxis, while the recipients of the other kidney and the pancreas were not. To the best of our knowledge, no other recipient of this donor's organs is infected with *Scedosporium* spp. The other centers were advised by the CDC to commence voriconazole prophylaxis for an undetermined duration. Expert opinion for the management of our patient's scedosporiosis was voriconazole targeting a trough of 2–4 mcg/mL. Additionally, immunosuppression was to be limited or discontinued to improve infection clearance.

S. apiospermum is inherently resistant to amphotericin B, including the lipid formulations. Of the newer triazole antifungals, data on the *in vitro* activity of voriconazole is most robust, showing activity against *S. apiospermum* with MICs of 0.12 to 0.5 mcg/mL in clinical isolates [30]. Because of poor activity with single agents, various antifungal combinations have been examined for efficacy against *S. apiospermum*. Strong synergy was found *in vitro* between voriconazole and terbinafine against clinical isolates of *Scedosporium* spp. [30]. Combination of micafungin and voriconazole has demonstrated a synergistic effect against several fungi *in vitro* including *Scedosporium* spp. The synergistic mechanism may include reorganization of the cell wall allowing increased exposure of beta-glucan to the immune system [44].

In addition to antifungal agents, GM-CSF has been studied with some success [44, 45]. While antifungal therapy remains crucial to recovery, the treatment of scedosporiosis infections depends on the function of the host's innate immune system, in particular, polymorphonuclear cells (PMNs). The mechanism of GM-CSF increases the antifungal action of PMNs *in vitro* [45].

Despite good allograft function, our patient did not survive disseminated infection with *S. apiospermum* after combined kidney and liver transplantation. The exact mode of transmission and acquisition of *S. apiospermum* in this patient remains uncertain. We suspect donor to recipient transmission as the donor was the victim of a near-drowning event and had chest radiographs suspicious for pneumonia; however, we cannot rule out recipient colonization or nosocomial infection after the transplant.

Infections caused by *Scedosporium* spp. following solid organ transplant, while not common, are often fatal for recipients. There are no standards of practice for prophylaxis for patients at risk for developing scedosporiosis, such as recipients of organs from nearly drowned donors. Considering our case and the scedosporiosis mortality rate over 50% and the low rate of nearly drowned donors, we recommend screening for *Scedosporium* spp. when donated organs originate from a near-drowning victim.

Competing Interests

The authors declare that there is no significant conflict of interests regarding the publication of this paper.

References

[1] L. S. Johnson, R. K. Shields, and C. J. Clancy, "Epidemiology, clinical manifestations, and outcomes of scedosporium infections among solid organ transplant recipients," *Transplant Infectious Disease*, vol. 16, no. 4, pp. 578–587, 2014.

[2] B. Bose, S. Sharma, P. Derrington, and D. Divi, "Scedosporium apiospermum peritonitis in a patient undergoing peritoneal dialysis," *Nephrology*, vol. 17, no. 5, pp. 521–522, 2012.

[3] A. Malini, N. S. Madhusudan, S. P. Sinhasan, and B. C. Harthimath, "A masquerading subcutaneous swelling caused by Scedosporium apiospermum: an emerging pathogen," *Indian Journal of Pathology and Microbiology*, vol. 58, no. 1, pp. 115–117, 2015.

[4] H. L. Wilson and K. J. Kennedy, "*Scedosporium apiospermum* brain abscesses in an immunocompetent man with silicosis," *Medical Mycology Case Reports*, vol. 2, no. 1, pp. 75–78, 2013.

[5] J. M. Schaenman, D. B. DiGiulio, L. F. Mirels et al., "Scedosporium apiospermum soft tissue infection successfully treated with voriconazole: potential pitfalls in the transition from intravenous to oral therapy," *Journal of Clinical Microbiology*, vol. 43, no. 2, pp. 973–977, 2005.

[6] T. J. Walsh, A. Groll, J. Hiemenz, R. Fleming, E. Roilides, and E. Anaissie, "Infections due to emerging and uncommon medically important fungal pathogens," *Clinical Microbiology and Infection*, vol. 10, supplement 1, pp. 48–66, 2004.

[7] K. J. Cortez, E. Roilides, F. Quiroz-Telles et al., "Infections caused by Scedosporium spp," *Clinical Microbiology Reviews*, vol. 21, no. 1, pp. 157–197, 2008.

[8] P. T. Ender and M. J. Dolan, "Pneumonia associated with near-drowning," *Clinical Infectious Diseases*, vol. 25, no. 4, pp. 896–907, 1997.

[9] A. Katragkou, J. Dotis, M. Kotsiou, M. Tamiolaki, and E. Roilides, "*Scedosporium apiospermum* infection after near-drowning," *Mycoses*, vol. 50, no. 5, pp. 412–421, 2007.

[10] P. A. Kowacs, C. E. Soares Silvado, S. Monteiro de Almeida et al., "Infection of the CNS by *Scedosporium apiospermum* after near drowning. Report of a fatal case and analysis of its confounding factors," *Journal of Clinical Pathology*, vol. 57, no. 2, pp. 205–207, 2004.

[11] M. S. Patel, A. J. Wright, R. Kohn, J. F. Markmann, C. N. Kotton, and P. A. Vagefi, "Successful long-term management of invasive cerebral fungal infection following liver transplantation," *Mycoses*, vol. 58, no. 3, pp. 181–186, 2015.

[12] S.-H. Kim, Y. E. Ha, J.-C. Youn et al., "Fatal scedosporiosis in multiple solid organ allografts transmitted from a nearly-drowned donor," *American Journal of Transplantation*, vol. 15, no. 3, pp. 833–840, 2015.

[13] K. Hoetzenecker, H. J. Ankersmit, G. Lang et al., "Considerations on infectious complications using a drowned lung for transplantation," *Transplant International*, vol. 23, no. 7, pp. e32–e34, 2010.

[14] S. Kusne, S. Ariyanayagam-Baksh, D. C. Strollo, and J. Abernethy, "Invasive *Scedosporium apiospermum* infection in a heart transplant recipient presenting with multiple skin nodules and a pulmonary consolidation," *Transplant Infectious Disease*, vol. 2, no. 4, pp. 194–196, 2000.

[15] M. Tamm, M. Malouf, and A. Glanville, "Pulmonary scedosporium infection following lung transplantation," *Transplant Infectious Disease*, vol. 3, no. 4, pp. 189–194, 2001.

[16] B. Castiglioni, D. A. Sutton, M. G. Rinaldi, J. Fung, and S. Kusne, "Pseudallescheria boydii (Anamorph scedosporium apiospermum) infection in solid organ transplant recipients in a tertiary medical center and review of the literature," *Medicine*, vol. 81, no. 5, pp. 333–348, 2002.

[17] E. L. Campagnaro, K. J. Woodside, M. G. Early et al., "Disseminated Pseudallescheria boydii (Scedosporium apiospermum) infection in a renal transplant patient," *Transplant Infectious Disease*, vol. 4, no. 4, pp. 207–211, 2002.

[18] M. Montejo, M. L. Muñiz, S. Zárraga et al., "Infection due to Scedosporium apiospermum in renal transplant recipients: a report of two cases and literature review of central nervous system and cutaneous infections by Pseudoallescheria boydii/Sc. apiospermum," *Mycoses*, vol. 45, no. 9-10, pp. 418–427, 2002.

[19] R. Raj and A. E. Frost, "Scedosporium apiospermum fungemia in a lung transplant recipient," *Chest*, vol. 121, no. 5, pp. 1714–1716, 2002.

[20] T. R. Talbot, J. Hatcher, S. F. Davis, R. N. Pierson III, R. Barton, and S. Dummer, "*Scedosporium apiospermum* pneumonia and sternal wound infection in a heart transplant recipient," *Transplantation*, vol. 74, no. 11, pp. 1645–1647, 2002.

[21] J. Fortún, P. Martín-Dávila, M. A. Sánchez et al., "Voriconazole in the treatment of invasive mold infections in transplant recipients," *European Journal of Clinical Microbiology and Infectious Diseases*, vol. 22, no. 7, pp. 408–413, 2003.

[22] J. Ahmed, D. M. Ditmars, T. Sheppard, R. Del Busto, K. K. Venkat, and R. Parasuraman, "Recurrence of Scedosporium

apiospermum infection following renal re-transplantation," *American Journal of Transplantation*, vol. 4, no. 10, pp. 1720–1724, 2004.

[23] D. Reimann, E. Büssemaker, and P. Gross, "Successful treatment due to vacuum seal technique of a severe Scedosporium apiospermum skin infection in a renal transplant recipient," *Nephrology Dialysis Transplantation*, vol. 19, no. 1, pp. 245–248, 2004.

[24] M. R. Vagefi, E. T. Kim, R. G. Alvarado, J. L. Duncan, E. L. Howes, and J. B. Crawford, "Bilateral endogenous Scedosporium prolificans endophthalmitis after lung transplantation," *American Journal of Ophthalmology*, vol. 139, no. 2, pp. 370–373, 2005.

[25] S. Husain, P. Muñoz, G. Forrest et al., "Infections due to *Scedosporium apiospermum* and *Scedosporium prolificans* in transplant recipients: clinical characteristics and impact of antifungal agent therapy on outcome," *Clinical Infectious Diseases*, vol. 40, no. 1, pp. 89–99, 2005.

[26] F. Symoens, C. Knoop, M. Schrooyen et al., "Disseminated Scedosporium apiospermum infection in a cystic fibrosis patient after double-lung transplantation," *Journal of Heart and Lung Transplantation*, vol. 25, no. 5, pp. 603–607, 2006.

[27] C. Farina, E. Gotti, F. Suter, and A. Goglio, "*Scedosporium apiospermum* soft-tissue infection: a case report and review of kidney transplant literature," *Transplantation Proceedings*, vol. 38, no. 5, pp. 1333–1335, 2006.

[28] M. Musk, D. Chambers, W. Chin, R. Murray, and E. Gabbay, "Successful treatment of disseminated Scedosporium infection in 2 lung transplant recipients: review of the literature and recommendations for management," *Journal of Heart and Lung Transplantation*, vol. 25, no. 10, pp. 1268–1272, 2006.

[29] P. G. Rogasi, M. Zanazzi, J. Nocentini et al., "Disseminated *Scedosporium apiospermum* infection in renal transplant recipient: long-term successful treatment with voriconazole: a case report," *Transplantation Proceedings*, vol. 39, no. 6, pp. 2033–2035, 2007.

[30] H. Sahi, R. K. Avery, O. A. Minai et al., "Scedosporium apiospermum (Pseudoallescheria boydii) Infection in lung transplant recipients," *Journal of Heart and Lung Transplantation*, vol. 26, no. 4, pp. 350–356, 2007.

[31] J. Y. Z. Li, T. Y. Yong, D. I. Grove, and P. T. H. Coates, "Successful control of *Scedosporium prolificans* septic arthritis and probable osteomyelitis without radical surgery in a long-term renal transplant recipient," *Transplant Infectious Disease*, vol. 10, no. 1, pp. 63–65, 2008.

[32] K. Ezzedine, K. M. Wissing, F. Jacobs, H. Rodriguez, D. Malvy, and T. Simonart, "Recurrent *Scedosporium apiospermum* skin infection in a renal transplant recipient," *Journal of the European Academy of Dermatology and Venereology*, vol. 23, no. 1, pp. 95–96, 2009.

[33] F. Morio, D. Horeau-Langlard, F. Gay-Andrieu et al., "Disseminated *Scedosporium/Pseudallescheria* infection after double-lung transplantation in patients with cystic fibrosis," *Journal of Clinical Microbiology*, vol. 48, no. 5, pp. 1978–1982, 2010.

[34] B. Luijk, M. B. Ekkelenkamp, P. A. De Jong et al., "Effective prolonged therapy with voriconazole in a lung transplant recipient with spondylodiscitis induced by *Scedosporium apiospermum*," *Case Reports in Infectious Diseases*, vol. 2011, Article ID 460313, 4 pages, 2011.

[35] S. Hirschi, V. Letscher-Bru, J. Pottecher et al., "Disseminated *Trichosporon mycotoxinivorans, Aspergillus fumigatus*, and *Scedosporium apiospermum* coinfection after lung and liver transplantation in a cystic fibrosis patient," *Journal of Clinical Microbiology*, vol. 50, no. 12, pp. 4168–4170, 2012.

[36] F. Miraldi, M. Anile, F. Ruberto et al., "*Scedosporium apiospermum* atrial mycetomas after lung transplantation for cystic fibrosis," *Transplant Infectious Disease*, vol. 14, no. 2, pp. 188–191, 2012.

[37] C. Hartmann, C. Müller, H. Weißbrodt et al., "Successful prevention of scedosporiosis after lung transplantation in a cystic fibrosis patient by combined local and systemic triazole therapy," *Medical Mycology Case Reports*, vol. 2, no. 1, pp. 116–118, 2013.

[38] D. M. Sayah, B. S. Schwartz, J. Kukreja, J. P. Singer, J. A. Golden, and L. E. Leard, "Scedosporium prolificans pericarditis and mycotic aortic aneurysm in a lung transplant recipient receiving voriconazole prophylaxis," *Transplant Infectious Disease*, vol. 15, no. 2, pp. E70–E74, 2013.

[39] M. Rathi, S. Gundlapalli, R. Ramachandran et al., "A rare case of cytomegalovirus, scedosporium apiospermum and mycobacterium tuberculosis in a renal transplant recipient," *BMC Infectious Diseases*, vol. 14, article 259, 2014.

[40] K. Uno, K. Kasahara, S. Kutsuna et al., "Infective endocarditis and meningitis due to *Scedosporium prolificans* in a renal transplant recipient," *Journal of Infection and Chemotherapy*, vol. 20, no. 2, pp. 131–133, 2014.

[41] M. E. Clement, E. K. Maziarz, J. N. Schroder, C. B. Patel, and J. R. Perfect, "*Scedosporium apiosermum* infection of the 'Native' valve: fungal endocarditis in an orthotopic heart transplant recipient," *Medical Mycology Case Reports*, vol. 9, pp. 34–36, 2015.

[42] A. Sharma and D. Singh, "*Scedosporium apiospermum* causing brain abscess in a renal allograft recipient," *Saudi Journal of Kidney Diseases and Transplantation*, vol. 26, no. 6, pp. 1253–1256, 2015.

[43] Deceased Donors Recovered in the U.S. by Mechanism of Death: Transplant Data 1988–2015, Department of Health and Human Services, Health Resources and Services Administration, Healthcare Systems Bureau, Division of Transplantation, Rockville, MD; United Network for Organ Sharing, Richmond, VA; University Renal Research and Education Association, Ann Arbor, MI.

[44] C. Goldman, M. J. Akiyama, J. Torres, E. Louie, and S. A. Meehan, "Scedosporium apiospermum infections and the role of combination antifungal therapy and GM-CSF: a case report and review of the literature," *Medical Mycology Case Reports*, vol. 11, pp. 40–43, 2016.

[45] M. J. Abzug and T. J. Walsh, "Interferon-γ and colony-stimulating factors as adjuvant therapy for refractory fungal infections in children," *Pediatric Infectious Disease Journal*, vol. 23, no. 8, pp. 769–773, 2004.

19

Yersinia enterocolitica Infection Simulating Lymphoproliferative Disease, after Liver Transplant

E. Jakobovich,[1] B. Koplewitz,[2] E. Marva,[3] and E. Granot[1,4]

[1] *Kaplan Medical Center, Rehovot, Israel*
[2] *Department of Medical Imaging, Hadassah Hebrew University Medical Center, Jerusalem, Israel*
[3] *Central Laboratory, Ministry of Health, Jerusalem, Israel*
[4] *Hebrew University, Hadassah Medical School, Jerusalem, Israel*

Correspondence should be addressed to E. Jakobovich; einatjmd@gmail.com

Academic Editor: Piero Boraschi

We describe a 14-year-old girl, who was 13 y after liver transplantation for biliary atresia with an unremarkable postoperative course. She presented with fever of up to 40°C, extreme fatigue, malaise, anorexia, and occasional vomiting. On physical examination the only finding was splenomegaly. Lab results showed hyperglobulinemia and an elevated sedimentation rate. Liver function tests were normal except for mild elevation of γGTP. Abdominal U/S and CT demonstrated an enlarged spleen with retroperitoneal and mesenteric lymph nodes enlargement. An exhaustive evaluation for infectious causes, autoimmune conditions, and malignancy was negative. A full recovery after 5 months prompted testing for self-limited infectious etiologies. *Yersinia enterocolitica* infection was diagnosed.

1. Introduction

In an immune suppressed host, prolonged fever in association with splenomegaly as the sole abnormal finding on physical exam may pose a difficult diagnostic challenge.

Late complications of post liver transplantation include chronic rejection, infections, autoimmune disorders, and malignancy [1]. All these can present with prolonged fever as their major symptom.

Of the infectious causes which have been described, including bacteria, viruses, fungi, and parasitic infection comprehensive reviews in immune suppressed posttransplant patients fail to include *Y. enterocolitica* among these diverse infectious etiologies [2].

We report a 14-year-old girl (13 years after liver transplantation) who presented with prolonged fever, extreme fatigue, malaise, and anorexia. On physical exam the only abnormal finding was splenomegaly. Following an extensive evaluation Yersinia infection was diagnosed.

2. Case Report

A 14-year-old girl, 13 years after orthotopic liver transplantation for biliary atresia, with an unremarkable posttransplant course, on maintenance immunosuppression with tacrolimus, presented with daily fever of up to 40°C, extreme fatigue, and malaise during the preceding 3 weeks. She complained of loss of appetite and occasional vomiting, without diarrhea, abdominal pain, or arthralgia.

Physical exam was unremarkable except for an enlarged spleen (4 cm below the costal margin).

Laboratory results at that time included WBC 12,000 k/ul with a neutrophil count of 84%, hemoglobin 10.7 g% with normal indices, and platelets 298,000 k/ul, as well as ESR 53 mm/h and CRP 16 mg/L ($N \leq 0.6$) which increased over a period of 3 weeks to 151 and 127, respectively.

Transaminases (GOT and GPT) were normal with minimal elevation of γGTP to 60–80 IU/mL (normal < 45 IU/mL). Bilirubin was normal, total protein 8.9 g%, and albumin 3.5 g%.

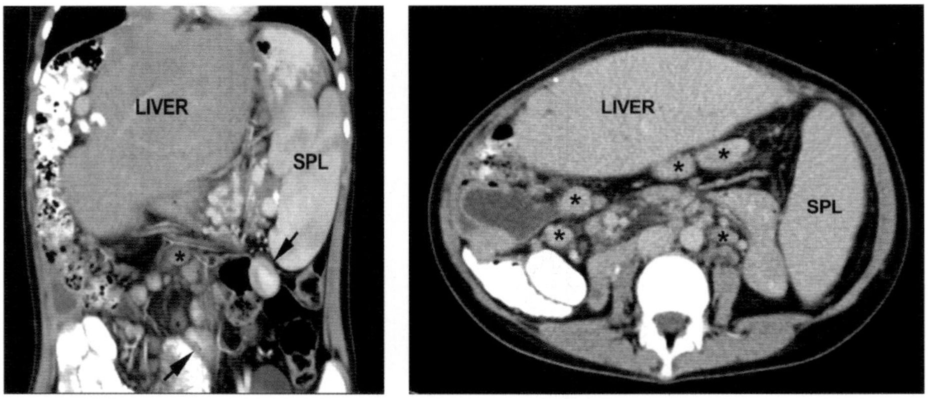

(a) (b)

FIGURE 1: Axial (a) and coronal reformats of contrast-enhanced abdominal CT showing marked enlargement of the spleen and transplanted liver, multiple moderately enlarged mesenteric and gastrohepatic ligament lymph nodes (∗), and focal small bowel wall thickening (arrows).

Blood and urine cultures were negative; stool was negative for culture, parasites, and occult blood.

Serology was negative for EBV (EBV-PCR 184 copies/mL), CMV, parvovirus, Q fever, cat scratch, *Legionella*, and *Brucella*. Autoimmune markers including ANA, antismooth muscle antibody, and anti-LKM were negative.

Chest radiograph was normal; abdominal sonography demonstrated enlarged retroperitoneal and mesenteric lymph nodes (up to 1.8 cm) with an enlarged inhomogeneous spleen.

On abdominal CT the enlarged lymph nodes were observed in the retroperitoneum and mesentery but none were easily accessible for needle biopsy (Figure 1).

PET-CT (FDG) (Figure 2) showed no increased pathological activity in any of the lymph nodes and therefore no further attempt was made, at that time, to surgically remove a lymph node.

The PET-CT demonstrated diffuse increased pathological uptake in bone marrow of sternum, vertebral bodies, and pelvic bones.

Following this finding a bone marrow aspiration and biopsy were performed. The aspirate was sent for cultures and staining for *Leishmania* Donovan bodies.

The bone marrow histology was normal with normal representation of all cell lines. No pathological cells were observed and bone marrow culture and staining for *Leishmania* Donovan bodies were negative.

Over the following two months her fever gradually decreased but she continued to suffer from intermittent elevations of fever up to 38.5°C. Complaints of severe fatigue and anorexia persisted. A repeat abdominal sonography showed persistent splenomegaly and a slight decrease in lymph node size.

Over the next 3 months symptoms gradually continued to resolve, the spleen was no longer palpable, and laboratory results including ESR, CRP, hyperglobulinemia, and γGTP levels gradually returned to normal.

An abdominal sonographic examination five months after initial onset of symptoms was normal with complete resolution of lymphadenopathy and splenomegaly.

Clinical recovery prompted a further attempt at a diagnostic search for an infectious, self-limiting etiology.

Serology was again sent for a multitude of infectious causes. This time testing also included *Y. enterocolitica* serology.

Y. enterocolitica serology was found to be positive. Antibodies of the IgG class against purified virulence factors from *Y. Enterocolitica* strain 0 : 3. (ELISA kit El 2173, Euroimmun AG) were elevated. On a blood sample obtained one month later, the antibody titer had increased twofold.

3. Discussion

In immune competent hosts, *Y. enterocolitica* may cause illness ranging from self-limited enteritis to infrequent life threatening infections [3]. It appears to be a common cause of diarrhea among children in Europe and Canada and has been recognized as an important seasonal gastroenteritis in certain cities in the United States. It is an infrequent infection in warm climates and is therefore rarely encountered in Israel.

In young children it usually presents as an acute diarrheal illness whereas in older children and adolescents the classic clinical presentation is that of a terminal ileitis with mesenteric lymphadenitis (pseudoappendicitis) which resolves over a 1-2-week period [4]. Septicemia caused by *Y. enterocolitica* has been rarely reported in children.

Yersinia enterocolitica is not commonly included in the differential diagnosis of infectious complications after liver transplantation.

In immunocompromised patients it can present as necrotizing pneumonia [5], sepsis [6], endocarditis [7], osteomyelitis [8], and bacteremia [9]. These infectious episodes are rare and are reported as isolated case reports.

Our patient had no gastrointestinal symptoms except for occasional vomiting. In retrospect the small bowel wall thickening, noted on abdominal CT coupled with the mesenteric lymphadenopathy were valuable clues to the diagnosis.

At the time of presentation the most likely diagnosis in our patient was posttransplant lymphoproliferative disorder, despite absence of evidence of EBV infection (EBV-PCR

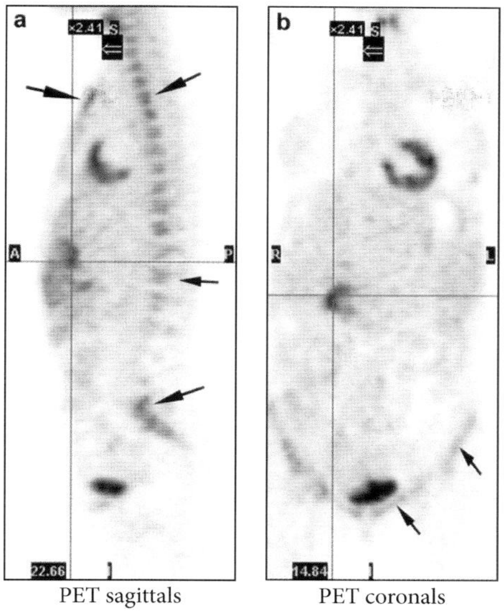

(a) (b)

Figure 2: PET-CT (FDG) diffuse increased uptake (arrows) in bone marrow of the sternum and vertebral bodies (a) as well as pelvic bones (b). No pathological uptake in lymph nodes or spleen.

negative). The enlarged abdominal lymph nodes which were not accessible for needle biopsy were not surgically removed as they showed no pathological uptake on PET-CT and were therefore not likely to represent lymphoma.

We have found one report describing a similar clinical presentation of *Yersinia enterocolitica*. The patient was a 50-year-old woman who similarly to our patient also had prolonged fever, splenomegaly, and retroperitoneal lymph nodes. The diagnosis of *Y. enterocolitica* infection was also established only after symptoms had resolved. It is noteworthy that the patient reported was not immune suppressed [10].

Although lymphoproliferative disease remains the primary etiology in the differential diagnosis of a patient with prior liver transplantation and recent onset of prolonged fever, splenomegaly, abdominal lymphadenopathy and hyperglobulinemia, unusual infectious etiologies should also be considered. As exemplified by our patient *Y. enterocolitica* infection can simulate posttransplant lymphoproliferative disease.

References

[1] J. C. Bucuvalas and F. C. Ryckman, "Long-term outcome after liver transplantation in children," *Pediatric Transplantation*, vol. 6, no. 1, pp. 30–36, 2002.

[2] H. Lee and J. P. Vacanti, "Liver transplantation and its long-term management in children," *Pediatric Clinics of North America*, vol. 43, no. 1, pp. 99–124, 1996.

[3] N. M. Abdel-Haq, B. I. Asmar, W. M. Abuhammour, and W. J. Brown, "Yersinia enterocolitica infection in children," *Pediatric Infectious Disease Journal*, vol. 19, no. 10, pp. 954–958, 2000.

[4] J. R. Murphy and G. P. Heresi, "Yersinia," in *NELSON Textbook of Pediatrics*, section 16, chapter 186, pp. 1202–1204, 18th edition, 2007.

[5] J. N. Greene, P. Herndon, J. P. Nadler, and R. L. Sandin, "Case report: yersinia enterocolitica necrotizing pneumonia in an immunocompromised patient," *American Journal of the Medical Sciences*, vol. 305, no. 3, pp. 171–173, 1993.

[6] J. Jouquan, D. Mottier, Y. Pennec et al., "Yersinia enterocolitica septicemia acquired within a hospital. Report of a case with septic shock in an immunocompromised patient," *Semaine des Hopitaux*, vol. 60, no. 1, pp. 47–48, 1984.

[7] G. Karachalios, G. Bablekos, G. Karachaliou, A. K. Charalabopoulos, and K. Charalabopoulos, "Infectious endocarditis due to Yersinia enterocolitica," *Chemotherapy*, vol. 48, no. 3, pp. 158–159, 2002.

[8] J. T. Sinnott 4th., H. Multhoop, J. Leo, and G. Rechtine, "Yersinia enterocolitica causing spinal osteomyelitis and empyema in nonimmunocompromised host," *Southern Medical Journal*, vol. 82, pp. 399–400, 1989.

[9] X. Nicolas, R. Le Berre, S. Ansart et al., "Bacteremia and pneumonia due to Yersinia enterocolitica serotype O:3 in an immunocompetent patient," *Medecine et Maladies Infectieuses*, vol. 35, no. 6, pp. 370–373, 2005.

[10] G. Trommer, A. Bewer, and S. Kösling, "Mesenteric lymphadenopathy in patient with Yersinia enterocolitica infection: a differential diagnosis to abdominal lymphoma," *Radiologe*, vol. 38, no. 1, pp. 37–40, 1998.

20

Cardiac Failure after Liver Transplantation Requiring a Biventricular Assist Device

Rita Jermyn,[1] Eiei Soe,[2] David D'Alessandro,[3] Julia Shin,[1] William Jakobleff,[3] Daniel Schwartz,[4] Milan Kinkhabwala,[2] and Paul J. Gaglio[2]

[1] *Division of Heart Failure, Department of Cardiology, Montefiore Medical Center, Albert Einstein College of Medicine, Bronx, NY, USA*
[2] *Division of Hepatology, Department of Gastroenterology, Montefiore Medical Center, Albert Einstein College of Medicine, Bronx, NY, USA*
[3] *Department of Cardiothoracic Surgery, Montefiore Medical Center, Albert Einstein College of Medicine, Bronx, NY, USA*
[4] *Department of Pathology, Montefiore Medical Center, USA*

Correspondence should be addressed to Rita Jermyn; rjermyn@montefiore.org

Academic Editor: Frieder Keller

Increased hepatic iron load in extrahepatic organs of cirrhotic patients with and without hereditary hemochromatosis portends a poorer long term prognosis after liver transplant. Hepatic as well as nonhepatic iron overload is associated with increased infectious and postoperative complications, including cardiac dysfunction. In this case report, we describe a cirrhotic patient with alpha 1 antitrypsin deficiency and nonhereditary hemochromatosis (non-HFE) that developed cardiogenic shock requiring mechanical circulatory support for twenty days after liver transplant. Upon further investigation, she was found to have significant iron deposition in both the liver and heart biopsies. Her heart regained complete and sustained recovery following ten days of mechanical biventricular support. This case highlights the importance of preoperatively recognizing extrahepatic iron deposition in patients referred for liver transplantation irrespective of etiology of liver disease as this may prevent postoperative complications.

1. Introduction

Patients with the heterozygous gene mutation for HFE or human hemochromatosis protein may demonstrate extrahepatic iron overload leading to organ impairment, particularly when associated with additional etiologies of chronic liver disease [1]. It has been observed that steatohepatitis and viral hepatitis may also contribute to abnormalities in control of iron homeostasis [1]. As an example, iron accumulation in extrahepatic sites such as the heart has been described in a series of patients with non-HFE associated iron overload [2]. This phenomenon has been associated with fatal cardiovascular complications after liver transplant [3]. Further exacerbating the complexity of extrahepatic iron overload is the potential for increased predisposition to infection with diminished cardiac output in the setting of stress or sepsis [1]. We report a patient with non-HFE hemochromatosis who developed profound heart failure after liver transplantation; this represents the first described case of cardiac iron deposition contributing to prolonged cardiogenic shock requiring mechanical circulatory support with eventual complete and sustained biventricular recovery.

2. Case Report

The patient is a 46-year-old Caucasian female with a history of non-HFE hemochromatosis, alpha 1 antitrypsin deficiency, and cavernous transformation of the portal vein, who presented to our institution for orthotopic liver transplantation. Pretransplant liver biopsy was not performed due to the patient's severe portal hypertension and risk of bleeding. Gene testing revealed she was compound heterozygous for the HFE gene (C282Y-H63D) with a low alpha 1 antitrypsin level, and Hepatitis B DNA and Hepatitis C RNA were negative. Serum iron was 104 mg/dL (normal

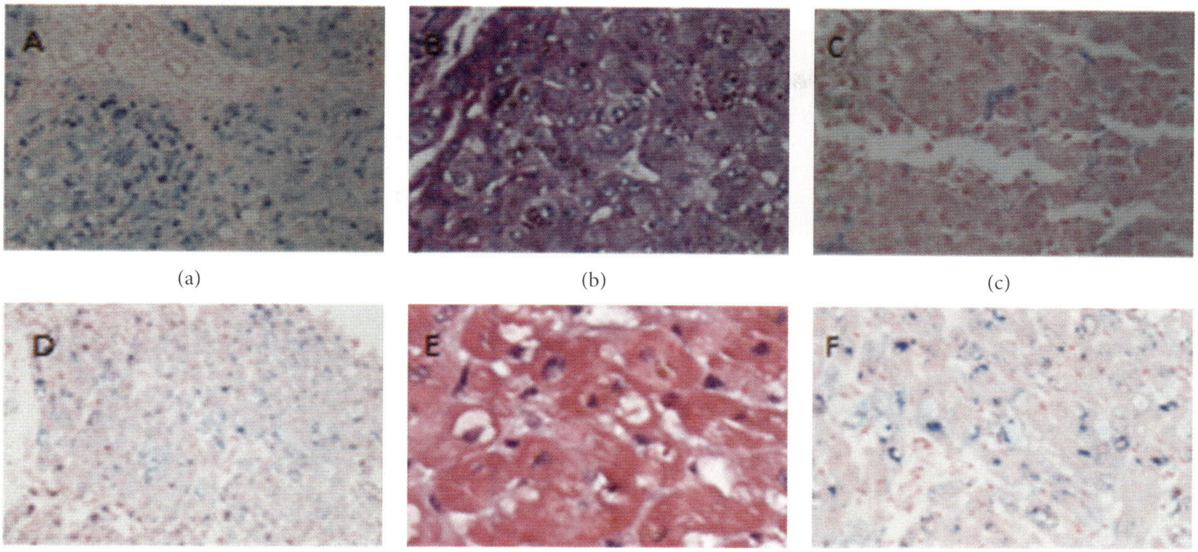

(a) (b) (c)

(d) (e) (f)

FIGURE 1: (a) Prussian-Blue stain showing iron granules in hepatocytes and bile duct epithelium in the explanted liver. (b) PAS-Diastase stain showing alpha 1 antitrypsin globules in periportal hepatocytes in the explanted liver. (c) Prussian-Blue stain showing iron granules in Kuppfer cells in the transplanted liver. (d) Prussian-Blue stain with extensive cytoplasmic iron in cardiac myocytes. (e) Hematoxylin and Eosin stain with intracytoplasmic hemosiderin in myocytes. (f) Prussian-Blue stain high power view of cytoplasmic iron in cardiac myocytes.

range 55–155 mg/dL), transferrin was 136 mg/dL, ferritin was 1240 ng/mL, and percent iron saturation was 61% (normal range 15–50%). She underwent uncomplicated orthotopic liver transplantation; however 72 hours postoperatively she developed multidrug resistant *E. coli* and MRSA peritonitis. Her blood cultures remained negative. Liver explant showed 3+ iron predominantly within hepatocytes and occasional Kupffer cells with intracytoplasmic alpha-1 antitrypsin globules on periodic acid-Schiff staining, indicative of both iron overload and alpha 1 antitrypsin deficiency (Figure 1). Approximately 72 hours postoperatively, she developed hypotension required reintubation and vasopressor support. An echocardiogram revealed severe, nondilated biventricular failure with an ejection fraction of 10 percent. Prior cardiac workup included a dobutamine stress echocardiogram done six months prior to liver transplantation which showed no ischemia, normal ventricular anatomy, and a normal ejection fraction. The patient also had a transthoracic echocardiogram done two months preoperatively to assess portopulmonary hypertension after she was admitted for volume overload and dyspnea. This revealed a normal pulmonary artery pressure; however, her ejection fraction was moderately diminished globally to 45% percent. Additional cardiac assessment following transplantation revealed that the patient had a peak Troponin T of 0.15 ug/L, CPK 108 IU/L, and her EKG did not reveal any ST segment abnormalities or q waves. Serum ferritin was increased to 5800 ng/mL.

Following intubation and the initiation of vasopressor support, the patient continued to deteriorate with multiorgan failure, with continued depression of her cardiac function with an EF of ten percent. The patient was started on venoarterial ECMO support, and repeat echocardiogram revealed significant mitral regurgitation with poor LV unloading. After ten days of VA ECMO support, the patient did not appear to have any myocardial recovery on transthoracic echo. She was taken back to the operating room for temporary biventricular support. Cannulas were placed from right ventricular to pulmonary artery and left ventricle to the aorta. This device supports the right and left ventricles with a centrifugal pump that is magnetically levitated to reduce afterload of the failing left ventricle and provide preload from the failing right ventricle. The ECMO circuit was decannulated and the left ventricular apex was excised and sent for pathology. Pathology revealed abundant cytoplasmic iron demonstrated as hemosiderin. Biventricular support was continued for an additional seven days. On post-op day twenty-six her bedside transthoracic echocardiogram showed a dramatic improvement in left ventricular ejection fraction and EF of forty-five percent. The patient returned to the operating room for decannulation of her bivad where intraoperative TEE revealed only mildly reduced left ventricular and right ventricular ejection. After explantation of the bivad, the patient remained hemodynamically stable and a bedside transthoracic echocardiogram one week later revealed an ejection fraction of 55% with mild apical akinesis and normal right ventricular function. She is currently forty-five days post-op from orthotopic liver transplant and her cardiac functions remain normal (Figure 2).

3. Discussion

The cause of cardiogenic shock in this patient five days after orthotopic liver transplant appeared to be related to

Transplant shock	VA ECMO	BIVAD	EF 45%	EF 55%
72 hours	10 days	7 days	26 days	45 days

Figure 2: Timeline.

several contributing factors, potentially due to extrahepatic iron deposition and myocardial stunning from septic shock. This case demonstrates successful biventricular recovery after ECMO and bivad mechanical circulatory support. When analyzing the phenomenon of cardiogenic shock in this patient, the etiology and pattern were unclear. Typically, sepsis induced cardiomyopathy produces reversibility within seven to ten days and the typical pattern of remodeling on echocardiogram is that of anterior wall akinesis [4]. Our patient's cardiac recovery took significantly longer. In addition, we do not believe that the patient had significant intrinsic cardiac dysfunction preoperatively as pretransplantation dobutamine stress echocardiogram did not reveal any significant abnormalities, although on reanalysis her immediate preoperative echocardiogram began to display a slight decrease in left ventricular ejection fraction, potentially due to iron overload.

Iron overload has been classified as primary as in hereditary hemochromatosis or secondary due to chronic transfusion therapy and ineffective erythropoiesis. After identification of the human hemochromatosis protein (HFE) in 1996, it was noted that only a minority of patients were homozygous for the C282Y mutation, indicative of hereditary hemochromatosis [5]. However, it has been observed that patients with a heterozygous HFE gene mutation may also experience hepatic iron overload, particularly in the setting of other etiologies of liver disease. A number of theories have been proposed to explain enhanced iron deposition in this setting including increased absorption of iron because of ineffective erythropoiesis, hemolysis, and currently unrecognized mutations affecting iron metabolism. Intrahepatic portosystemic shunts have also been shown to result in hepatic iron overload [6]. Often alcoholic liver disease or chronic hepatitis C can be associated with hepatic iron overload. This is thought to be related to decreased hepcidin expression [7]. It has also been observed that individuals who display compound heterozygosity for the HFE gene mutation (C282Y/H63D) may develop hepatic as well as extrahepatic iron overload, the mechanism potentially related to additional gene mutations such as S65C mutation [8]. Any mutation in HFE causes increased transferrin which the intestines misinterpret as iron deficiency resulting in further increase in absorption of iron. The HFE gene also affects production of hepcidin in the liver which can further exacerbate inappropriate iron loading [8].

Iron overload may portend a poor prognosis following liver transplantation. Several studies have shown the 1- as well as 5-year survival after liver transplant is lower than expected in patients with severe iron overload when compared to patients without iron overload [9]. It has been hypothesized that iron deposition compromises the function of other organs such as the heart, pancreas, and brain. In addition, iron overload may predispose the patient to an increased risk of infection which is clearly problematic in an already immunocompromised host [9]. The pathophysiology of iron associated cardiac dysfunction has been well documented; by free radical mediated pathways, labile iron exceeds cellular antioxidant mechanisms and peroxidation of membrane lipids, cellular protein, and nucleic acids occurs [10]. Persistent free radicals affect the sarcoplasmic reticulum and mitochondria leading to calcium leakage into the cytoplasm [10]. Iron deposition in the heart first occurs in the ventricular followed by atrial myocardium. Increased ferrous iron transport through the L-type calcium channels of the heart results in impaired excitation-contraction coupling which may cause the systolic dysfunction appreciated in iron overload patients [9].

We hypothesize that our patient was already displaying subtle signs of cardiac dysfunction due to iron deposition preoperatively as she displayed mildly decreased left ventricular function on transthoracic echocardiogram. The most common cardiac manifestations associated with hereditary hemochromatosis are dilated cardiomyopathies and ventricular arrhythmias [9]. However, our patient was unusual in that, postoperatively, she displayed nondilated biventricular failure and was genotype negative for the homozygous HFE gene. Perhaps as a result of the already compromised myocardial function preoperatively due to iron, the patient was at greater risk of decompensation in the setting of sepsis induced myocardial stunning. This phenomenon of depressed myocardial function due to sepsis was first described by Maeder and Hunziker in 2009 [11]. A transiently decreased left ventricular ejection fraction with preserved stroke volume was often described in these patients with the average duration of abnormal function lasting four days and rebounding to normal by seven days. Patients with profound unremitting shock requiring mechanical circulatory support for twenty days exclusively due to sepsis are an extreme rarely reported condition [11]. Another potential factor in our patient to consider would be the physiologic circulatory state in some patients with portal hypertension, described as "cirrhotic cardiomyopathy" [12]. This phenomenon is most commonly but not exclusively seen in patients with alcoholic cirrhosis, characterized by elevated filling pressure, ventricular arrhythmias, and eventually systolic dysfunction. Diastolic dysfunction may be present in up to 25% of these patients after liver transplantation [12]. Given the frequency of preexisting cardiac disease and potential perioperative complications in cirrhotic patients, all patients considered for liver transplant undergo at minimum a noninvasive cardiac workup [12]. Our patient had no evidence of ischemia on dobutamine stress echo or elevated pulmonary pressure six months prior to transplant and thus cirrhotic cardiomyopathy was unlikely.

Therapy of cardiac iron overload has been previously described. For patients with acquired cardiac siderosis and systolic dysfunction, most frequently occurring in patients requiring chronic transfusions, there is literature showing there may be an improvement in ejection fraction with oral iron chelators. However, this was mostly reported in case reports and included both oral and intravenous chelation therapy in addition to typical heart failure medications for a minimum of 12 months [13].

This case was unusual for several reasons; it was remarkable that the patient was able to maintain a normal ejection fraction intra- and immediately postoperatively despite the dramatic circulatory changes that occur during and after liver transplantation. When the patient developed sepsis postoperatively, she developed profound biventricular failure, with eventual recovery using a combination of ECMO and biventricular mechanical support. This experience highlights the importance of recognizing hepatic iron deposition preoperatively as a risk factor for extrahepatic iron accumulation in end stage cirrhotic patients awaiting transplant. Iron deposition can enhance the risk of infection in immunocompromised patients and may lead to severe cardiac complications postoperatively. The role of preoperative chelation in patients with non-HFE associated iron overload needs to be explored.

Abbreviations

Non-HFE: Nonhereditary hemochromatosis
HFE: Human hemochromatosis protein
VA ECMO: Venoarterial extracorporeal membrane oxygenation
BIVAD: Biventricular Assist Device.

References

[1] S. J. Cotler, M. P. Bronner, R. D. Press et al., "End-stage liver disease without hemochromatosis associated with elevated hepatic iron index," *Journal of Hepatology*, vol. 29, no. 2, pp. 257–262, 1998.

[2] S. C. Eng, S. L. Taylor, V. Reyes, S. Raaka, J. Berger, and K. V. Kowdley, "Hepatic iron overload in alcoholic end-stage liver disease is associated with iron deposition in other organs in the absence of HFE-1 hemochromatosis," *Liver International*, vol. 25, no. 3, pp. 513–517, 2005.

[3] A. Y. O'Glasser, D. L. Scott, C. L. Corless et al., "Hepatic and cardiac iron overload among patients with end-stage liver disease referred for liver transplantation," *Clinical Transplantation*, vol. 24, no. 5, pp. 643–651, 2010.

[4] O. Court, A. Kumar, and J. E. Parrillo, "Clinical review: myocardial depression in sepsis and septic shock," *Critical Care*, vol. 6, no. 6, pp. 500–508, 2002.

[5] K. Kowdley, B. Tung, S. Han et al., "Prevalence of hepatic iron overload and HFE mutations among orthotopic liver transplant recipients; preliminary results from the National Hemochromatosis Transplant Registry," AASLD, 2001.

[6] D. J. Brandhagen, W. Alvarez, T. M. Therneau et al., "Iron overload in cirrhosis—HFE genotypes and outcome after liver transplantation," *Hepatology*, vol. 31, no. 2, pp. 456–460, 2000.

[7] J. Ludwig, E. Hashimoto, M. K. Porayko, T. P. Moyer, and W. P. Baldus, "Hemosiderosis in cirrhosis: a study of 447 native livers," *Gastroenterology*, vol. 112, no. 3, pp. 882–888, 1997.

[8] M. Vujić Spasić, J. Kiss, T. Herrmann et al., "HFE acts in hepatocytes to prevent hemochromatosis," *Cell Metabolism*, vol. 7, no. 2, pp. 173–178, 2008.

[9] B. Y. Tung, F. J. Farrell, T. M. McCashland et al., "Long-term follow-up after liver transplantation in patients with hepatic iron overload," *Liver Transplantation and Surgery*, vol. 5, no. 5, pp. 369–374, 1999.

[10] D. Kremastinos and D. Farmakis, "Iron overload cardiomyopathy in clinical practice," *Circulation*, vol. 124, no. 20, pp. 2253–2263, 2011.

[11] M. T. Maeder and P. Hunziker, "Sepsis-associated myocardial dysfunction: from bedside to bench," *Journal of Organ Dysfunction*, vol. 5, no. 2, pp. 79–90, 2009.

[12] P. J. Gaglio Jr. and P. J. Gaglio Sr., "Complications in patients with alcohol-associated liver disease who undergo liver transplantation," *Clinics in Liver Disease*, vol. 16, no. 4, pp. 865–875, 2012.

[13] R. Origa, P. Bina, A. Agus et al., "Combined therapy with deferiprone and desferrioxamine in thalassemia major," *Haematologica*, vol. 90, no. 10, pp. 1309–1314, 2005.

21

Urgent Splenectomy after Partial Splenic Embolization in Liver-Transplanted Patient

Jorge Herrador Benito,[1] M. G. Zunzarren,[1] T. Pozancos de Simón,[1] L. Tortolero,[1] R. Latorre Fragua,[1] J. Nuño,[2] and E. Lobo[1]

[1] *Department of General and Digestive Surgery, Ramón y Cajal Hospital, Cra. Colmenar Km 9, 1, 28034 Madrid, Spain*
[2] *Liver Transplantation Unit, Department of General and Digestive Surgery, Ramón y Cajal Hospital, Cra. Colmenar Km 9, 1, 28034 Madrid, Spain*

Correspondence should be addressed to Jorge Herrador Benito, jorge.herrador@gmail.com

Academic Editors: C. F. Classen, C. Costa, and J. Jazbec

We describe a 51-year-old-male. Three months after liver transplantation due to hepatitis C virus (HCV) hepatopathy, an HCV relapse was detected, and partial splenic embolization (PSE) was performed prior to antiviral treatment. Eleven days after PSE emergency splenectomy was performed due to the development of a splenic abscess, which is a rare but severe complication of PSE. Between May 2002 and March 2012, 18 PSEs have been performed in transplant patients in our centre. The patient presented here is the only case of splenic abscess and the only one who has needed surgery after complications of PSE.

1. Introduction

Approximately 20–30% of patients who receive a liver transplant due to hepatitis c virus hepatopathy develop cirrhosis before 5 years, and up to 14% experience a serious relapse in the first year after transplantation [1–3]. Hypersplenism in these patients results in decreased platelet levels, which does not allow treatment with pegylated interferon (Peg-IFN) and ribavirin because these drugs are associated with hematological toxicity, especially thrombocytopenia in the case of Peg-IFN. Partial splenic embolization (PSE) is an effective alternative to splenectomy in these patients to correct platelet levels if antiviral treatment is necessary [4–7].

2. Case Report

We describe a 51-year-old male who received a liver transplant secondary to HCV liver cirrhosis. Immunosuppression received was Tacrolimus 6 mg/12 h and Methylprednisolone 20 mg. During the postoperative period the patient presented with right pleural effusion, mild renal failure, and mild preservation injury with minimal graft dysfunction compatible with preservation cholestasis.

Three months after liver transplantation a serious HCV relapse was detected by the presence of serious lobular hepatitis in a liver biopsy, with a total bilirubin of 6 mg/dL, HCV viral load of 100,000,000 UI/mL, and hyperglycemia associated with the relapse. Platelet levels were 44,600 cells/mm^3 (see Table 1).

To correct the blood platelet levels prior to antiviral treatment, splenic embolization was performed for approximately 90% of the parenchyma, preserving only a central hilar area and another area in the upper pole (see Figure 1). The technique was distal superselective catheterization of the splenic artery through the femoral artery with the injection of particles of polyvinyl alcohol in solution with penicillin, gentamicin, and iodinated contrast. The patient was discharged 6 days after embolization, after a period of time without complications.

Three days later, the patient arrived at the emergency department with a fever of 38.5°C and diffuse abdominal pain, primarily in the left upper quadrant. An urgent CT scan showed free fluid in the pelvis and paracolic gutters,

Table 1: The evolution of blood platelet levels.

	Platelets (cells/mm^3)
Prembolization levels (70 days post-transplant)	44,600
Postembolization levels (15 days post-PSE)	318,000
Postsplenectomy (38 days after splenectomy)	466,000

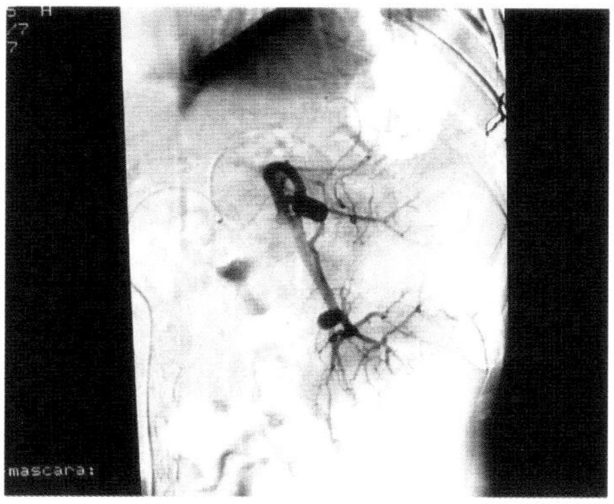

Figure 1: Splenic arteriography.

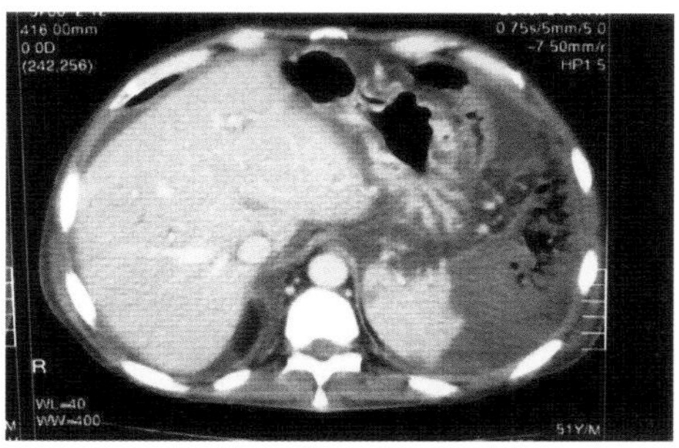

Figure 2: CT scan.

with uptake of contrast medium in the peritoneum. The spleen was enlarged with gas bubbles compatible with the embolization.

We decided to initiate empiric antibiotic and antimycotic treatment (meropenem, tobramycin, and fluconazole). Over the following days, the clinical course included torpidity, development of renal failure, leukocytosis above 30,000, and persisting malaise with abdominal pain and fever. At all times the patient was hemodynamically stable with no need for vasoactive drugs and without respiratory support. *Bacteroides fragilis* was isolated in blood culture. Eleven days after admission, a new CT scan showed multiple splenic collections of gas compatible with a splenic abscess secondary to the PSE. In addition, adjacent hemoperitoneum was observed, and the splenic capsule was ruptured (Figure 2).

Emergency surgery found roughly 3.5 liters of reddish-brown peritoneal fluid. Splenectomy was performed and blood products transfused. After 3 days in the ICU, the patient required a prolonged stay and was discharged at postoperative day 40. Regarding the evolution of graft function from the time of embolization, the analytical figures were gradually normalized, reaching the following levels: AST = 43, ALT = 16, FA = 202, and GGT = 296.

3. Discussion

The morbidity of PSE is well known. Almost 100% of patients develop the so-called "postembolization syndrome" (fever, abdominal pain, nausea) caused by splenic infarction and the release of proinflammatory cytokines. Other "minor" complications were pleural effusion, the development of neutrophilic ascites, which is usually transient and responsive to diuretic therapy, and splenic or portal thrombosis. The most serious complications are the development of splenic abscess and distal pancreatitis. Splenic abscess formation is not a infrequent and severe complication of PSE that occurs in 5–15% of PSE. Like other complications, abscess formation is related to the volume of parenchyma that is embolized, occurring with volumes greater than 70%. The treatment of choice is urgent splenectomy; though medical treatment support, antibiotics, and occasional percutaneous drainage can be attempted in patients with major functional impairment, it often provides worse results [8–10].

Between May 2002 and March 2012, 74 PSEs have been performed in our centre, including 18 procedures in transplant patients. The patient presented here is the only case of splenic abscess, and the only one who has required surgery after complications of PSE, assuming 1.4% for total PSE and 5.6% among transplant patients.

References

[1] R. Bárcena, A. Moreno, J. R. Foruny et al., "Partial splenic embolization and peg-IFN plus RBV in liver transplanted patients with hepatitis C recurrence: safety, efficacy and long-term outcome," *Clinical Transplantation*, vol. 24, no. 3, pp. 366–374, 2010.

[2] E. Otón, R. Bárcena, J. M. Moreno-Planas et al., "Hepatitis C recurrence after liver transplantation: viral and histologic response to full-dose peg-interferon and ribavirin," *American Journal of Transplantation*, vol. 6, no. 10, pp. 2348–2355, 2006.

[3] I. Fernández, J. C. Meneu, F. Colina et al., "Clinical and histological efficacy of pegylated interferon and ribavirin therapy of recurrent hepatitis C after liver transplantation," *Liver Transplantation*, vol. 12, no. 12, pp. 1805–1812, 2006.

[4] B. Sangro, I. Bilbao, I. Herrero et al., "Partial splenic embolization for the treatment of hypersplenism in cirrhosis," *Hepatology*, vol. 18, no. 2, pp. 309–314, 1993.

[5] M. A. Amin, M. M. El Gendy, I. E. Dawoud, A. Shoma, A. M. Negm, and T. A. Amer, "Partial splenic embolization versus splenectomy for the management of hypersplenism in cirrhotic patients," *World Journal of Surgery*, vol. 33, no. 8, pp. 1702–1710, 2009.

[6] M. Takahara, Y. Miyake, H. Miyatake et al., "Partial splenic embolization facilitates the adherence to peginterferon in chronic hepatitis C with thrombocytopenia," *Internal Medicine*, vol. 50, no. 22, pp. 2731–2736, 2011.

[7] N. Sohara, H. Takagi, S. Kakizaki, K. Sato, and M. Mori, "The use of partial splenic artery embolization made it possible to administer interferon and ribavirin therapy in a liver transplant patient with fibrosing cholestatic hepatitis C complicated with thrombocytopenia," *Transplant International*, vol. 19, no. 3, pp. 255–257, 2006.

[8] H. Yoshida, Y. Mamada, N. Taniai, and T. Tajiri, "Partial splenic embolization," *Hepatology Research*, vol. 38, no. 3, pp. 225–233, 2008.

[9] J. R. Foruny, R. Bárcena, A. Moreno et al., "Benefit of pegylated interferon-α-2a/ribavirin in a patient with common variable immunodeficiency and hepatitis C virus cirrhosis after liver transplantation and splenic embolization," *Transplantation*, vol. 82, no. 2, pp. 289–290, 2006.

[10] A. Petermann, P. Chabrot, L. Cassagnes et al., "Hypersplenism due to portal hypertension: retrospective evaluation of 17 patients treated by splenic embolization," *Diagnostic and Interventional Imaging*, vol. 93, no. 1, pp. 30–36, 2012.

22

Cutaneous Metastases from Primary Hepatobiliary Tumors as the First Sign of Tumor Recurrence following Liver Transplantation

Adam T. Hauch,[1] Joseph F. Buell,[1] Margit McGowan,[2] Parisha Bhatia,[1] Eleanor Lewin,[3] Mary Killackey,[1] Nathan J. Shores,[4] Luis A. Balart,[4] Martin Moehlen,[4] Bob Saggi,[1] and Anil S. Paramesh[1]

[1] *Tulane Transplant Institute, Tulane University School of Medicine, 1415 Tulane Avenue, HC-5, New Orleans, LA 70112, USA*
[2] *Department of Hematology and Oncology, Tulane University School of Medicine, New Orleans, LA 70112, USA*
[3] *Department of Pathology, Tulane University School of Medicine, New Orleans, LA 70112, USA*
[4] *Department of Gastroenterology, Section of Hepatology, Tulane University School of Medicine, New Orleans, LA 70112, USA*

Correspondence should be addressed to Anil S. Paramesh; aparames@tulane.edu

Academic Editor: Piero Boraschi

Cutaneous metastasis from hepatobiliary tumors is a rare event, especially following liver transplantation. We report our experience with two cases of cutaneous metastases from both hepatocellular carcinoma and mixed hepatocellular/cholangiocarcinoma following liver transplantation, along with a review of the literature.

1. Introduction

Cutaneous metastases from internal malignancies occur in 0.6%–10.4% of cancer patients and represent just 2% of all skin tumors [1, 2]. They often present with variable clinical appearance, which may result in a delay and failure in making their diagnosis, impacting morbidity, prognosis, and treatment [2]. Furthermore, they may represent the first sign of cancer recurrence and hence require a high index of suspicion for making the diagnosis.

Skin metastases from primary hepatobiliary malignancies, such as hepatocellular carcinoma (HCC) or cholangiocarcinoma, are exceedingly rare events described mostly in case reports [3–7]. It is estimated that cutaneous metastasis from HCC represents only 0.2%–2.7% of all cutaneous metastases [8], and metastatic lesions to the skin secondary to cholangiocarcinoma are even more infrequent with less than thirty documented reports in the literature [7].

Although rare, cutaneous metastases may represent the first sign of HCC or cholangiocarcinoma recurrence. To date, there has been only one documented case describing skin metastasis from HCC in a patient who underwent liver transplantation [9]. In this report, we will describe our experience with the diagnosis and management of cutaneous hepatobiliary metastases in two patients following liver transplantation.

2. Case 1

The patient is a 60-year-old Caucasian male who underwent liver transplantation on 1/24/2011 for cirrhosis secondary to Hepatitis C virus (HCV) infection, with a biopsy proven Stage II HCC (3.2 cm single lesion). He underwent chemoembolization prior to transplant. Surgical pathology of the native liver explant demonstrated a residual 2 cm well-differentiated HCC with no lymphovascular invasion and negative margins.

The patient initially had good liver function but developed recurrent HCV liver disease about one year after transplant and was initiated on antiviral therapy with an interferon, ribavirin, and boceprevir protocol. In December 2013 the patient developed several violaceous, painful, firm, immobile skin lesions on his right anterior chest wall,

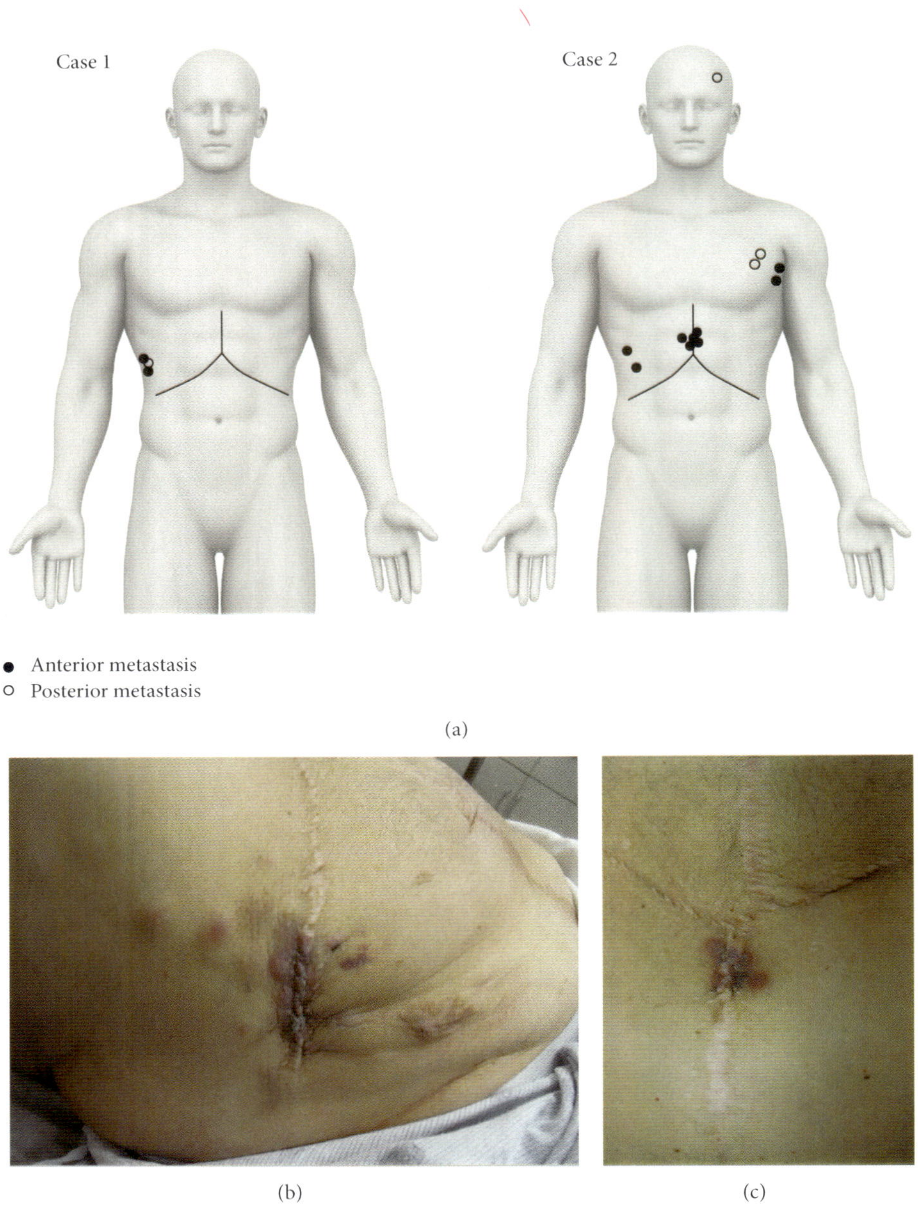

Figure 1: (a) Illustration demonstrating locations of cutaneous metastases for patients of Case 1 and Case 2. (b and c) Multiple erythematous-violaceous metastatic lesions with irregular borders representing mixed HCC/cholangiocarcinoma found at the previous incision site of the patient in Case 2.

several inches from his transplant incision (Figure 1(a)). These lesions were biopsied and demonstrated subcutaneous metastatic well-differentiated HCC (Figure 2(a)). Immunohistochemical staining was positive for HepPar-1 (Figure 2(b)). Interestingly, imaging did not reveal any evidence of intrahepatic or pulmonary HCC recurrence. The patient had undergone a percutaneous biopsy of his HCC pretransplant, but this had been done in October of 2010, more than three years earlier. His alpha-fetoprotein (AFP) levels were never elevated.

With clinically and radiographically localized disease, the patient underwent metastectomy with wide local excision and mesh reconstruction in January 2014. Surgical pathology revealed three nodules, the largest measuring 3.7 cm, with each revealing a moderately differentiated HCC. Lymphovascular invasion was also present. After resection, the patient's immunosuppression was changed from a tacrolimus-based to an everolimus-based regimen, due to its potential antitumor properties, and sorafenib therapy was initiated.

3. Case 2

The second patient is a 55-year-old Caucasian male who underwent orthotopic liver transplantation on 4/7/2012 for HCV-associated cirrhosis and biopsy proven well-differentiated Stage II HCC (4.9 cm single lesion). He underwent chemoembolization of this mass prior to transplant.

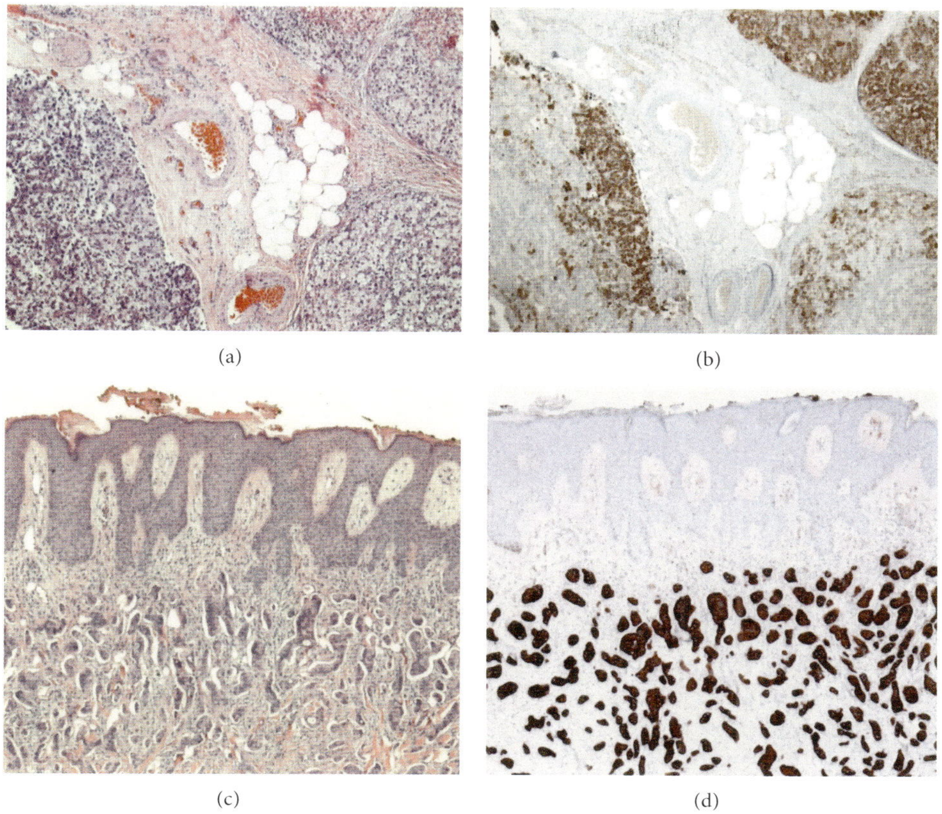

Figure 2: (a) H&E staining of abdominal wall excisional biopsy showing nodules of tumor cells with intervening entrapped soft tissue. Tumor cells demonstrate large variation in size with moderate nuclear pleomorphism; many tumor cells show cytoplasmic clearing. (b) Tumor cells show strong focal cytoplasmic reactivity for HepPar-1 supporting a diagnosis of metastatic HCC. (c) H&E staining of punch biopsy of skin showing tumor cells in the dermis streaming in cords and trabeculae with occasional gland-like formations. Tumor cells are hyperchromatic with increased nuclear-to-cytoplasmic ratio. (d) Tumor cells highlighted by CK7 immunohistochemistry (brown), showing diffuse strong cytoplasmic reactivity. Tumor cells were also positive for EMA and focally positive for mucicarmine; CK20, HepPar-1, CDX-2, and PSA were negative. The immunoprofile (CK7(+), CK20(−), and HepPar-1(−)) supports biliary over hepatic origin but is not definitive.

Posttransplant surgical pathology of the native liver explant revealed a minimal focus (0.5 cm) of residual HCC at the previous chemoembolization site, as well as another 2.5 cm adenocarcinoma in the perihilar region of the liver, which was suggestive by morphologic appearance and immunophenotypic profiling (positive for CK7, CK20, and mCEA) to be consistent with a mixed HCC/cholangiocarcinoma. This tumor demonstrated microscopic lymphatic, vascular, and perineural invasion with bile duct dysplasia. The lesion had not been seen on pretransplant imaging studies or during his hepatic angiogram during chemoembolization. Because of this, he was maintained with a low-dose immunosuppression regimen and closely monitored for recurrence.

In December 2013, eighteen months following transplant, the patient developed numerous painful skin nodules on his abdomen along the lateral and superior aspects of his previous incision site, chest wall, and scalp (Figure 1). A biopsy and histopathologic examination of one of the skin lesions revealed tumor cells which were positive for CK7 and EMA immunostains and which were morphologically compatible with metastatic cholangiocarcinoma/HCC (Figures 2(c) and 2(d)). Again, imaging did not reveal any evidence of intrahepatic tumor recurrence, or any other site of metastasis. His AFP levels remained normal as they had been before transplant, but his CA19-9 level in January 2014 was markedly elevated at 5600 U/mL (not done before transplant).

This patient's immunosuppression was also changed from a tacrolimus- to an everolimus-based regimen. He was treated with palliative electron beam radiation therapy to the skin lesions (250 cGy/d given as 14 fractions to 3500 cGy) and was initiated on a systemic chemotherapy regimen of gemcitabine (1000 mg/m^2 IV on days 1 and 8) and cisplatin (25 mg/m^2 IV on days 1 and 8) every 21 days with the goal of completing six cycles in total. In March 2014, he developed a large pleural effusion, which thoracentesis confirmed as malignant. Due to a rapidly deteriorating performance status, chemotherapy was discontinued and hospice services were initiated.

4. Discussion

The incidence of hepatocellular carcinoma is increasing in the United States and Europe, and it is the third highest cause of cancer-related death globally [10]. HCC is one of the few indications of a tumor that may be potentially cured with liver transplantation, by elimination of both the tumor and the preneoplastic background of underlying liver cirrhosis.

Patients within the Milan criteria (defined as no gross vascular invasion with either a single tumor ≤5 cm or three tumors with the largest lesion <3 cm; up to Stage II tumors) are given priority on transplant waiting lists following workup to rule out metastases [11]. Although recurrence of HCC following liver transplantation has significantly declined since the adoption of the Milan criteria, 8–12% of patients will still develop recurrence with the majority of these patients developing advanced forms of multifocal and extrahepatic metastases. The most common metastatic sites are lung, bones, lymph node, and adrenal glands; cutaneous metastases occur much less frequently [4].

Cutaneous metastases from HCC are estimated to represent only 0.2%–2.7% of all cutaneous metastases [8]. Cholangiocarcinoma tends to spread to adjacent organs with less than thirty cases of cutaneous metastases described in the literature [7].

Metastasis to the skin may occur by several different pathways, including hematogenous and lymphatic spread, direct contiguous tissue invasion, and iatrogenic implantation [8]. Cutaneous metastases from HCC most commonly occur in the face, scalp, chest, and shoulders and appear as single or multiple 1–5 cm lesions, which are often firm and reddish blue. Ulceration is often absent and rapid growth is common [4, 8]. These skin lesions may resemble pyogenic granulomas [5] or subcutaneous abscesses [4] or have a hemangiomatous morphology with profuse bleeding due to tumor hypervascularity [6]. Cutaneous metastases from cholangiocarcinoma may also occur in the scalp and face, but they are more often located on the abdominal wall (i.e., at the exit-site of a percutaneous biliary drain) [8].

In our first case, the etiology of the cutaneous metastases is unclear. The original tumor did not appear to have any lymphatic invasion although this may be due to the ablative chemoembolization. The patient had a CT guided biopsy at an outside institution, and it is possible that the site of metastases may have been the site of needle insertion. Still, this biopsy occurred three years earlier making the diagnosis of needle tracking less likely. There was no tumor spillage in either of the cases.

Histopathology of cutaneous HCC demonstrates a bottom heavy architecture, with the main infiltrate located in the deep dermis, and the presence of trabecular and pseudoglandular patterns composed of acidophilic cells [3, 8]. Tumor necrosis and vascular invasion are common findings. Furthermore, Mallory bodies (intracytoplasmic inclusion bodies found in hepatocytes) strongly suggest HCC and the presence of bile is confirmative [3, 8]. Cutaneous metastasis from cholangiocarcinoma presents with a nonspecific pattern of diffuse involvement of the dermis by pleomorphic epithelial cells with poorly preserved glandular architecture [8].

Immunohistochemical studies have added great value to the establishment of a pathologic diagnosis for these diseases. Neoplastic hepatocyte cells express immunoreactivity for polyclonal carcinoembryonic antigen (CEA), AFP, cytokeratins (CK) 8 and 18, and hepatocyte paraffin-1 (HepPar-1) (an antigen of the hepatocyte mitochondria) monoclonal antibody, which has been considered as the most specific and sensitive marker of normal and neoplastic hepatocytes [3, 8]. Although there is no characteristic panel of antibodies that are pathognomonic for cholangiocarcinoma, tumors of biliary epithelial origin tend to express CK7 and sometimes CK20 although they lack CDX2 expression [7, 8]. These immunohistochemical markers can thus be helpful in initially narrowing the diagnosis.

To date, there have been no reports of metastatic cholangiocarcinoma to the skin and only one case of metastatic HCC to the skin following liver transplantation [9]. In the report by Alonso-González, HCC recurrence was identified within the liver, lungs, and lymph nodes. The patient died just 6 weeks following their diagnosis of skin metastases. We present two cases of cutaneous metastases from hepatobiliary primaries, representing both HCC and mixed HCC/cholangiocarcinoma, as the first sign of tumor recurrence in two liver transplant recipients. Intrahepatic recurrence or metastases elsewhere were not identified in either case profile.

Skin metastases from liver cancers represent a dismal prognosis for most patients, with overall survival varying between a few weeks and six months [4, 9]. The patient who underwent abdominal wall resection and mesh reconstruction is doing well at the time of the publication of this paper, six months since diagnosis, while the other patient suffered a precipitous decline in his health with malignant pleural fluid and poorly controlled pain and died just three months following diagnosis. The first patient has been started on sorafenib, an oral multikinase inhibitor of the vascular endothelial growth factor receptor, the platelet-derived growth factor receptor β, and Raf, which has been shown to inhibit tumor-cell proliferation and angiogenesis and increase the rate of tumor-cell apoptosis in advanced cases of hepatocellular carcinoma and other tumors [12]. Two large randomized control trials have demonstrated that it can increase survival of patients with advanced HCC by approximately 2 to 3 months, and the Food and Drug Administration approved it in 2007 for this patient population [12, 13]. Recent case-control studies have demonstrated similar modest survival benefit in patients with recurrent HCC following liver transplantation [14, 15], and based on current data, algorithms that integrate sorafenib into the management of posttransplant HCC recurrence are emerging [16].

Additionally, both patients underwent modifications in immunosuppression and have been switched to everolimus due to the potential antitumor activities of this drug through its ability to inhibit the mTOR pathway, a key regulator of cellular proliferation and angiogenesis, the activation of which has been linked to a variety of malignancies [17]. Despite the potentially beneficial effects of mTOR inhibitors on HCC recurrence following liver transplantation, there are currently only retrospective and uncontrolled clinical trials available from which to draw supportive evidence [17]. Fortunately, a prospective, randomized open-label trial examining the application of mTOR inhibitors for the prevention of

HCC recurrence following liver transplantation is currently underway [18].

In summary, the present report demonstrates that cutaneous metastases from hepatobiliary cancers may occur following liver transplantation. This may be the first sign of recurrence and a high degree of suspicion is warranted. Although skin metastases generally portend a grim prognosis, palliative options may include surgery, radiotherapy, immunosuppressant adjustments, and systemic chemotherapy.

Disclosure

The authors of this paper have no conflicts of interest to disclose. The final version of the paper has been read and approved by all of the authors. The authors take full responsibility for the integrity and accuracy of the information presented in this paper. This paper was not prepared or funded by any commercial organization, and it has not been submitted elsewhere.

References

[1] D. P. Lookingbill, N. Spangler, and K. F. Helm, "Cutaneous metastases in patients with metastatic carcinoma: a retrospective study of 4020 patients," *Journal of the American Academy of Dermatology*, vol. 29, no. 2, pp. 228–236, 1993.

[2] D. Nashan, F. Meiss, M. Braun-Falco, and S. Reichenberger, "Cutaneous metastases from internal malignancies," *Dermatologic Therapy*, vol. 23, no. 6, pp. 567–580, 2010.

[3] T. Terada and H. Maruo, "Unusual extrahepatic metastatic sites from hepatocellular carcinoma," *International Journal of Clinical and Experimental Pathology*, vol. 6, no. 5, pp. 816–820, 2013.

[4] A. Amador, N. G. Monforte, N. Bejarano et al., "Cutaneous metastasis from hepatocellular carcinoma as the first clinical sign," *Journal of Hepato-Biliary-Pancreatic Surgery*, vol. 14, no. 3, pp. 328–330, 2007.

[5] Y. Kubota, T. Koga, and J. Nakayama, "Cutaneous metastasis from hepatocellular carcinoma resembling pyogenic granuloma," *Clinical and Experimental Dermatology*, vol. 24, no. 2, pp. 78–80, 1999.

[6] D. Ackerman, R. J. Barr, and A. N. Elias, "Cutaneous metastases from hepatocellular carcinoma," *International Journal of Dermatology*, vol. 40, no. 12, pp. 782–784, 2001.

[7] K. L. West, M. A. Selim, and P. K. Puri, "Cutaneous metastatic cholangiocarcinoma: a report of three cases and review of the literature," *Journal of Cutaneous Pathology*, vol. 37, no. 12, pp. 1230–1236, 2010.

[8] I. Alcaraz, L. Cerroni, A. Rütten, H. Kutzner, and L. Requena, "Cutaneous metastases from internal malignancies: a clinicopathologic and immunohistochemical review," *The American Journal of Dermatopathology*, vol. 34, no. 4, pp. 347–393, 2012.

[9] J. Alonso-González, D. Sánchez-Aguilar, and J. Toribio, "Multiple cutaneous metastases from hepatocellular carcinoma as the first sign of tumor recurrence in a transplant patient," *Actas Dermo-Sifiliograficas*, vol. 103, no. 4, pp. 339–341, 2012.

[10] D. M. Parkin, F. Bray, J. Ferlay, and P. Pisani, "Global cancer statistics, 2002," *Cancer Journal for Clinicians*, vol. 55, no. 2, pp. 74–108, 2005.

[11] V. Mazzaferro, E. Regalia, R. Doci et al., "Liver transplantation for the treatment of small hepatocellular carcinomas in patients with cirrhosis," *The New England Journal of Medicine*, vol. 334, no. 11, pp. 693–699, 1996.

[12] J. M. Llovet, S. Ricci, V. Mazzaferro et al., "Sorafenib in advanced hepatocellular carcinoma," *New England Journal of Medicine*, vol. 359, no. 4, pp. 378–390, 2008.

[13] A. L. Cheng, Y. K. Kang, Z. Chen et al., "Efficacy and safety of sorafenib in patients in the Asia-Pacific region with advanced hepatocellular carcinoma: a phase III randomised, double-blind, placebo-controlled trial," *The Lancet Oncology*, vol. 10, no. 1, pp. 25–34, 2009.

[14] A. Waghray, B. Balci, G. El-Gazzaz et al., "Safety and efficacy of sorafenib for the treatment of recurrent hepatocellular carcinoma after liver transplantation," *Clinical Transplantation*, vol. 27, no. 4, pp. 555–561, 2013.

[15] C. Sposito, L. Mariani, A. Germini et al., "Comparative efficacy of sorafenib versus best supportive care in recurrent hepatocellular carcinoma after liver transplantation: a case-control study," *Journal of Hepatology*, vol. 59, no. 1, pp. 59–66, 2013.

[16] C. Toso, G. Mentha, and P. Majno, "Integrating sorafenib into an algorithm for the management of post-transplant hepatocellular carcinoma recurrence," *Journal of Hepatology*, vol. 59, no. 1, pp. 3–5, 2013.

[17] K. Chen, K. Man, H. J. Metselaar, H. L. Janssen, M. P. Peppelenbosch, and Q. Pan, "Rationale of personalized immunosuppressive medication for hepatocellular carcinoma patients after liver transplantation," *Liver Transplantation*, vol. 20, pp. 261–269, 2014.

[18] A. A. Schnitzbauer, C. Zuelke, C. Graeb et al., "A prospective randomised, open-labeled, trial comparing sirolimus-containing versus mTOR-inhibitor-free immunosuppression in patients undergoing liver transplantation for hepatocellular carcinoma," *BMC Cancer*, vol. 10, article 190, 2010.

23

Domino Liver Transplantation from a Child with Propionic Acidemia to a Child with Idiopathic Fulminant Hepatic Failure

Marina Moguilevitch and Ellise Delphin

Department of Anesthesiology, Montefiore Medical Center, Albert Einstein College of Medicine, Bronx, NY 10463, USA

Correspondence should be addressed to Marina Moguilevitch; mmoguile@montefiore.org

Academic Editor: Piero Boraschi

Domino liver transplant has emerged as a viable strategy to increase the number of grafts available for transplantation. In the domino transplant organs explanted from one patient are transplanted into another patient. The first successful domino liver transplant was performed in Portugal in 1995. Since then this innovative concept has been applied to several genetic or biochemical disorders that are treated by liver transplantation. An important consideration during this operation is that such livers can pose a risk of the de novo development of the disease in the recipient. That is why this surgical procedure requires careful planning, proper selection of the patients, and informed consent of both donor and recipient.

1. Introduction

With the ever-present shortage of liver grafts available for transplantation, new methods to expand the donor pool are being employed. In addition to split liver and living donors, the concept of "domino liver transplantation" (DLT) has been described as a way of utilizing an organ that would be discarded otherwise. Morphologically normal livers from donors with metabolic diseases can be used for select recipients. Usually, the metabolic disease of the donor should not produce symptoms in the DLT recipients for many years. In order to gather information on the DLT procedures an international register was created in 1999. By the end of 2015 a total 1112 domino transplantations were registered. They were reported from 63 different hospitals in 21 countries. There are no reports of use of the whole liver donor graft from the patient with propionic acidemia (PA).

2. Case Presentation

We would like to share our unique experience with the successful domino liver transplantation from a child with propionic acidemia to a young teenager with idiopathic fulminant hepatic failure. A 20 kg, O positive, 4-year-old female developed metabolic acidosis at birth and was diagnosed with PA by newborn screening. She required a protein restricted diet supplemented with Propimex formula and daily L-carnitine therapy for management. She had multiple propionic acidemia flares with hospital admissions for ammonia and urinary ketones elevation as well as dehydration secondary to poor oral intake. As a result of PA, she was developmentally delayed with impaired motor and verbal skills. Upon admission for possible transplantation, she was in her usual state of health with elevated ammonia level (73.9 μmol/L) and urinary ketones (6.8 μmol/L). The rest of the laboratory values including all liver function tests and coagulation studies were within normal limits.

When a cadaveric liver became available for this child there was a 14-year-old, blood type A positive, 50 kg male in the pediatric intensive care unit (PICU) with fulminant hepatic failure secondary to hepatitis of unknown etiology. Upon admission he had complaints of nausea and vomiting and on exam had scleral icterus. His admission laboratory values were notable for total bilirubin of 314.5 μmol/L, direct bilirubin 217 μmol/L, alkaline phosphatase 5.7 ukat/L, alanine aminotransferase 52.4 ukat/L, aspartate aminotransferase 64.4 ukat/L, international normalized ratio (INR) 2.1, and prothrombin time (PT) 32.3 seconds.

His course rapidly progressed to grade IV encephalopathy and fulminant hepatic failure necessitating intubation. His liver function deteriorated significantly with total bilirubin increase to 405 μmol/L, ammonia 10.6 μmol/L, INR 3.8, and PT 38 seconds. CT of the brain did not show any signs of edema. He was listed as a status 1 and an urgent liver transplant would be his only life-saving opportunity. Prior to the time of his listing a cadaveric liver graft offer had already been given to the child with propionic acidemia and no other suitable grafts were available. The team was concerned about rapidly deteriorating neurologic status of the patient. Temporizing measures of blood purification known to improve coagulation status but not proven to guarantee reversal of encephalopathy were discussed with the family. After waiting for about 24 hours parents were presented with the option of using the liver from the patient with propionic acidemia. The family had full understanding that a missing mitochondrial enzyme is also present in other organs of the body but the liver remains primary source of it. A careful review of the risks for a liver transplantation in critically ill patient as well as lack of data associated with transplanting the liver from the patient with propionic acidemia was conducted with the family. The family expressed full understanding and gave consent for the surgery. The family of the child with propionic acidemia was also approached with the permission to use the explanted liver. After obtaining informed consent for the surgery from both families domino liver transplant was performed. Donor liver was procured using classic technique. Venous outflow reconstruction was accomplished by end-to-side cavocaval anastomosis. To overcome a common problem of the short venous cuffs a bridge venoplasties technique between donor and recipient hepatic veins was utilized.

During the postoperative period the recipient with the transplanted propionic acidemia liver had received careful monitoring of his metabolic profile on monthly schedule, particularly urinary ketones and serum ammonia levels. His protein intake was initially restricted but ultimately liberalized and he was discharged to a rehabilitation facility tolerating a regular diet. His outpatient follow-up has been uneventful for two years with recommended checkup every 2 to 3 months. The family was presented with an option of possible retransplantation in the future in case of the development of propionic acidemia. Our 4-year-old patient with PA had one minor complication, an increase in liver function tests approximately 3 weeks after transplantation, causing concern about rejection. Liver biopsy showed scattered inflammation with neutrophils and lymphocytes consistent with infection rather than rejection, which eventually resolved. The patient was discharged home and is doing well.

3. Discussion

In 1995 domino liver transplantation emerged as a viable strategy to relieve the organ shortage. The first reported case came from Portugal where the liver from a patient with familial amyloidotic polyneuropathy (FAP) was used for non-FAP patient [1]. The domino approach can be considered for patients with some genetic or biochemical disorders that today are treated by liver transplantation. With the increasing need for organs, livers explanted from patients with primary hyperoxaluria (PH), acute intermittent porphyria (AIP), maple syrup urine disease (MSUD), and homozygous familial hypercholesterolemia (HFHC) are being used for DLT. The outcomes of these transplantations are variable: they are better in cases of MSUD and HFHC and are not as favorable in cases of PH and AIP. One of the latest developments in this area is the use of the grafts in neonates as a bridging therapy; this allows babies to grow until they can receive a size-compatible liver. The main risk of these surgeries includes de novo development of the genetic disorders in the recipients. Other important aspects to consider are the donors' survival as well as a need to keep mortality and morbidity of the recipients to a minimum [2].

This procedure raises very unique ethical issues. The most important one is informed consent of both donor and recipient with emphasis on the possibility of the recipient developing a metabolic disorder in the future. A hepatectomy procedure on a domino donor should meet the demands of the suitable graft and should not expose a donor to additional surgical risks. With the growing experience in DLT the main indication for the recipients remains hepatocellular carcinoma (HCC). Other possible indications listed in Domino Liver Transplant Registry are metastatic hepatic malignancy, cirrhosis secondary to hepatitis B and hepatitis C, alcoholic cirrhosis, and retransplantation.

To date, there have been no published case reports regarding the use of whole liver from patients with propionic academia (PA) for a DLT. PA is an autosomal recessive disease classified as a branched chain organic aminoacidemia. It is caused by a reduction in the activity of enzyme propionyl coenzyme A carboxylase (PCC). This occurs during the β-oxidation of odd chain fatty acids, catabolism of methionine, leucine, isoleucine, threonine, and valine, or metabolism of the cholesterol side chain. This altered metabolism leads to metabolic acidosis and hyperammonemia. There are two clinical phenotypes: (1) neonatal, the most common, and (2) late onset, less common. Clinical manifestations of the disease are poor feeding, vomiting, lethargy, and developmental delay leading to rapid neurologic deterioration, failure to thrive, and cardiomyopathy. PCC is also being produced in extrahepatic locations, mainly gut and central nervous system, which makes these patients not ideal candidates for liver transplantation as a potential cure for the disease [3]. The use of liver transplantation for patients with PA has been described in several case study series as one of the potential treatment modalities in reducing the risks of metabolic decompensation, neurocognitive dysfunction, and quality of life [4, 5]. The domino reuse of livers affected by propionic acidemia should provide hepatic rescue therapy for the recipient and theoretically avoid metabolic crisis because of enzyme production in extrahepatic sites [6]. According to the literature, DLT using grafts affected by a metabolic disorder could be an option for recipients who fulfill at least one of the following criteria: presence of normal systemic enzyme activity that can compensate for the genetic defect transmitted by the graft; an expected interval before the onset of the acquired metabolic disease that is longer than expected survival without liver transplantation; a bridge therapy while waiting for the healthy graft [7].

Postoperative management of the recipient of the PA liver involves initially restricting protein intake, as one would do in a patient with PA. Close follow-up of metabolic profile, particularly urinary ketones and serum ammonia, is very important. Liver transplantation plays a major role in survival as well as quality of life improvement of patients suffering from propionic acidemia. The ideal timing of transplantation for patients with this metabolic disorder is still unknown. There is ongoing debate about prioritization of these candidates on transplant list. We still do not know what quality of organ is acceptable for these non-life-saving transplantations. At this point in time it behooves us to report every new experience in transplantation for patients with metabolic disorders and especially the successful use of explanted liver from these patients as donors. This will expand our knowledge in the relatively new area of domino liver transplantation and allow this novel strategy to be used to increase the number of liver grafts available.

We report this as one of the first DLT procedures utilizing a liver from a patient with PA that resulted in salvage and recovery of a patient with fulminant hepatic failure.

Disclosure

This case report has been partially presented at the 2017 ILTS meeting.

References

[1] A. Furtado, L. Tomé, F. J. Oliveira, E. Furtado, J. Viana, and R. Perdigoto, "Sequential liver transplantation," *Transplantation Proceedings*, vol. 29, no. 1-2, pp. 467-468, 1997.

[2] G. Tincani, E. Hoti, P. Andreani et al., "Operative risks of domino liver transplantation for the familial amyloid polyneuropathy liver donor and recipient: A double analysis," *American Journal of Transplantation*, vol. 11, no. 4, pp. 759–766, 2011.

[3] K. A. Chapman and M. L. Summar, "Propionic acidemia consensus conference summary," *Molecular Genetics and Metabolism*, vol. 105, no. 1, pp. 3-4, 2012.

[4] N. R. Barshes, J. M. Vanatta, A. J. Patel et al., "Evaluation and management of patients with propionic acidemia undergoing liver transplantation: A comprehensive review," *Pediatric Transplantation*, vol. 10, no. 7, pp. 773–781, 2006.

[5] R. Vara, C. Turner, H. Mundy et al., "Liver transplantation for propionic acidemia in children," *Liver Transplantation*, vol. 17, no. 6, pp. 661–667, 2011.

[6] S. Govil, N. P. Shanmugam, M. S. Reddy, G. Narasimhan, and M. Rela, "A metabolic chimera: Two defective genotypes make a normal phenotype," *Liver Transplantation*, vol. 21, no. 11, pp. 1453-1454, 2015.

[7] A. Schielke, F. Conti, C. Goumard, F. Perdigao, Y. Calmus, and O. Scatton, "Liver transplantation using grafts with rare metabolic disorders," *Digestive and Liver Disease*, vol. 47, no. 4, pp. 261–270, 2015.

24

Colonic Diffuse Large B-Cell Lymphoma in a Liver Transplant Patient with Historically Very Low Tacrolimus Levels

Christopher M. Moore,[1] Ihab Lamzabi,[2] Anne K. Bartels,[1] Shriram Jakate,[2] and David H. Van Thiel[1]

[1] *Section of Hepatology, Rush University Medical Center, Chicago, IL 60612, USA*
[2] *Section of Pathology, Rush University Medical Center, Chicago, IL 60612, USA*

Correspondence should be addressed to Christopher M. Moore, christopher_moore@rush.edu

Academic Editors: S. Faenza, R. L. Heilman, and R. Zhang

Posttransplant lymphoproliferative disorders (PTLDs) comprise a wide spectrum of hematologic malignancies that are found increasingly in orthotopic liver transplant (OLT) patients given the rising frequency of these surgeries and their long-term success. PTLDs are highly correlated with both the Epstein-Barr virus (EBV) infection and the degree of immunosuppression involved. Herein is reported a case of a 53-year-old male with successfully treated hepatitis C virus genotype 4 and hepatocellular carcinoma who underwent OLT and developed symptoms of weakness and poor appetite 4 years later while on tacrolimus 3 mg b.i.d. with historically very low plasma levels. He was found to be anemic and colonoscopy revealed a 4.5 cm cecal diffuse large B-cell lymphoma (DLBCL). Further workup revealed mesenteric lymph node enlargement consistent and nodal DLBCL dissemination. He was treated with cyclophosphamide-hydroxyldaunorubicin-oncovin-prednisone-rituximab (CHOP-R) chemotherapy and his tacrolimus dose was lowered. Additionally, he manifested PTLD-associated cryoglobulinemia leading to acute kidney injury. After a prolonged hospitalization he was discharged with close followup.

1. Introduction

Orthotopic liver transplantation (OLT) is a definitive therapy for fulminant liver failure and advanced chronic liver disease including hepatitis C virus (HCV) and alcoholic cirrhosis [1]. OLT incurs the cost of chronic immunosuppressive therapy-associated renal injury and posttransplant lymphoproliferative disorders (PTLDs) [2]. With the increased frequency of OLT and prolonged survival of these patients through (1) better patient allocation, (2) improvement in both surgical technique, and (3) post-OLT immunosuppressive therapies, the concern for and treatment of PTLD has increased.

PTLDs are a diverse group of potentially lethal neoplasms whose incidence is 1.2% for all solid organ transplants and 0.9% for OLT specifically [2]. PTLDs are highly correlated, and distinguished from lymphomas, by the association with Epstein-Barr virus (EBV) infection, the duration and intensity of immunosuppressive therapies, and type of organ transplanted [3]. Reduction in immunosuppressive therapy may lead to regression in a proportion of cases whereas others may progress to lymphoma [4].

Depending upon the initial site of the PTLD, the clinical presentation can range from lymphadenopathy and "B-symptoms" to renal failure and gastrointestinal hemorrhage and/or obstruction. The treatment is based upon location, extent, and metastasis and can include surgery, radiation, or chemotherapy [3].

Herein is a case report of an OLT patient with colonic PTLD diffuse large B-cell lymphoma (DLBCL) presenting with symptomatic anemia and cryoglobulin-induced acute kidney injury (AKI).

2. Case Presentation

A 53-year-old Egyptian male with HCV genotype 4 cirrhosis and hepatocellular carcinoma (HCC), who was successfully treated with antiviral HCV therapy prior to OLT in 2007,

Table 1: Key laboratory data during hospitalizations*.

	10/12/11	2/17/12[α]	2/27/12	3/1/12^	3/7/12[†]	3/9/12	3/16/12	Normal range
BUN (mg/dL)	33	63	88	92	129	123	99	8–21
Cr (mg/dL)	2.1	4.9	4.02	3.4	3.8	4.6	3.6	0.75–1.20
Alb (g/dL)	3.7	2.6	3.1	3.8	2.8	2.9	2.2	3.5–5.0
TB (mg/dL)	0.2	0.2	0.3	0.3	0.7	0.5	0.3	0.2–1.3
AP (U/L)	44	41	38	17	21	23	53	30–125
AST (U/L)	15	12	16	10	8	8	10	3–44
ALT (U/L)	9	6	7	6	7	7	9	0–40
INR (no units)	—	1.2	1.2	—	1.3	—	—	0.83–1.2
WBC ($10^3/\mu$L)	4.5	3.5	4.1	2.3	0.55	6.0	5.5	4.0–10.0
HGB (g/dL)	9.7	7.6	8.1	8.3	10.4	9.4	7.8	13.5–17.5
PLT ($10^3/\mu$L)	210	246	248	225	109	82	204	150–399
Tac (ng/mL)	6.6	3.1	—	3.7	4.3	6.6	3.0	No range

BUN: blood urea nitrogen; Cr: creatinine; alb: albumin; TB: total bilirubin; AP: Alkaline phosphatase; AST: aspartate aminotransferase; alanine aminotransferase; INR: international normalized ratio; WBC: white blood cells; HGB: hemoglobin; PLT: platelets; Tac: tacrolimus; —: no lab drawn that day. [α]Day of admission; ^2 days after chemotherapy; [†]first day of hemodialysis.

was admitted to the hospital in February 2012 for increasing weakness and poor appetite in the past month. His comorbid diseases included diabetes mellitus and chronic kidney disease (CKD). His immunosuppressive regimen was tacrolimus 3 mg bid, at a stable dose, with an admission plasma level of 3.1 ng/mL. He was noted to have had both chronically normal liver injury tests and very low tacrolimus plasma levels (<5 ng/mL) during outpatient visits.

Upon presentation his blood laboratory specimens revealed a number of abnormalities (see Table 1). His hemoglobin (hgb) levels had decreased from 9.7 (baseline) to 7.6 g/dL. His WBC was $3.5 \times 10^3/\mu$L with a 60% lymphocyte differential. He had denied any overt bleeding in recent memory and was not on any anticoagulants. Notably his creatinine (Cr) levels had risen from a baseline of approximately 2 to 4.9 mg/dL upon admission; he was still producing urine with noted proteinuria (~7 g/day) and hematuria. Ultrasound of the kidneys was consistent with CKD. On day 7 he underwent a kidney biopsy displaying refractile eosinophilic hyaline globules in glomerular capillary lumen suggestive of cryoglobulin deposits. Serum cryoglobulin precipitate levels for IgG were 122 mg/dL, IgM 113 mg/dL, IgA < 1.0 mg/dL, and RF > 650 IU/mL. His Cr at that time was 4.3 mg/dL, having received daily IV fluids in the interval. He was started on plasmapharesis (to receive six total treatments during this hospitalization) and oral prednisone starting on hospital day 8, to continue until discharge home. His liver-injury parameters including total bilirubin (TB), alkaline phosphatase (AP), and transaminases were normal, as was the INR upon admission and it remained so throughout the hospitalization. A liver biopsy on day 7 displayed no signs of viral inclusions, immune rejection, nor signs of fibrosis or lymphoma. Serum HCV-RNA was less than 12 IU/mL at admission.

Given his anemia he underwent colonoscopy which revealed a 4.5 cm nodular and friable mass in the cecum (see Figure 1); biopsy diagnosed it as a DLBCL (see Figures 2, 3 and 4). Histologically, the mass showed a dense monomorphic infiltrate of abnormal lymphoid cells. Immunoprofile was typical of B-cell lymphoma (CD20 positive and negative for CD3, CD5, CD10, and cyclin D1). BCL6 showed patchy positivity suggestive of potential preexistent follicular lymphoma. EBV-encoded small RNA (EBER) *in situ* hybridization for EBV was negative (see Figure 5). Prognostically, the DLBCL had multiple favorable markers including germinal center origin (MUM-1 negative and BCL6 positive), low proliferative index (Ki-67 positive for only 25% of tumor cells), enhanced T-cell immune response (>60% CD3 positive cells), and low staining for P53 (only 10% of tumor cells). EBV blood level was ~ 1200 copies/mL; CMV blood level was <300 copies/mL. Prior EBV and CMV levels from 2010 were <250 and 300 copies/mL, respectively. Noted were the serum C3 < 5 mg/dL, C4 < 1 mg/dL, and RF > 2000 IU/mL at admission; CH50 was not checked. Computed tomography (CT) of his head, chest and abdomen, and pelvis was only relevant for enlarged mesenteric lymph nodes. A bone marrow biopsy on day 12 displayed no evidence for malignant infiltration. On day 12 he received his first dose of cyclophosphamide-hydroxyldaunorubicin-oncovin-prednisone (CHOP) chemotherapy.

His Cr level reached its nadir of 3.4 mg/dL on day 14. By day 22, his BUN and Cr values were 123 mmol/L and 4.6 mg/dL, respectively, and his clinical status warranted the use of hemodialysis (HD). By hospital day 29 he completed 6 courses of plasmapheresis, received a dose of rituximab to complement his initial one time CHOP chemotherapy, and his electrolytes had stabilized in the setting of good urinary output such that HD could be discontinued. He was discharged on a dose of tacrolimus 0.5 mg bid.

At 2 months after hospitalization a repeat colonoscopy did not show any further evidence of lymphoma and EBV levels were <250 copies/mL. A CT scan at 3 months displayed decrease in size of his mesenteric lymphadenopathy, but he still had positive serum cryoprecipitate levels. At 4 months he had completed 6 cycles of CHOP-R therapy. Currently his

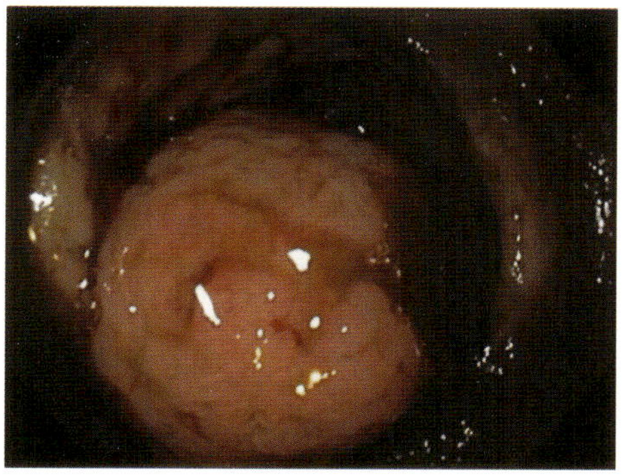

Figure 1: Colonoscopy image showing the polypoid cecal mass.

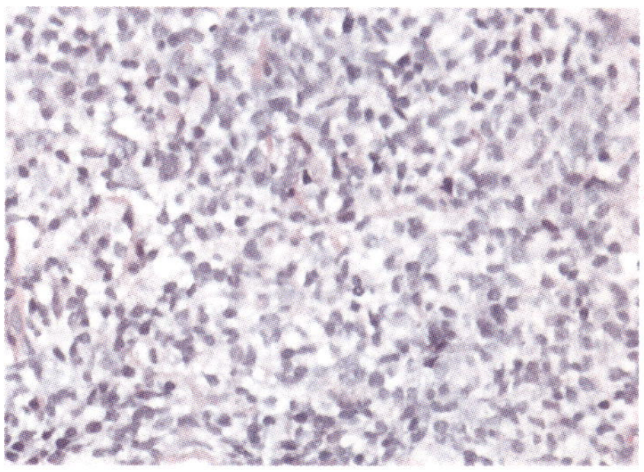

Figure 2: Diffuse proliferation of medium sized to large lymphoid cells, intermixed with few small lymphocytes.

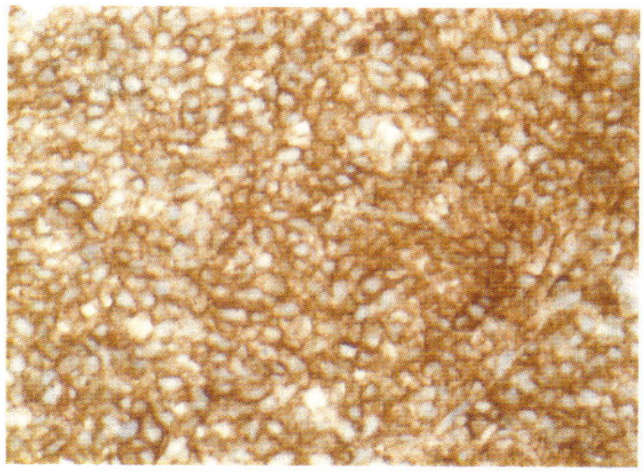

Figure 3: Tumor cells express CD20.

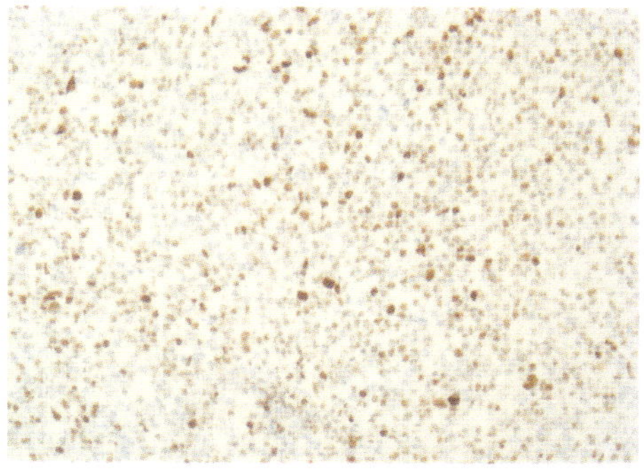

Figure 4: Most tumor cells are positive for BCL-6.

serum Cr remains around 3 mg/dL and is being evaluated for renal transplant. He continues on tacrolimus 0.5 mg bid and prednisone 20 mg daily immunosuppression and valacyclovir for prophylaxis. All liver enzyme and INR values are normal.

3. Discussion

OLT has proven to be a successful therapy for fulminant liver failure and advanced chronic liver disease [1]. Nevertheless, given the necessary use of immunosuppressive therapies, such as tacrolimus, and the increasing survival rates of these patients, the frequency of PTLD has increased [3, 5]. PTLD comprises a spectrum of diseases and is highly associated EBV infection in 90% of documented cases. PTLD tends to occur at a median of 7–10 months post-OLT and the clinical presentation can range from typical "B-symptoms" of fevers and weakness to gastro-intestinal symptoms [3, 5, 6].

In the current report, a 53-year-old male with pre-transplant treated HCV and HCC developed a cecal 4.5 cm DLBCL with mesenteric nodal dissemination approximately 4 years after OLT complicated by cryoglobulin-induced AKI. Cryoglobulinemia in this case was more likely driven by the PTLD B cells than his HCV, the latter which was successfully treated prior to OLT. His PTLD and associated AKI were treated with CHOP-R chemotherapy and plasmapharesis, and the tacrolimus dosage was lowered by the time of discharge.

This patient's case brings up a number of interesting points. The presentation of PTLD is typically much earlier for OLT patients than as presented here, although this particular presentation is not unexpected either. His symptomatic anemia is also consistent with a gastrointestinal presentation of PTLD. Interesting is the negative EBV immunostain of the cecal mass but positive EBV blood levels which may indicate the poor sensitivity of the former and the high sensitivity of the later test. EBV-negative PTLD tends to occur later than EBV positive cases, is more likely to be monomorphic, such as in this case, and is more common in adults [7, 8].

Given the known reversibility of these PTLD lesions to cessation and/or reduction in immunosuppression therapies, his tacrolimus dose was reduced [2, 3]. Other options include switching to the non-calcineurin inhibitor, sirolimus, a mammalian target of rapamycin (mTOR) inhibitor, which has less renal toxicity [3]. Given the (1) long-term normal levels of his liver injury tests and the absence of any fibrosis or rejection on recent liver biopsy, (2) the duration after OLT and the known degree of chimerism that takes place vis a vis the host immune system and the allograft, and (3) his clinical tolerance of tacrolimus, dose reduction rather than switching to another medication seemed a sensible first maneuver. This method has produced satisfactory results in the author's (David H. Van Thiel) own experience and is similar to others [4]. It is rather interesting that historically his tacrolimus plasma levels were not simply within recommended ranges,

Figure 5: EBER *in situ* hybridization negative for EBV.

but chronically quite lower (2-3 ng/mL in the preceding 3 years) with still excellent immunosuppression (chronically normal liver injury tests and biopsies).

Furthermore, the presentation of a colonic PTLD renews concerns for the utility of colonoscopic surveillance after OLT. For instance, in patients with primary sclerosing cholangitis (PSC) and inflammatory bowel disease, the known intrinsic risk for colonic malignancy is quite real and thus colonoscopic surveillance every 1-2 years has been advocated regardless of OLT status. One study looked at otherwise healthy non-PSC OLT patients comparatively and their risk for colonic malignancy and has suggested that these patients follow standard screening and surveillance protocols similar to those without OLT [9]. Thus beyond the finding of alarm signs and symptoms, such as anemia seen in this presentation, accelerated rates of after OLT endoscopic surveillance are likely not cost-effective.

In summary, PTLD represents a not uncommon occurrence in OLT patients, and is highly correlated with EBV infection, and the duration and intensity of immunosuppressive therapies. This patient presented with a less common location, that is, the colon, of DLBCL, with features of symptomatic anemia and cryoglobulin-induced AKI, despite historically very low tacrolimus levels. This case highlights the concern and utility for further research into screening (serologically and/or endoscopically) for PTLD in OLT patients.

References

[1] K. F. Murray and R. L. Carithers, "AASLD practice guidelines: evaluation of the patient for liver transplantation," *Hepatology*, vol. 41, no. 6, pp. 1407–1432, 2005.

[2] V. R. Dharnidharka, A. H. Tejani, P. L. Ho, and W. E. Harmon, "Post-transplant lymphoproliferative disorder in the United States: young Caucasian males are at highest risk," *American Journal of Transplantation*, vol. 2, no. 10, pp. 993–998, 2002.

[3] D. G. Koch, L. Christiansen, J. Lazarchick, R. Stuart, I. R. Willner, and A. Reuben, "Posttransplantation lymphoproliferative disorder—the great mimic in liver transplantation: appraisal of the clinicopathologic spectrum and the role of Epstein-Barr virus," *Liver Transplantation*, vol. 13, no. 6, pp. 904–912, 2007.

[4] T. V. Cacciarelli, M. Green, R. Jaffe et al., "Management of posttransplant lymphoproliferative disease in pediatric liver transplant recipients receiving primary tacrolimus (FK506) therapy," *Transplantation*, vol. 66, no. 8, pp. 1047–1052, 1998.

[5] W. K. Kremers, H. C. Devarbhavi, R. H. Wiesner, R. A. F. Krom, W. R. Macon, and T. M. Habermann, "Post-transplant lymphoproliferative disorders following liver transplantation: incidence, risk factors and survival," *American Journal of Transplantation*, vol. 6, no. 5, part 1, pp. 1017–1024, 2006.

[6] M. J. Kim, S. H. Yun, H. K. Chun, W. Y. Lee, and Y. B. Cho, "Post-transplant lymphoproliferative disorder localized in the colon after liver transplantation: report of a case," *Surgery Today*, vol. 39, no. 12, pp. 1076–1079, 2009.

[7] I. M. Ghobrial, T. M. Habermann, M. J. Maurer et al., "Prognostic analysis for survival in adult solid organ transplant recipients with post-transplantation lymphoproliferative disorders," *Journal of Clinical Oncology*, vol. 23, no. 30, pp. 7574–7582, 2005.

[8] B. P. Nelson, M. A. Nalesnik, D. W. Bahler, J. Locker, J. J. Fung, and S. H. Swerdlow, "Epstein-Barr virus-negative post-transplant lymphoproliferative disorders: a distinct entity?" *American Journal of Surgical Pathology*, vol. 24, no. 3, pp. 375–385, 2000.

[9] M. A. Silva, P. S. Jambulingam, and D. F. Mirza, "Colorectal cancer after orthotopic liver transplantation," *Critical Reviews in Oncology/Hematology*, vol. 56, no. 1, pp. 147–153, 2005.

25

Unusual Case of Severe Lactic Acidosis in a Liver Transplant Patient

Shweta Yemul Golhar,[1] Michael S. Green,[1] and Stephen Guy[2]

[1]*Department of Anesthesiology, Drexel University College of Medicine/Hahnemann University Hospital, Philadelphia, PA, USA*
[2]*Department of Surgery, Drexel University College of Medicine/Hahnemann University Hospital, Philadelphia, PA, USA*

Correspondence should be addressed to Michael S. Green; msg37@drexel.edu

Academic Editor: Ryszard Grenda

Lactic acidosis is a standard indicator for oxygen debt and some other very significant causes. We describe a case of liver transplant patient presenting with vague abdominal pain and lactic acidosis without any liver dysfunction/failure/ischemia/rejection or sepsis. The imaging studies showed vague bowel edema and normal hepatic perfusion. The patient continued to deteriorate with rising lactic acidosis when a repeat CT abdomen eventually showed signs of lymphomatosis peritonei. Biopsy revealed the unusual diagnosis of posttransplant lymphoproliferative disorder. Immediate discontinuation of immunosuppression and initiation of chemotherapy led to clinical improvement. Our intention of presenting this case is to increase awareness of posttransplant lymphoma and propose lactic acidosis as not only an indicator of liver dysfunction or rejection but also an aid for diagnosis of this unusual but fatal and potentially curable condition.

1. Introduction

Lactic acidosis is a universally accepted marker for adequacy of perfusion. It is the end product of anaerobic metabolism and thus is commonly used as an indicator for oxygen debt. Lactic acid serves as a marker of mortality risk and a target for therapy [1, 2]. Lactic acidosis in a liver transplant patient holds profound implications. It is an indicator of early organ dysfunction, organ failure or rejection, infections, or severe sepsis and hence early detection can help initiate treatment and potentially alter the course of the condition [3]. However, there are some uncommon but very significant causes of severe lactic acidosis. We discuss a case of severe lactic acidosis in a liver transplant patient with an unusual cause and an ambiguous presentation.

2. Case Report

A 68-year-old male with past medical history of orthoptic liver transplant secondary to NASH cirrhosis 4 years earlier and chronic kidney disease, presented with vague abdominal pain, weight loss, and fatigue. Mycophenolate and tacrolimus provided immunosuppression. Upon admission liver function tests (AST, ALT, and ALP), CBC, and tacrolimus level were all within normal limits. Additionally, the patient had an unremarkable RUQ ultrasound. He had some raised s. creatinine (1.58) compared to baseline of 1.28 due to poor oral intake. Patient was afebrile and vitals were stable, with no evidence of infection or sepsis. Hydration brought the creatinine down to baseline. A CT scan showed nonspecific bowel edema (Figure 1). Stool heme/WBC and culture, fungal culture, gram stain, AFB quantiferon, AFB culture, Yersinia, and urine culture were sent. LFTs and coagulation were still normal. Stool WBC was negative. Patient was still afebrile, without bandemia.

Colonoscopy showed an area at the distal ileum which was inflamed, granular, and necrotic, biopsy of which was consistent with nonspecific/ischemic ileitis. Antibiotics (ciprofloxacin and metronidazole) were started empirically due to ischemic changes in pathology. Later that day patient started complaining of increased abdominal pain concerning for bowel perforation; hence an immediate diagnostic laparoscopy was done which showed edematous bowel but no other significant abnormalities and ruled out ischemic

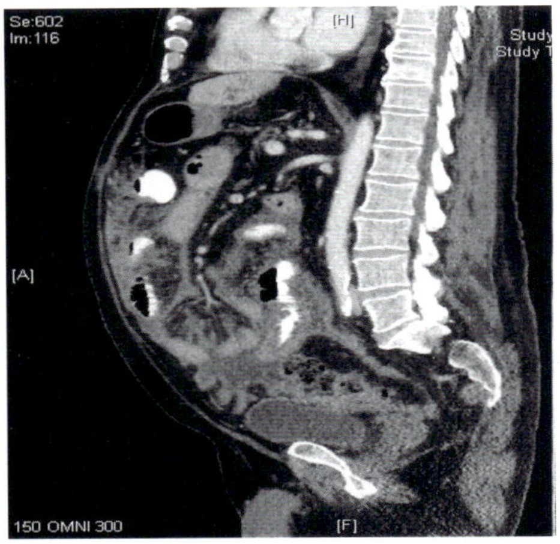

Figure 1: Diffuse nonspecific bowel edema.

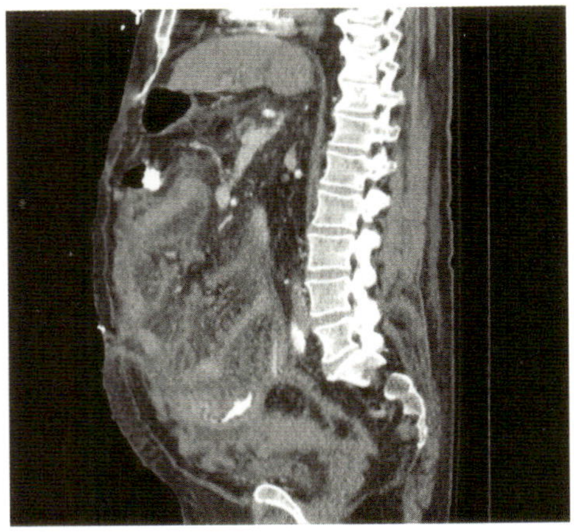

Figure 2: Mesenteric stranding and peritoneal thickening diagnostic for peritoneal lymphoma.

bowel. Ascitic fluid gram stain was negative; ascitic fluid and peritoneal cultures were sent.

Intraoperatively, the patient suffered from severe metabolic acidosis with a pH of 7.08 and became hemodynamically stable. The lactate levels remained high despite therapy and the pH further dropped to 6.9 despite fluid resuscitation. In ICU, sodium bicarbonate infusion and hemodialysis with bicarbonate dialysate was initiated to correct the acidosis and electrolyte abnormality. Vasoactive medications were initiated. Despite extensive efforts the lactate levels remained elevated. At this time, acute liver rejection, sepsis, portal/mesenteric arteriovenous thrombosis, or CMV infection were high on the differential diagnosis. However, liver enzymes remained normal and CT angiogram revealed patent vessels ruling out liver rejection/failure or any arteriovenous thrombosis. Mycophenolate was discontinued suspecting CMV ileitis. CMV PCR was sent. Urine analysis was normal. C. difficile toxin and EBV PCR laboratory evaluation was completed. Blood culture, sputum gram stain, CRE, stool WBC, and anaerobic blood culture were negative. PTLD was suspected. Tacrolimus was discontinued. Micafungin was added empirically considering fungemia as possibility. Pressors were tapered off slowly; LA peaked to 14 and then gradually came to 4–6 but never below that.

Repeat CT abdomen in a few days showed extensive bowel edema, mesenteric thickening, and stranding (Figure 2). Immediately, the patient was reexplored. At laparotomy, there was diffuse thickening of all bowel, mesentery, and peritoneum with several discrete lesions in the small bowel and mesentery. The surface was variegated and pebble like (Figure 3).

The peritoneal/omental and bowel biopsy was consistent with monomorphic Burkitt's lymphoma. Immediately, immunosuppression was held and chemotherapy was initiated. Rituximab and prednisone started initially and then Vincristine and cyclophosphamide. After the initiation of chemotherapy, the lactic acidosis started to resolve (Figure 4). Vasoactive medications were weaned and the patient was

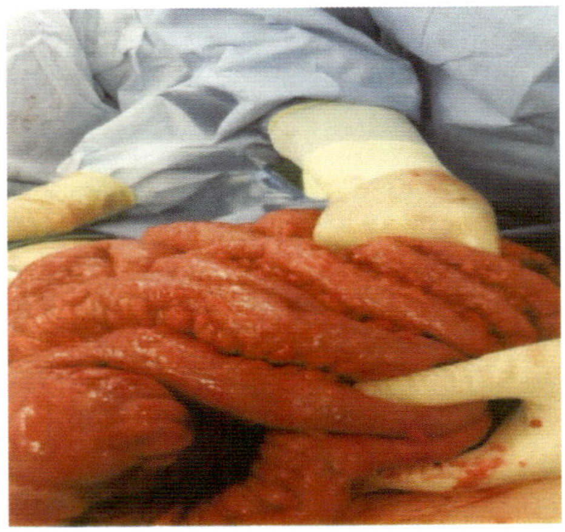

Figure 3: Variegated and pebble like peritoneum and bowel.

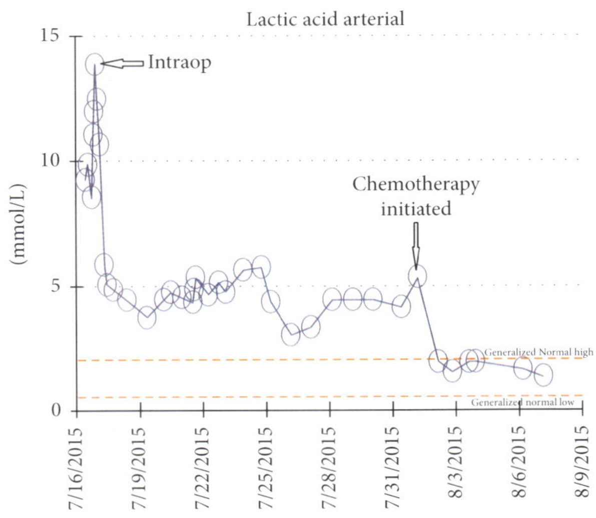

Figure 4: Lactic Acid Level timeline.

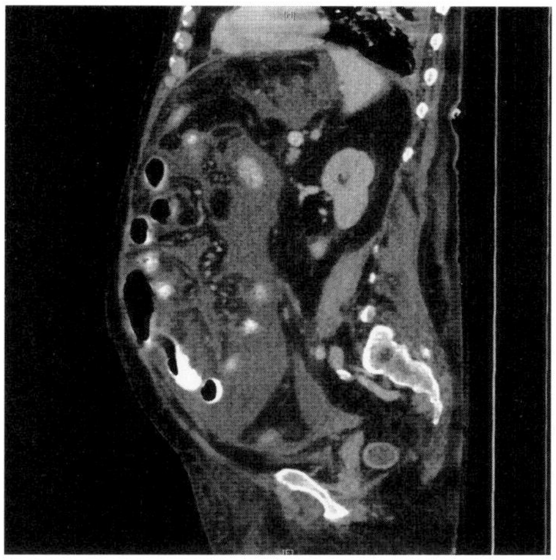

FIGURE 5: Resolution of the mesenteric and the peritoneal thickening after initiation of chemotherapy.

extubated. Repeat CT scan one week later showed tremendous improvement in the mesenteric thickening (Figure 5).

Following clinical improvement, unfortunately, the patient developed complications of chemotherapy associated pneumonia leading to sepsis and finally suffered pulmonary embolism. The patient deteriorated over next two weeks and care was withdrawn.

3. Discussion

Posttransplant lymphoproliferative disorder (PTLD) is a very grave complication of immunosuppression in transplant patients. PTLD is defined as the unrestrained growth of B cells in the face of T cell suppression. PTLD presents as both localized involvement or a more potent generalized disease. The UNOS database reports a 1.2% incidence in organ-transplant recipients [4]. The incidence is rising because of more potent immunosuppression and is higher in thoracic organs, hemopoietin stem cell, and intestine transplant and seems to increase with each passing year of transplant. Incidence of lymphoma in transplant recipients is 40 times higher than the general population [5]. The involvement can be nodal or extranodal with the most common sites being lymph nodes, liver, lung, kidney, and bone marrow [6]. Less common sites include the oral cavity and skin or subcutaneous lesions. Peritoneal involvement is extremely rare.

Most clinical symptoms are nonspecific and include fever, weight loss, lymphadenopathy, bowel obstruction, or mass effect. Extranodal disease is common but symptoms are very vague and presentation is very subtle. This can cause further delay in diagnosis which occurred in the patient presented [7]. There is a 6.8–24 times more association between EBV infection and lymphoproliferative disease [8]. However, EBV negative PTLD is more aggressive, has later presentation, and has poorer prognosis as was seen in our patient who was EBV negative. This explains the rapid fulminant spread within weeks and the aggressive nature of this disease. High lactic acid levels and a rapid fall after initiation of chemotherapy are indicators of high tumor load and remission, respectively.

Diagnosis of posttransplant lymphoma is made with the utilization of routine tests. No specific tests will yield a complete picture but many help contribute to the final diagnosis. CT scan, MRI, CXR, ultrasound, CSF if neurological involvement is suspected, bone marrow aspirate, PET scan, EBV viral load immunoglobulins, colonoscopy, biopsy of suspected lesion, cell markers like CD 20, immunohistochemistry, and LMP1 antigen all will provide valuable information. Our patient presented with normal liver function tests and negative EBV serology. The CT scan showed a very nonspecific edema of the bowel initially and subsequent biopsy was nondiagnostic. However, within the span of a week the repeat CT showed characteristic findings of peritoneal PTLD which includes mesenteric thickening and stranding. CT diagnosis of this condition especially without lymphadenopathy or any mass is challenging and unfortunately a late finding [9]. We believe that the disease was peritoneal to begin with and very rapidly spread to the peritoneum and that was the reason for negative biopsy at colonoscopy.

Mathur et al. reported a case of severe multiple organ failure in a patient following renal transplant. The patient presented with nonspecific symptoms and progressed to gradual failure of organs and severe lactic acidosis with liver failure. Reduction in immunosuppression did not alter the course and the patient expired. The diagnosis was made at autopsy which showed widely disseminated PTLD. This patient also showed very severe lactic acidosis without any response to treatment. In this case however, the liver failure also contributed to the high lactic acidosis, which was not the case in our patient [7].

Early diagnosis is the cornerstone of treatment as early reduction or discontinuation of immunosuppression allows the patient's natural immunity to recover and gain control over proliferating B cells. Other treatment modalities consist of chemotherapy, antiviral therapy, intravenous gamma globulin therapy, alpha interferon, radiation therapy, monoclonal antibodies, and cytotoxic T lymphocytes.

Lactic acidosis is an indicator of oxygen debt and is of 2 types. Type A is due to blood supply and demand becoming imbalanced. Type B is when the oxidative phosphorylation is hindered by toxins, drugs and inborn errors of metabolism. Lactic acidosis in a liver transplant patient is an ominous sign and is an indicator of liver dysfunction due to ischemia, congestion, liver cell failure due to early rejection, or infection/sepsis. Other unusual causes of lactic acidosis include malignancies, especially acute leukemia and high grade lymphoma. These generally have very poor prognosis. The cause of high lactic acidosis in lymphoma is mostly thought to be liver dysfunction, sepsis, and SIRS associated with these malignancies [10]. Overexpression of type II hexokinase or increased IGF-binding protein (IGFBP) activity has been implicated in the increased glycolysis in cancer cells [11, 12].

Weil and Afifi reviewed 20 case reports and found that a reduction in lactic acidosis in leukemia or lymphoma after initiation of chemotherapy was a good indicator for remission. In our case chemotherapy was initiated and lactic acid levels decreased. Severe lactic acidosis, even with maximal therapy, has a very high mortality of 60–90% and is an indicator for poor prognosis [13].

With increasing immunosuppression, use of more potent drugs, use of organs from extended criteria donors, and the increasing longevity of the transplant patients, the complications due to immunosuppression are occurring more frequently. The liver is a vital organ and unfortunately without any effective artificial replacement yet; hence diagnosis of early rejection or failure after liver transplant is extremely important. Use of lactic acidosis as an early indicator of liver dysfunction is very significant.

Our aim in reporting this case is to raise awareness of this rare but life threatening and potentially treatable cause of lactic acidosis in the liver transplant patients. PTLD should be included in any posttransplant patient with elevated lactic acid.

Disclosure

This case was presented at a resident research conference as a poster case report. No portion of the report has been published. The conference was for the benefit of those who attended and for residents to learn the skill of presentation.

References

[1] O. Kruse, N. Grunnet, and C. Barfod, "Blood lactate as a predictor for in-hospital mortality in patients admitted acutely to hospital: a systematic review," *Scandinavian Journal of Trauma, Resuscitation and Emergency Medicine* , vol. 19, article 74, 2011.

[2] C. Barfod, L. H. Lundstrøm, M. M. Lauritzen et al., "Peripheral venous lactate at admission is associated with in-hospital mortality, a prospective cohort study," *Acta Anaesthesiologica Scandinavica*, vol. 59, no. 4, pp. 514–523, 2015.

[3] L. W. Andersen, J. Mackenhauer, J. C. Roberts, K. M. Berg, M. N. Cocchi, and M. W. Donnino, "Etiology and therapeutic approach to elevated lactate levels," *Mayo Clinic Proceedings*, vol. 88, no. 10, pp. 1127–1140, 2013.

[4] V. R. Dharnidharka, A. H. Tejani, P.-L. Ho, and W. E. Harmon, "Post-transplant lymphoproliferative disorder in the United States: Young Caucasian males are at highest risk," *American Journal of Transplantation*, vol. 2, no. 10, pp. 993–998, 2002.

[5] G. Opelz and R. Henderson, "Incidence of non-Hodgkin lymphoma in kidney and heart transplant recipients," *The Lancet*, vol. 342, no. 8886-8887, pp. 1514–1516, 1993.

[6] D. Jagadeesh, B. A. Woda, J. Draper, and A. M. Evens, "Post transplant lymphoproliferative disorders: Risk, classification, and therapeutic recommendations," *Current Treatment Options in Oncology*, vol. 13, no. 1, pp. 122–136, 2012.

[7] R. V. Mathur, G. Kudesia, K. Suvarna, and W. McKane, "Fulminant post-transplant lymphoproliferative disorder presenting with lactic acidosis and acute liver failure," *Nephrology Dialysis Transplantation* , vol. 19, no. 7, pp. 1918–1920, 2004.

[8] T. Haque, J. A. Thomas, K. I. Falk et al., "Transmission of donor Epstein-Barr virus (EBV) in transplanted organs causes lymphoproliferative disease in EBV-seronegative recipients," *Journal of General Virology*, vol. 77, no. 6, pp. 1169–1172, 1996.

[9] F. C. Cabral, K. M. Krajewski, K. W. Kim, N. H. Ramaiya, and J. P. Jagannathan, "Peritoneal lymphomatosis: CT and PET/CT findings and how to differentiate between carcinomatosis and sarcomatosis," *Cancer Imaging*, vol. 13, no. 2, pp. 162–170, 2013.

[10] J. J. Glasheen and M. D. Sorensen, "Burkitt's lymphoma presenting with lactic acidosis and hypoglycemia - A case presentation," *Leukemia & Lymphoma*, vol. 46, no. 2, pp. 281–283, 2005.

[11] E. M. Sillos, J. L. Shenep, G. A. Burghen, C.-H. Pui, F. G. Behm, and J. T. Sandlund, "Lactic acidosis: A metabolic complication of hematologic malignancies: Case report and review of the literature," *Cancer*, vol. 92, no. 9, pp. 2237–2246, 2001.

[12] F. H. Chan, D. Carl, and L. J. Lyckholm, "Severe lactic acidosis in a patient with B-cell lymphoma: a case report and review of the literature," *Case Reports in Medicine*, vol. 2009, Article ID 534561, 6 pages, 2009.

[13] M. H. Weil and A. A. Afifi, "Experimental and clinical studies on lactate and pyruvate as indicators of the severity of acute circulatory failure (shock)," *Circulation*, vol. 41, no. 6, pp. 989–1001, 1970.

26

Aspergillus Tracheobronchitis Causing Subtotal Tracheal Stenosis in a Liver Transplant Recipient

Sonia Radunz, Carmen Kirchner, Jürgen Treckmann, Andreas Paul, and Fuat H. Saner

Department of General, Visceral, and Transplantation Surgery, Essen University Hospital, 45122 Essen, Germany

Correspondence should be addressed to Sonia Radunz; sonia.radunz@uk-essen.de

Academic Editors: C. F. Classen, S. Faenza, G. Forrest, S. Pinney, and G. Schlaf

Invasive aspergillosis is recognized as one of the most significant opportunistic infections after liver transplantation. Diagnosis of invasive aspergillosis in transplant recipients has been proven to be challenging, and optimal approach to the treatment of invasive aspergillosis is still controversial. We here present an unusual case of *Aspergillus* tracheobronchitis in the setting of liver transplantation. A 47-year-old female patient with persistent dry cough after liver transplantation developed respiratory insufficiency and was readmitted to the intensive care unit 55 days after liver transplantation. A CT scan revealed subtotal tracheal stenosis; bronchoscopy was performed, and extended white mucus coverings causative of the tracheal stenosis were removed. Microbiological assessment isolated *Aspergillus fumigatus*. The diagnosis was obstructive *Aspergillus* tracheobronchitis. The patient was started on a treatment of voriconazole 200 mg orally twice daily, adjusted to a trough level of 1–4 mg/L. For further airway management, a tracheal stent had to be implanted. The patient is alive and well 28 months after liver transplantation. Invasive aspergillosis should be considered a possible etiology in liver transplant patients presenting with unspecific symptoms such as persistent dry cough. Optimal strategies for improved and early diagnosis as well as prophylaxis need to be defined.

1. Introduction

Invasive aspergillosis is one of the most significant opportunistic infections in solid-organ transplant recipients, and its diagnosis carries a high mortality rate [1]. Early diagnosis of invasive aspergillosis has been proven to be challenging, and the optimal approach to the treatment of invasive aspergillosis is still controversial.

Aspergillus tracheobronchitis is a rare but severe form of invasive pulmonary aspergillosis in which the infection is entirely or predominantly confined to the tracheobronchial tree. Up to now, approximately 150 cases have been published in the English literature since 1985 [2]. Approximately 75% of patients with *Aspergillus* tracheobronchitis are immunocompromised. Of the reported cases, approximately 45% were solid-organ transplant recipients with a median time between transplantation and symptom onset of three months. Initial symptoms are generally deceptively mild. Patients often present with nonspecific respiratory symptoms for example, cough, dyspnea, stridor, or wheezing, and radiographic images frequently reveal no relevant findings. Delay of diagnosis and delayed initiation of targeted treatment remain critical for patient outcome. Approximately 30% of patients develop acute respiratory distress. Overall hospital mortality is approximately 40%.

Denning proposed a classification and a unified terminology consisting of three types of *Aspergillus* tracheobronchitis [3]. Ulcerative *Aspergillus* tracheobronchitis is characterized by focal, ulcerative processes with histological invasion of *Aspergillus* species. Pseudomembranous *Aspergillus* tracheobronchitis is characterized by a membrane containing *Aspergillus* species overlaying the mucosa of the entire tracheobronchial tree. Obstructive *Aspergillus* tracheobronchitis is characterized by thick mucous plugs containing *Aspergillus* species without relevant bronchial inflammation.

We describe here the case of a 47-year-old female patient suffering from persistent dry cough 40 days after liver transplantation. To our knowledge, this is the first report of *Aspergillus* tracheobronchitis in a liver transplant recipient, although random cases of *Aspergillus* tracheobronchitis in thoracic organ recipients and hematopoietic stem cell recipients have previously been reported.

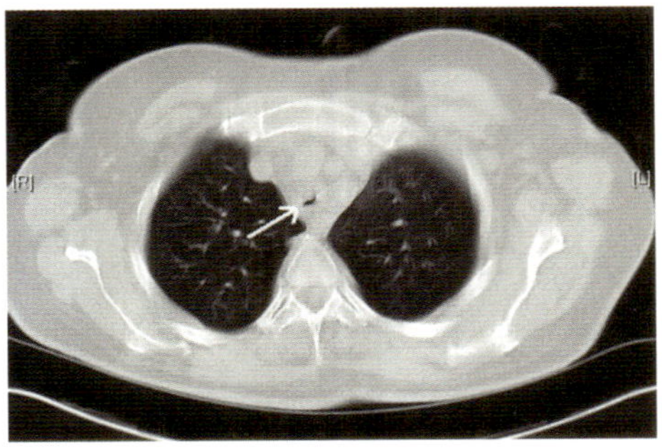

Figure 1: CT scan revealing tracheal stenosis.

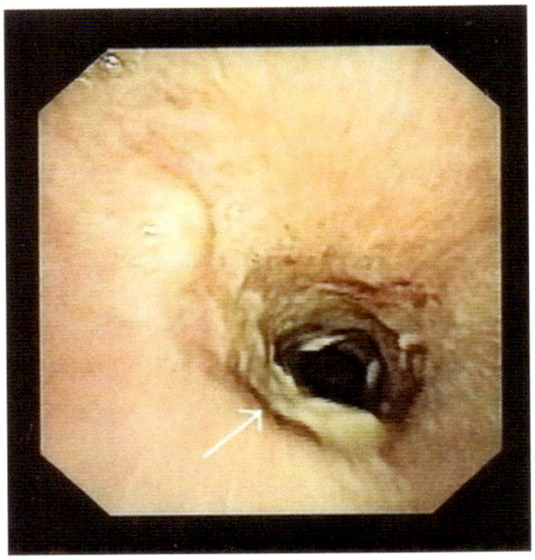

Figure 2: Bronchoscopy revealing extended white mucus coverings causative of the tracheal stenosis.

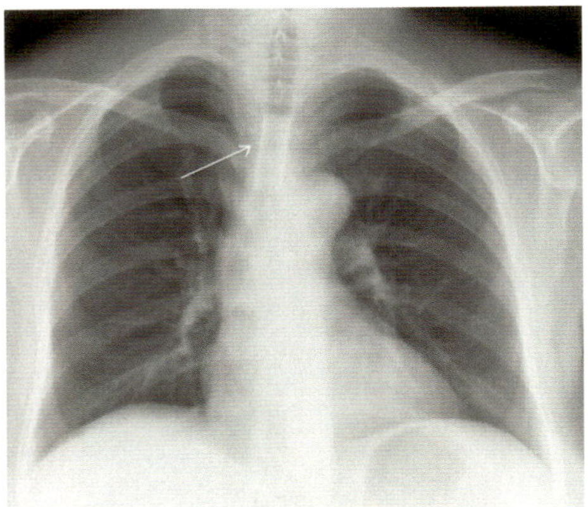

Figure 3: Chest X-ray with tracheal stent in place.

2. Case Presentation

A 47-year-old female patient was admitted to our department with acute-on-chronic liver failure in the setting of chronic hepatitis B and autoimmune hepatitis. Her past medical history included arterial hypertension and insulin-dependent diabetes mellitus type 2. Initially, she received supportive treatment for liver failure. Due to progressive liver failure resulting in a lab-MELD score of 32, she underwent orthotopic liver transplantation ten days after admission to the hospital. Because of primary nonfunction of the graft, the patient underwent retransplantation within two days.

Immunosuppression consisted of prednisolone 10 mg/kg intraoperatively. Postoperatively, the patient received triple immunosuppression, consisting of tacrolimus 0.1 mg/kg adjusted to a trough level of 8–10 ng/mL, prednisolone 20 mg tapered and withdrawn within six weeks, and mycophenolate mofetil 1 g orally twice daily. For prophylaxis of cytomegalovirus infection, valganciclovir was administered.

The postoperative course was complicated by dialysis-dependent acute renal failure in the setting of initial primary nonfunction of the graft. Due to expected long-term artificial ventilation, tracheotomy was performed on postoperative day (POD) 4. In the further clinical course, kidney function recovered, and dialysis treatment could be stopped. Twelve days after retransplantation, the patient was decannulated and four days later she was transferred to a surgical ward in good clinical condition.

The further postoperative course was unremarkable, except for a persistent dry cough. Regularly performed auscultation did not reveal any abnormal findings; especially no wheezing was detected. A chest X-ray showed no pathological results. Laboratory assessments revealed leucopenia, which was judged to be a side effect of mycophenolate mofetil. Mild laryngitis was diagnosed, and symptomatic treatment with dexpanthenol inhalation was started.

On POD 55, the patient developed respiratory insufficiency and was readmitted to the intensive care unit. Tracheal stenosis was diagnosed by CT scan (Figure 1). Emergency bronchoscopy was performed, and extended, thick, and white mucous coverings causative of the tracheal stenosis were removed (Figure 2). There were no signs of relevant bronchial inflammation. Microbiological assessments of the removed mucous plugs isolated *Aspergillus fumigatus*. The serum galactomannan index was <0.5. The diagnosis was obstructive *Aspergillus* tracheobronchitis.

The patient was started on a treatment of voriconazole 200 mg orally twice daily, adjusted to a trough level of 1–4 mg/L. Voriconazole was maintained for five months. In the setting of severe infection, mycophenolate mofetil was paused, and tacrolimus dosage was adjusted accordingly because of drug interaction to a trough level of 5–7 ng/mL [4].

The persistent dry cough subsided, and a follow-up bronchoscopy on POD 59 showed a clearance of the extended white mucus coverings. On POD 71, an emergency bronchoscopy had to be performed again due to inspiratory stridor. For further airway management, a tracheal stent was implanted because of residual tracheal stenosis (Figure 3). On POD 80, the patient was discharged in good clinical condition. Twenty-eight months after liver transplantation, the patient is alive and well. The tracheal stent was removed after five months. For follow-up, the patient is seen in our outpatient clinic. The patient is routinely treated endoscopically for ischemic-type biliary lesion.

3. Discussion

Infections are a common cause of morbidity and mortality in solid-organ transplant recipients. Invasive aspergillosis is recognized as one of the most significant opportunistic infections in these patients. *Aspergillus spp.* have been isolated from approximately 9%–34% of patients with invasive fungal infection after liver transplantation [1, 5]. Risk factors for invasive aspergillosis in liver transplant recipients include pretransplant hepatic failure, primary graft dysfunction or nonfunction, retransplantation, dialysis treatment, and high transfusion requirement [6].

Aspergillus tracheobronchitis is a rare finding with deceptively mild symptoms and absence of radiographic abnormalities; therefore, early diagnosis is challenging. The reported incidence is much higher in lung transplant recipients, and so far no cases have been reported after liver, pancreas, or intestine transplantation [2, 7].

Besides a persistent dry cough, there were no findings suspicious of any infection in our patient. The differential diagnosis of persistent dry cough is broad and includes upper respiratory tract infection ("common cold"), allergic asthma, psychogenic cough, drug side effects (ACE inhibitors), (atypical) pneumonia, and lung cancer. In our patient, possible causative allergens were eliminated, and there were no clinical signs of infection or malignancy. Therefore, simply symptomatic treatment was initiated. A final diagnosis of invasive aspergillosis was only possible when the patient became severely symptomatic, and microbiological assessment of samples collected during bronchoscopy revealed *Aspergillus fumigatus*.

The galactomannan test failed to demonstrate invasive aspergillosis in our patient. The definitive role of the galactomannan test in early diagnosis of invasive aspergillosis without lung parenchyma involvement still has to be established. The galactomannan test was evaluated in hematopoietic stem cell patients with conflicting results [8–12]. In a study with lung transplant patients, the test detected only 29% of patients with invasive aspergillosis and failed to detect patients with *Aspergillus* tracheobronchitis [13]. A subsequent study in lung transplant patients indicated that a higher cutoff for the galactomannan antigen for aspergillosis of 1 in the bronchoalveolar lavage increases the specificity to 98% [14].

An optimal approach to the treatment of invasive aspergillosis is still controversial. Voriconazole is now regarded as the drug of choice for primary treatment of invasive aspergillosis, a recommendation endorsed by the Infectious Diseases Society of America (IDSA) for the treatment of invasive aspergillosis [15]. In a prospective randomized trial, the successful outcome and survival rate in the voriconazole group were significantly higher as compared with the amphotericin B deoxycholate group. Also, voriconazole-treated patients had fewer side effects, except for transient visual disturbances [16]. Caspofungin is currently the only echinocandin which is approved by the FDA for treatment of aspergillosis. Caspofungin was successfully used as first-line therapy in heart-lung transplant patients and as salvage therapy in invasive aspergillosis as a single agent [17, 18]. Posaconazole, a new extended-spectrum triazole, was successfully applied as rescue treatment for patients refractory or intolerant to conventional therapy in a prospective open-label study [19].

Increasingly, antifungal combination therapy is used despite limited data existence with regard to the clinical efficacy of combination therapy for invasive aspergillosis. Perea et al. investigated the *in vitro* interaction of caspofungin and voriconazole and their results indicated that a combination of caspofungin and voriconazole might be more effective against infections caused by *Aspergillus spp.* as compared with single treatment [20]. In a clinical trial with solid-organ transplant recipients with proven invasive aspergillosis, including liver transplant patients, Singh et al. prospectively assessed a combination therapy consisting of caspofungin and voriconazole in comparison with a historical control group which was treated with liposomal amphotericin B [21]. The overall 90-day survival rate was not different in both groups, but patients infected with *Aspergillus fumigatus* and patients with renal failure showed a significant better 90-day survival. Therefore, a combination of voriconazole and caspofungin might be considered as preferable therapy for certain subsets of organ transplant recipients with invasive aspergillosis. The latest IDSA guidelines recommend combination therapy as salvage treatment only [22].

Initial antifungal therapy in our patient included voriconazole alone. Reduction in immunosuppression and maintenance therapy with voriconazole as well as interventional therapy by tracheal stenting resulted in a favorable outcome. Final follow-up bronchoscopy and follow-up CT scan showed a significant decrease of the tracheal stenosis.

In conclusion, we need to be aware of *Aspergillus* tracheobronchitis as a potential diagnosis in transplant recipients and other immunocompromised patients with nonspecific respiratory symptoms and few radiographic abnormalities. Future studies should address optimal strategies for improved and early diagnosis as well as standardized treatment. Antifungal prophylaxis in high-risk liver transplant recipients may be warranted.

References

[1] S. Gabardi, D. W. Kubiak, A. K. Chandraker, and S. G. Tullius, "Invasive fungal infections and antifungal therapies in solid organ transplant recipients," *Transplant International*, vol. 20, no. 12, pp. 993–1015, 2007.

[2] M. Fernandez-Ruiz, J. T. Silva, R. San-Juan et al., "*Aspergillus* tracheobronchitis: report of 8 cases and review of the literature," *Medicine*, vol. 91, no. 5, pp. 261–273, 2012.

[3] D. W. Denning, "Commentary: unusual manifestations of aspergillosis," *Thorax*, vol. 50, no. 7, pp. 812–813, 1995.

[4] R. Venkataramanan, S. Zang, T. Gayowski, and N. Singh, "Voriconazole inhibition of the metabolism of tacrolimus in a liver transplant recipient and in human liver microsomes," *Antimicrobial Agents and Chemotherapy*, vol. 46, no. 9, pp. 3091–3093, 2002.

[5] M. J. Pacholczyk, B. Lagiewska, W. Lisik, D. Wasiak, and A. Chmura, "Invasive fungal infections following liver transplantation—risk factors, incidence and outcome," *Annals of Transplantation*, vol. 16, no. 3, pp. 14–16, 2011.

[6] M. Rosenhagen, R. Feldhues, J. Schmidt, T. Hoppe-Tichy, and H. K. Geiss, "A risk profile for invasive aspergillosis in liver transplant recipients," *Infection*, vol. 37, no. 4, pp. 313–319, 2009.

[7] A. Ramos, J. Segovia, M. Gómez-Bueno et al., "Pseudomembranous aspergillus tracheobronchitis in a heart transplant recipient: case report," *Transplant Infectious Disease*, vol. 12, no. 1, pp. 60–63, 2010.

[8] R. Herbrecht, V. Letscher-Bru, C. Oprea et al., "*Aspergillus* galactomannan detection in the diagnosis of invasive aspergillosis in cancer patients," *Journal of Clinical Oncology*, vol. 20, no. 7, pp. 1898–1906, 2002.

[9] J. Maertens, K. Theunissen, E. Verbeken et al., "Prospective clinical evaluation of lower cut-offs for galactomannan detection in adult neutropenic cancer patients and haematological stem cell transplant recipients," *British Journal of Haematology*, vol. 126, no. 6, pp. 852–860, 2004.

[10] J. Maertens, K. Theunissen, G. Verhoef, and J. Van Eldere, "False-positive *Aspergillus* galactomannan antigen test results," *Clinical Infectious Diseases*, vol. 39, no. 2, pp. 289–290, 2004.

[11] M. Siemann, M. Koch-Dörfler, and M. Gaude, "False-positive results in premature infants with the Platelia *Aspergillus* sandwich enzyme-linked immunosorbent assay," *Mycoses*, vol. 41, no. 9-10, pp. 373–377, 1998.

[12] P. E. Verweij, E. C. Dompeling, J. P. Donnelly, A. V. M. B. Schattenberg, and J. F. G. M. Meis, "Serial monitoring of *Aspergillus* antigen in the early diagnosis of invasive aspergillosis. Preliminary investigations with two examples," *Infection*, vol. 25, no. 2, pp. 86–89, 1997.

[13] S. Husain, E. J. Kwak, A. Obman et al., "Prospective assessment of PlateliaŮ *Aspergillus* galactomannan antigen for the diagnosis of invasive aspergillosis in lung transplant recipients," *American Journal of Transplantation*, vol. 4, no. 5, pp. 796–802, 2004.

[14] S. Husain, D. L. Paterson, S. M. Studer et al., "*Aspergillus* galactomannan antigen in the bronchoalveolar lavage fluid for the diagnosis of invasive aspergillosis in lung transplant recipients," *Transplantation*, vol. 83, no. 10, pp. 1330–1336, 2007.

[15] P. G. Pappas, C. A. Kauffman, D. Andes et al., "Clinical practice guidelines for the management of candidiasis: 2009 update by the Infectious Diseases Society of America," *Clinical Infectious Diseases*, vol. 48, no. 5, pp. 503–535, 2009.

[16] R. Herbrecht, D. W. Denning, T. F. Patterson et al., "Voriconazole versus amphotericin B for primary therapy of invasive aspergillosis," *The New England Journal of Medicine*, vol. 347, no. 6, pp. 408–415, 2002.

[17] J. Groetzner, I. Kaczmarek, T. Wittwer et al., "Caspofungin as first-line therapy for the treatment of invasive aspergillosis after thoracic organ transplantation," *Journal of Heart and Lung Transplantation*, vol. 27, no. 1, pp. 1–6, 2008.

[18] M. R. Carby, M. E. Hodson, and N. R. Banner, "Refractory pulmonary aspergillosis treated with caspofungin after heart-lung transplantation," *Transplant International*, vol. 17, no. 9, pp. 545–548, 2004.

[19] T. J. Walsh, I. Raad, T. F. Patterson et al., "Treatment of invasive aspergillosis with posaconazole in patients who are refractory to or intolerant of conventional therapy: an externally controlled trial," *Clinical Infectious Diseases*, vol. 44, no. 1, pp. 2–12, 2007.

[20] S. Perea, G. Gonzalez, A. W. Fothergill, W. R. Kirkpatrick, M. G. Rinaldi, and T. F. Patterson, "In vitro interaction of caspofungin acetate with voriconazole against clinical isolates of *Aspergillus* spp," *Antimicrobial Agents and Chemotherapy*, vol. 46, no. 9, pp. 3039–3041, 2002.

[21] N. Singh, A. P. Limaye, G. Forrest et al., "Combination of voriconazole and caspofungin as primary therapy for invasive aspergillosis in solid organ transplant recipients: a prospective, multicenter, observational study," *Transplantation*, vol. 81, no. 3, pp. 320–326, 2006.

[22] T. J. Walsh, E. J. Anaissie, D. W. Denning et al., "Treatment of aspergillosis: clinical practice guidelines of the infectious diseases society of America," *Clinical Infectious Diseases*, vol. 46, no. 3, pp. 327–360, 2008.

27

Replacement of Vena Cava up to the Right Atrium during Living Donor Liver Transplantation for *Echinococcus alveolaris*

Fahri Yetişir,[1,2] S. Murad Dogan,[2,3] Ruslan Mamedov,[2,4] Cuneyt Kayaalp,[2] and Sezayi Yilmaz[2]

[1] *General Surgery Department, Atatürk Research and Training Hospital, Turkey*
[2] *Liver Transplantation Institute, Inonu University, Malatya, Turkey*
[3] *General Surgery Department, İzmir Research and Training Hospital, Turkey*
[4] *Azerbaijan Medical University, Baku, Azerbaijan*

Correspondence should be addressed to Fahri Yetişir; drfahriyetisir@hotmail.com

Academic Editor: Giuseppe Orlando

Management of advanced stage of *Echinococcus alveolaris* is a very difficult procedure. Surgical treatment like resection and liver transplantation is accepted procedure nowadays. Here we presented a case report of *Echinococcus alveolaris* which invaded the inferior vena cava up to the right atrium and surrounding tissues. This patient underwent living donor liver transplantation with replacement of inferior vena cava up to the right atrium with cryopreserved cadaveric aortic graft. This procedure is very difficult but it is a life-saving chance for patients in advanced cases of *Echinococcus alveolaris*.

1. Introduction

Human alveolar *Echinococcus* is a potentially fatal, chronic, and progressive disease [1–3]. The treatment of EA is very difficult, because patients are coming to surgical centers with advanced stages of disease. In these cases partial liver resection can be performed in only 35% of patients [3]. Liver transplantation is only life-saving treatment of advanced stages of *Echinococcus alveolaris* [4]. Living donor liver transplantation (LDLT) has been also used to treat advanced stage EA, because of the rarity of cadaveric liver donor. In most cases EA may invade surrounding tissues including major vessel. Because of that, in these cases resection and replacement of major vessel are often unavoidable. That could force the surgeon to perform complicated surgical technique [5].

Herein we report a case of a patient with advanced stage EA invading the surrounding tissues and IVC up to the right atrium. This patient was treated with living donor liver transplantation with replacement of inferior vena cava up to the right atrium with cryopreserved cadaveric aortic graft.

2. Case Report

A 25-year-old young man was referred to our center with serious abdominal asit, lower extremities edemas. Indirect echinococcal haemagglutination test was positive and INR level was 1.7. Abdominal computerized tomography (CT) showed that the liver which was compressing the other abdominal content was occupying the entire abdomen and pelvis, in size of (38 × 29 cm). A large mass in the liver was compressing and invading the inferior vena cava and completely obstructing retrohepatic IVC (Figure 1).

Because of advanced stage EA (wide spread parasitic dissemination and liver deficiency), living donor liver transplantation was chosen as the method of definitive treatment and the patient's brother decided to be the donor.

Benz incision was used. Large liver with alveolar disease extended to pelvis and had strong adhesions with the surrounding tissues, anterior abdominal wall, right hemidiaphragm, colon and small intestine, and the retrohepatic part of inferior vena cava up to the right atrium that made recipient hepatectomy more difficult than other cirrhotic livers

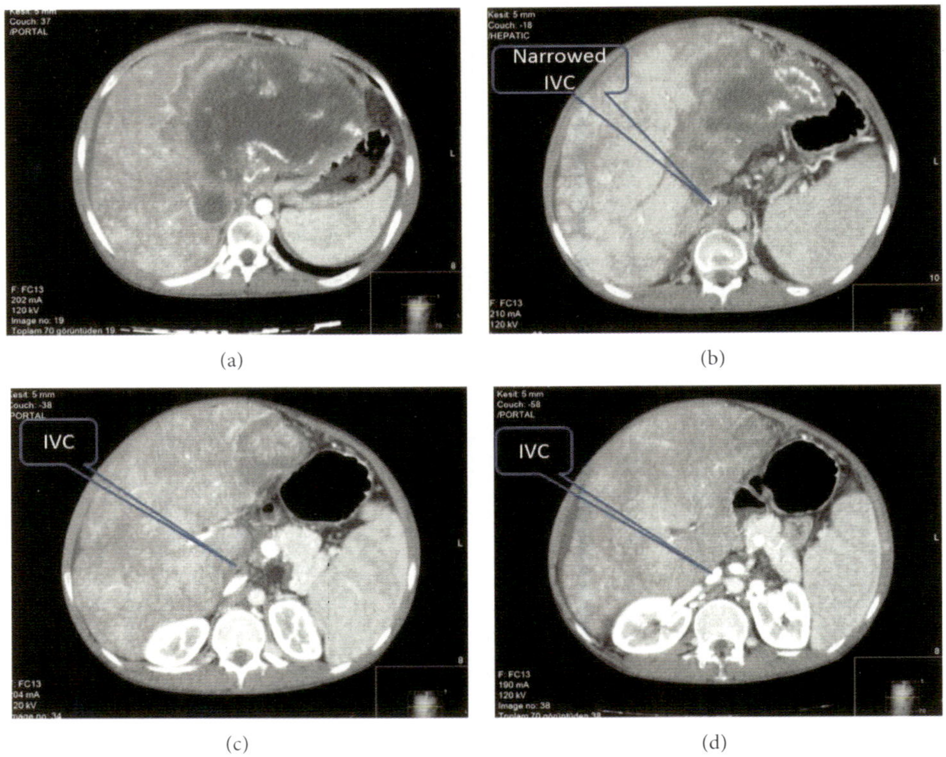

Figure 1: CT view of preoperative liver with (a) large mass filling almost all liver and IVC is nonvisible. (b) Invasion and compression of IVC by EA are seen. (c) Compression to surrounding tissues and organs by EA. (d) Compression and invasion of IVC extending up to renal vein level.

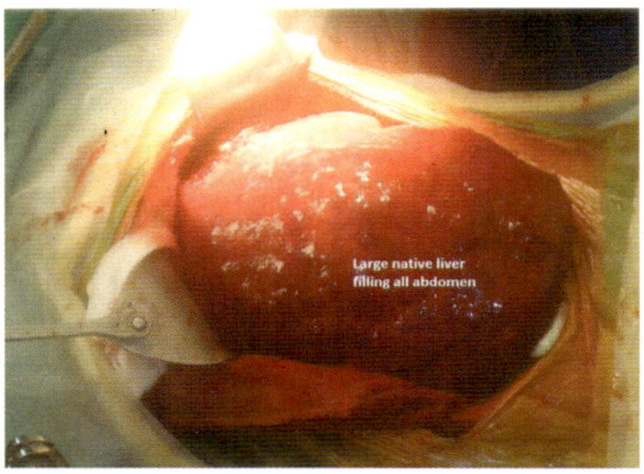

Figure 2: Large native liver filling the entire abdomen is seen.

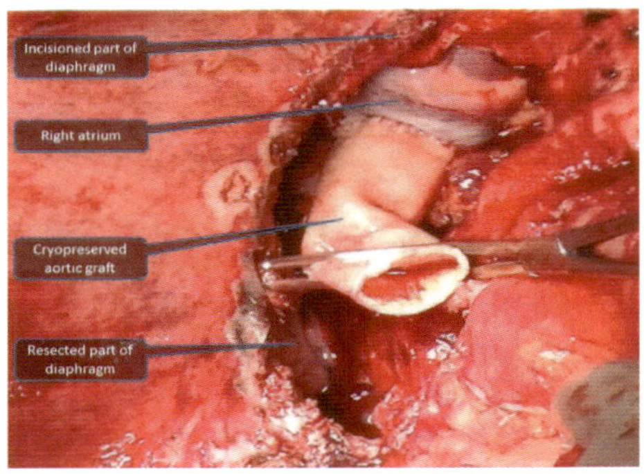

Figure 3: The view after diaphragm resection and the anastomosis between right atrium and first part of cadaveric aortic graft is seen.

(Figure 2). In particular, strong invasion to the diaphragm and inferior vena cava extending in cephalic destination forces us to perform caval vein resection until right atrium and resection a left suprahepatic part of diaphragm (Figure 3). After IVC resection deposits of EA were seen on upper end of IVC, upper clamp was reclamped from one more centimeter upper and reexcision of invaded part of IVC was performed. 4-5 minutes after this procedure, a quick decline in arterial blood pressure occurred and hart bate on left diaphragmatic side had not been felt. After conforming hemopericardium, pericardiotomy was performed in seconds. The hematoma was evacuated and reclamped from atrium. After all of them hemodynamic status of patient improved.

For performing this procedure, we needed to make a curvilinear incision through the tendinous part of the diaphragm near the excisioned part to get expose the pericardium. Replacement of inferior vena cava was done from the suprarenal part of IVC up to the right atrium by cryopreserved cadaveric aortic graft with end-to-end anastomosis (Figures 3 and 4). Defect in diaphragm was repaired with using mesh (Figures 5 and 6).

Donor's right lobe of liver with middle hepatic vein was transplanted and graft/recipient weight ratio was more

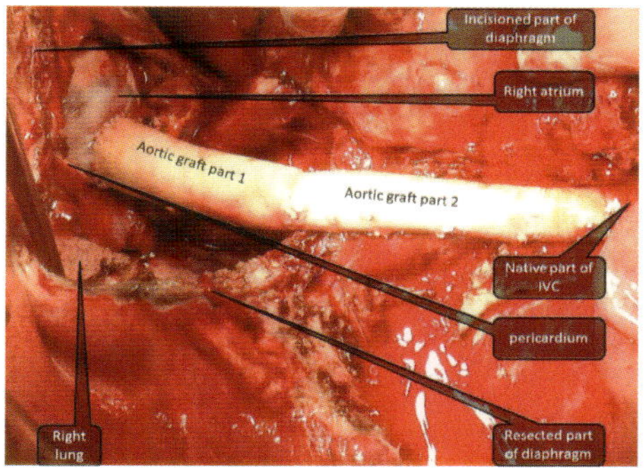

Figure 4: Incised pericardium and total replacement of retrohepatic part of vena cava (from renal vein to right atrium) are seen.

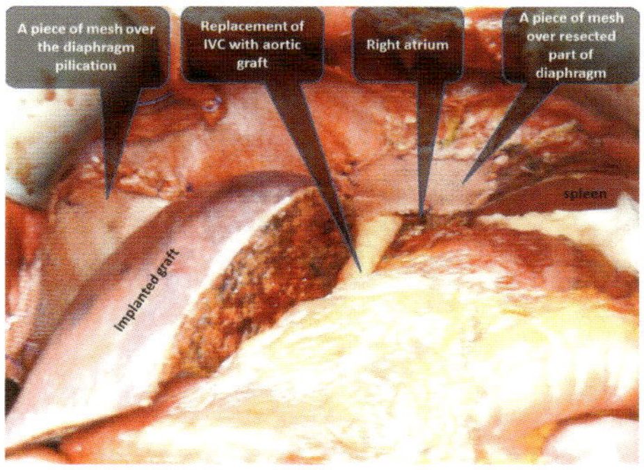

Figure 5: Final view after implantation. Diaphragm plication with mesh is seen.

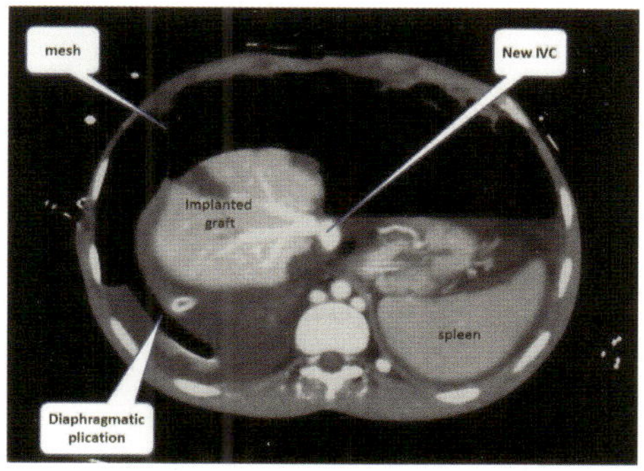

Figure 6: CT view after living donor liver transplantation. Diaphragmatic plication and new IVC are seen.

than 1%. Venous and arterial reconstructions were carried out with a standard method. During back-table procedure, we used cryopreserved venous graft surrounding middle and right hepatic veins with aim to make all-in-one orifice. This provided us an easier and large anastomosis with new vena cava. End-to-end portoportal anastomosis was done. Arterial anastomosis was performed with ×6.5 surgical loupes by separated sutures. Duct-to-duct biliary anastomosis was performed, with an external tube replacing through the cystic duct. Because of the large space after removing of native liver, the newly created arteries and portal vein was under tension. For resolving this problem we used retrohepatic part of diaphragm plication with mesh (Figures 5 and 6). He was discharged on day 25 after operation.

3. Discussion

Despite the available multiple treatments for advanced stage EA including medical therapy [6], the surgical technique remains the only radical treatment for this pathology. Radical surgical treatment like liver transplantation is more preferable for treatment of EA, because palliative resection does not offer advantages when compared with conservative treatment [3]. The more that palliative surgery is often done because of the impossibility of complete removal of the parasite due to the spread it on the irresectable structures [5, 7].

There are several reports for liver transplantation in patients with EA, especially from endemic regions. Thus in 2009 Moray et al. reported two cases of liver transplantation for advanced EA and one of them had operation with resection and replacement of IVC with PTFE graft [4]. In our center previously, we performed resection and replacement of IVC during living donor liver transplantation to treat Budd-Chiari syndrome associated with hydatid cyst. Retrohepatic part of IVC in this patient was also replaced with cadaveric aortic graft [5, 8]. This report is the third case of complicated stage EA, which was treated by living donor liver transplantation. The difference in this case from our previous case was extending invasion of IVC until the right atrium. There are some reports that describe surgical technique for replacement of IVC until the right atrium. Thus, in 2012 Wise et al. presented a case of a patient with giant primary synovial sarcoma with invasion to the inferior vena cava extending to the right atrium with caval reconstruction under cardiopulmonary bypass and circulatory arrest. They performed bovine pericardial patch reconstruction of the IVC [9].

In 2013 Mancuso et al. reported a case of a patient with Budd-Chiari syndrome with replacement of IVC including intrapericardial part with a caval homograft [10].

We used this technique for management of advanced stage of EA during living donor liver transplantation and we did not need to perform this operation under cardiopulmonary bypass and circulatory arrest. Additionally for resolving tension of anastomoses we made diaphragm plication with mesh. According to our knowledge, these are new techniques for management of advanced stage EA.

Ex vivo liver resection and autotransplantation have been used successfully in suitable EA cases, but in our case, there was no disease-free, healthy liver tissue present to be used in autotransplantation.

Although some authors think that shaping of the hepatic veins of the graft and reconstruction with right atrium without reconstruction of retrohepatic vena cava would not be necessary when the collateral circulation was sufficient for compensation, we preferred to reconstruct retrohepatic IVC.

4. Conclusion

Living donor liver transplantation with caval replacement up to the right atrium is a very difficult operation but it is a life-saving chance for patients with EA invading IVC up to the atrium.

References

[1] E. Moreno-Gonzalez, C. L. Segurola, M. A. G. Urena et al., "Liver transplantation for *Echinococcus granulosus* hydatid disease," *Transplantation*, vol. 58, no. 7, pp. 797–800, 1994.

[2] S. Bresson-Hadni, S. Koch, J. P. Miguet et al., "Indications and results of liver transplantation for *Echinococcus* alveolar infection: an overview," *Langenbeck's Archives of Surgery*, vol. 388, no. 4, pp. 231–238, 2003.

[3] G. Nunnari, M. R. Pinzone, S. Gruttadauria et al., "Hepatic echinococcosis: clinical and therapeutic aspects," *World Journal of Gastroenterology*, vol. 18, no. 13, pp. 1448–1458, 2012.

[4] G. Moray, R. Shahbazov, S. Sevmis et al., "Liver transplantation in management of alveolar echinococcosis: two case reports," *Transplantation Proceedings*, vol. 41, no. 7, pp. 2936–2938, 2009.

[5] I. Sakçak, C. Eriş, A. Ölmez, C. Kayaalp, and S. Yılmaz, "Replacement of the vena cava with aortic graft for living donor liver transplantation in Budd-Chiari syndrome associated with hydatid cyst surgery: a case report," *Transplantation Proceedings*, vol. 44, no. 6, pp. 1757–1758, 2012.

[6] B. Geramizadeh, S. Nikeghbalian, and S. A. Malekhosseini, "Alveolar echinococcosis of the liver: report of three cases from different geographic areas of iran," *Hepatitis Monthly*, vol. 12, no. 9, Article ID e6143, 2012.

[7] K. Buttenschoen, D. Carli Buttenschoen, B. Gruener et al., "Long-term experience on surgical treatment of alveolar echinococcosis," *Langenbeck's Archives of Surgery*, vol. 394, no. 4, pp. 689–698, 2009.

[8] R. Mamedov, N. Novruzov, A. Baskiran et al., "Living donor liver transplantation with replacement of vena cava for *Echinococcus alveolaris*: a case report," *International Journal of Surgery Case Reports*, vol. 5, no. 3, pp. 169–171, 2014.

[9] K. B. Wise, S. M. Said, C. J. Clark et al., "Resection of a giant primary synovial sarcoma of the inferior vena cava extending into the right atrium with caval reconstruction under cardiopulmonary bypass and circulatory arrest," *Perspectives in Vascular Surgery and Endovascular Therapy*, vol. 24, no. 2, pp. 95–101, 2012.

[10] A. Mancuso, L. Martinelli, L. De Carlis et al., "A caval homograft for Budd-Chiari syndrome due to inferior vena cava obstruction," *World Journal of Hepatology*, vol. 5, no. 5, pp. 292–295, 2013.

Hepatic Epithelioid Hemangioendothelioma Presenting as an Enlarging Vascular Lesion within the Spleen

Juliet A. Emamaullee,[1] Klaudia Nowak,[2] Marla Beach,[2] Julinor Bacani,[2] and A. M. James Shapiro[3]

[1]*Department of Surgery, University of Southern California, Los Angeles, CA, USA*
[2]*Department of Anatomic Pathology, University of Alberta, Edmonton, AB, Canada*
[3]*Department of Surgery, University of Alberta, Edmonton, AB, Canada*

Correspondence should be addressed to Juliet A. Emamaullee; juliet.emamaullee@med.usc.edu

Academic Editor: Federica Meloni

Epithelioid hemangioendothelioma (EHE) is a rare vascular neoplasm with variable malignant potential that most often presents within the liver. Many patients present with bilobar or extrahepatic disease, and the current treatment paradigm involves liver transplantation, with favorable long term results. Up to 25% of patients are diagnosed incidentally following imaging for other indications, and confirmation of diagnosis requires histologic analysis, as there are no classical imaging features to distinguish hepatic EHE (HEHE) from other solid hepatic lesions. Here we describe a case of microscopic HEHE that was diagnosed following splenectomy for an enlarging vascular tumor within the spleen. Due to the unexpected diagnosis of EHE within the spleen and coexisting but stable appearing liver hemangiomata, a left hepatic lobectomy was performed. Explant histology revealed benign hemangiomata and diffuse, microscopic HEHE. The patient ultimately underwent liver transplantation. HEHE can be a challenging diagnosis, and this case emphasizes that any enlarging vascular lesion, even within the spleen, should prompt a high index of suspicion for HEHE in the setting of known hemangiomata.

1. Introduction

Epithelioid hemangioendothelioma (EHE) is a rare vascular neoplasm that occurs more often in women than men and usually arises within the liver, but can also present within other tissues including lung, bone, or peritoneum [1]. The behavior of these tumors is variable, ranging from a relatively benign clinical course to rapidly progressive, metastatic disease [1–3]. More than 25% of patients are asymptomatic and diagnosed after incidental finding of a liver lesion [4]. The mainstay of treatment for hepatic epithelioid hemangioendothelioma (HEHE) is surgical resection or transplantation, and excellent long term outcomes have been reported [4, 5]. Typically, HEHE presents with bulky tumors, which may be multifocal and/or bilateral, and >30% of patients may present with extrahepatic disease [4]. In the present case report, we describe a patient with multiple benign, classical appearing hepatic hemangiomata and an atypical, enlarging vascular lesion within the spleen which lead to the diagnosis of microscopic HEHE and ultimately liver transplantation.

2. Case Report

A 49-year-old woman with no significant past medical history presented to her family physician in 2014 with vague right upper quadrant abdominal pain. Her vital signs were stable, her abdominal exam was unremarkable, and she had no palpable organomegaly. Her hemoglobin, platelet count, white cell count, liver function, and renal function tests were all within normal limits. She underwent abdominal ultrasound, which demonstrated multiple vascular lesions within the liver, with the appearance of hemangiomata. Her abdominal pain had since resolved, but due to the ultrasound findings, she received an MRI of the abdomen. This study

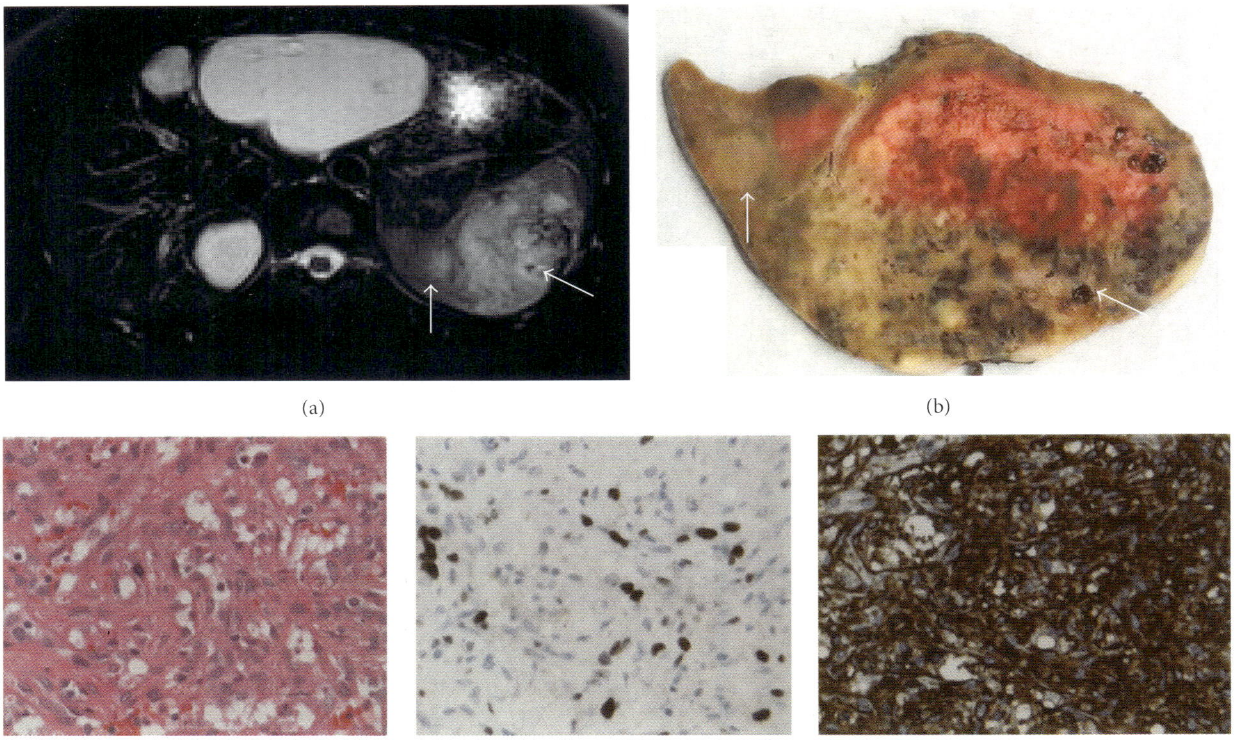

(a) (b) (c) (d) (e)

Figure 1: Epithelioid hemangioendothelioma arising within the spleen. (a) Axial MRI scan showing liver hemangiomata (white masses) and vascular splenic lesions. (b) Gross specimen following splenectomy. White arrows correspond to imaging findings in (a). (c) H&E staining demonstrated a highly cellular, atypical complex vascular lesion with rare mitotic figures. (d) MIB-1 staining illustrates a proliferation index of approximately 10%. (e) Immunophenotyping with CD31.

demonstrated multiple liver lesions with enhancement patterns consistent with hemangiomata. There was also a 4.6 × 3.1 × 2.8 cm vascular lesion within the body of the spleen that enhanced with features consistent of hemangioma, although it was less bright than the liver hemangiomata. She remained asymptomatic. These lesions were followed with serial MRI studies, and while the liver lesions remained stable in size and enhancement, follow-up imaging at two years demonstrated an interval enlargement in the splenic lesion to 7.1 × 5.0 × 6.3 cm, with four additional new nodules within the spleen (Figure 1(a), white arrows). The dominant lesion had heterogenous enhancement compared to the liver hemangiomata (white lesions within the liver in Figure 1(a)).

Due to the increase in size, new nodules, and heterogeneous enhancement, she was referred for surgical resection. She underwent an uncomplicated open splenectomy in September 2016. Gross pathology demonstrated an 8.0 × 5.8 × 4.5 cm lesion with a mottled appearance and focal hemorrhagic tissue which nearly replaced the splenic parenchyma (Figure 1(b)), which was consistent with preoperative imaging (Figure 1(a); white arrows correlate to similar areas in gross specimen in Figure 1(b)). Histological assessment demonstrated a highly cellular, atypical complex vascular lesion with rare mitotic figures on H&E staining (Figure 1(c)). MIB-1 staining illustrates a proliferation index of approximately 10% (Figure 1(d)). Immunophenotyping with CD31 (Figure 1(e)) and CD34 (not shown) confirmed the presence of vascular endothelium. Taken together, the morphological and immunophenotypic findings are consistent with a diagnosis of epithelioid hemangioendothelioma (EHE). Given this diagnosis, and the previously identified hepatic vascular lesions, she underwent a left hepatic lobectomy and nonanatomic resection of a segment 8 lesion to rule out HEHE in November 2016. Final pathology showed benign hemangiomata in the areas observed on imaging and multifocal, microscopic EHE within the liver parenchyma which was not appreciated on multiple previous imaging studies. Based on these findings, she was referred for liver transplantation. She was carefully evaluated by our multidisciplinary team and referred to medical oncology for consultation. She underwent full body imaging including a CT chest, abdomen, and pelvis, as well as abdominal and pelvis MRI, which did not demonstrate any new lesions or evidence of extrahepatic disease. The collective opinion based on multidisciplinary assessment was to proceed with liver transplantation as the best option for R0 resection. She ultimately underwent liver transplantation in early 2017, with evidence of multifocal HEHE in the explanted liver (Figure 2). There were no concerning lesions, nodules, or lymph nodes noted at the time of transplant, and no malignant periportal lymph nodes were identified within the explant. She received induction immunosuppression with basiliximab and maintenance therapy with tacrolimus and

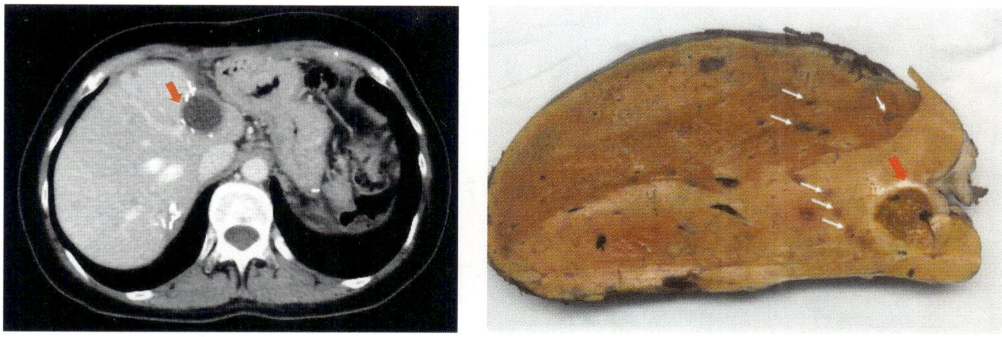

(a) (b)

FIGURE 2: Epithelioid hemangioendothelioma in explant following liver transplantation. (a) Axial CT scan showing liver hemangioma (dark mass) and no obvious additional lesions. Red arrow indicates known residual hemangioma following left lobectomy. (b) Gross specimen following hepatectomy and liver transplantation. White arrows indicate multifocal EHE which was not apparent on preoperative imaging studies. Red arrow indicates corresponding lesion from (a), which demonstrated microscopic EHE within hemangioma on microscopic examination (not pictured).

mycophenolate mofetil, which is the standard of care for most patients in our center. She has had an uncomplicated postoperative course with no evidence of recurrent EHE on follow-up imaging, with more than one year of follow-up to date.

3. Discussion

HEHE can be challenging to diagnose and also be a management dilemma, particularly in patients with multiorgan involvement. The case reported here is unique in that it appears as though the primary tumor developed within the spleen, with microscopic liver involvement. Historically, patients with multifocal disease have a more aggressive course and may not be considered good transplant candidates, although more recent data suggests that, with metastasectomy, these patients can have good outcomes [4]. It was somewhat surprising to diagnose microscopic HEHE in this patient, who had stable benign hepatic hemangiomata on imaging over more than two years. There are no pathognomonic imaging characteristics for EHE, and thus the gold standard for diagnosis is microscopic analysis. Histological features of EHE include high cellularity, rare mitoses, and evidence of endothelial markers including CD31 and CD34 [1]. Our group has previously reported vascular endothelial growth factor (VEGF) expression in EHE as well [6]. The mainstay of treatment for EHE remains surgical resection or liver transplantation, with excellent long term disease-free recurrence in most patients, at least within the context of HEHE [2, 4–6]. The present case illustrates that any enlarging vascular lesion, even within the spleen, should be referred for surgical evaluation and resection as it may represent a unique presentation of HEHE.

References

[1] A. Mehrabi, A. Kashfi, H. Fonouni et al., "Primary malignant hepatic epithelioid hemangioendothelioma: a comprehensive review of the literature with emphasis on the surgical therapy," *Cancer*, vol. 107, no. 9, pp. 2108–2121, 2006.

[2] A. Mehrabi, K. Hoffmann, K. H. Weiss et al., "Long term follow up after resection emphasizes the role of surgery in primary hepatic epithelioid hemangioendothelioma," *Annals of Medicine and Surgery*, vol. 11, pp. 1–4, 2016.

[3] H. R. Makhlouf, K. G. Ishak, and Z. D. Goodman, "Epithelioid hemangioendothelioma of the liver: a clinicopathologic study of 137 cases," *Cancer*, vol. 85, no. 3, pp. 562–582, 1999.

[4] T. E. Grotz, D. Nagorney, J. Donohue et al., "Hepatic epithelioid haemangioendothelioma: is transplantation the only treatment option?" *HPB*, vol. 12, no. 8, pp. 546–553, 2010.

[5] J. Cardinal, M. E. de Vera, J. W. Marsh et al., "Treatment of hepatic epithelioid hemangioendothelioma: a single-institution experience with 25 cases," *JAMA Surgery*, vol. 144, no. 11, pp. 1035–1039, 2009.

[6] J. A. Emamaullee, R. Edgar, C. Toso et al., "Vascular endothelial growth factor expression in hepatic epithelioid hemangioendothelioma: implications for treatment and surgical management," *Liver Transplantation*, vol. 16, no. 2, pp. 191–197, 2010.

A Symptomatic De Novo Pheochromocytoma 23 Years after Liver Transplantation

M. I. Montenovo,[1] F. G. Jalikis,[2] B. Hoch,[2] and R. Bakthavatsalam[1]

[1]*Division of Transplantation, Department of Surgery, University of Washington, Seattle, WA, USA*
[2]*Department of Anatomic Pathology, University of Washington, Seattle, WA, USA*

Correspondence should be addressed to M. I. Montenovo; martinm@uw.edu

Academic Editor: Marian Klinger

We report a case of subacute onset of headaches and tremors with a newly discovered adrenal pheochromocytoma 23 years after an orthotopic liver transplantation and provide a review of the scarce literature regarding endocrine malignancies in liver transplant recipients. We describe the clinical presentation, diagnostic work-up, and management. This is the second case report in the literature of a de novo pheochromocytoma after solid organ transplantation. It shows that new-onset common symptoms in transplant recipients are always challenging and deserve a very thorough work-up until the cause of the symptoms is elucidated. A broad differential diagnosis should always be included in the study of any abnormalities in this patient population.

1. Introduction

Headaches are a very common symptom in adult liver transplant recipients. Immunosuppressant medications must always be considered a possible etiology [1] when assessing the origins of this symptom in transplant patients.

In addition to having an increased risk of developing migraines, malignancy in recipients has emerged as a prevailing cause of late morbidity and mortality [2]. Skin cancer and posttransplant lymphoproliferative disease comprise the most common malignancies after liver transplantation, followed by other solid organ cancers. Endocrine tumors are exceedingly rare in this population. Only one case of de novo pheochromocytoma has been previously reported in a liver transplant recipient who presented with diabetes mellitus [3].

Classically, pheochromocytomas present with episodic headache, HTN, palpitations, and sweating.

In this case report we describe a patient who was diagnosed with pheochromocytoma in association with new onset of migraines 23 years after liver transplantation.

2. Case Report

A 61-year-old lady with a history of end-stage liver disease secondary to autoimmune hepatitis after orthotopic liver transplantation in 1990 presented at her annual check-up clinic with new-onset episodic tremors and debilitating migraines. She had a previous history of tremors immediately after the transplant which disappeared after several months. Over the last year she has developed recurrent episodic tremors which have significantly progressed in the last few months. She also developed a new onset of episodic severe headaches without aura for which she was started on sumatriptan with only partial relief. She denied any shortness of breath, palpitations, or hypertension. There was no other significant medical history. She denies any family history concerning pheochromocytoma or multiple endocrine neoplasia syndrome. For immunosuppression, she was on cyclosporine 100 mg QD, azathioprine 50 mg QD, and prednisone 1 mg QD. Her routine annual abdominal ultrasound protocol showed a new incidental heterogeneous mass measuring

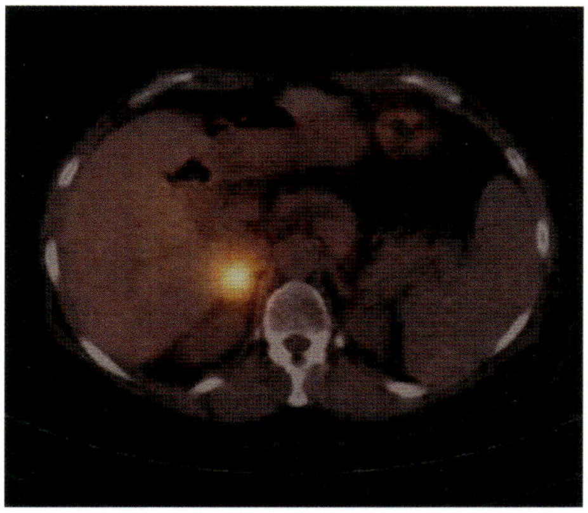

Figure 1: MIBG scan shows avid uptake of radiotracer in the right adrenal gland.

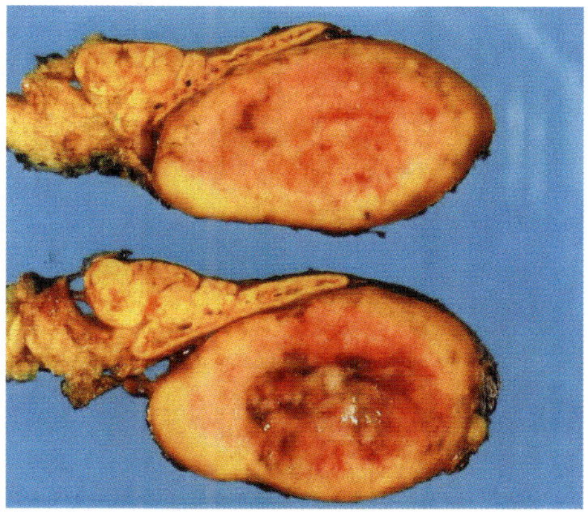

Figure 2: Gross appearance of the pheochromocytoma specimen.

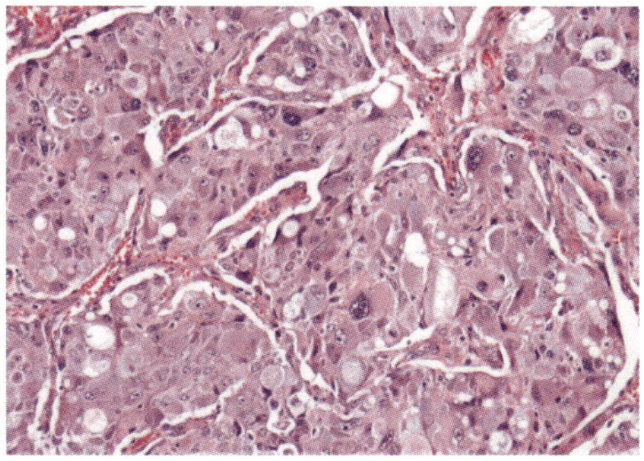

Figure 3: Histological examination revealed a neoplasm characterized by variably atypical cells exhibiting different growth patterns. Depicted here are pleomorphic neoplastic cells with intracytoplasmic hyaline globules (H&E stain, 20x).

3.1 cm × 2.2 cm × 2.6 cm in the right adrenal gland. A computed tomography with intravenous contrast demonstrated a 2.9 cm × 2.8 cm indeterminate nodule in the right adrenal mass of intermediate density (42 HU). A 24-hour urine collection demonstrated total urine metanephrines of 2,973 mcg/24 hr (reference <616 mcg/24 hr) and urine normetanephrine of 2,304 mcg/24 hr (reference <521 mcg/24 hr). An MIBG (iodine-123-meta-iodobenzylguanidine) scan showed avid uptake of radiotracer in the right adrenal gland with otherwise normal physiological distribution (Figure 1). The patient was started on phenoxybenzamine 10 mg BID ten days before the operation and titrated to orthostatic symptoms. She was admitted the day before the operation for appropriate hydration and underwent an uneventful open right adrenalectomy. She was discharged home on postoperative day 5, free of tremors and headaches. The final pathology report showed a pheochromocytoma (Figures 2 and 3).

She has remained asymptomatic and off antimigraine medication since discharge.

3. Discussion

Improved posttransplant patient and graft survival has been associated with an increased prevalence and incidence of posttransplant malignancies. Malignancies are a major cause of late death in liver transplant recipients [2]. The increased risk of cancer associated with duration and intensity of immunosuppression in organ transplant recipients [4] is well recognized. There is evidence of an increased incidence of skin, cervical, and lymphoid tumors after liver transplantation [5]. Endocrine tumors have rarely been reported in the medical literature. These case reports include a glucagonoma in a kidney transplant recipient, small cell neuroendocrine tumors of the small intestine in kidney, liver, and heart transplant recipients [6–8], and a pheochromocytoma in a liver transplant recipient [3].

In addition to the increased risk of tumors, transplant recipients also have an increased risk of new onset or exacerbation of headaches. Mild to severe headaches are a very common symptom in adult liver transplant recipients. Several conditions can lead to headaches and warrant special consideration. The neurotoxicity of immunosuppressants is commonly manifested as headaches [1]. Often, immunosuppressant-associated headaches are migraine-like and may occur de novo, or preexisting migraines may be exacerbated or may recur with immunosuppressant introduction. Patients susceptible to migraines experience increased severity and frequency of headaches when using calcineurin inhibitors, particularly tacrolimus. The incidence of headaches in patients treated with tacrolimus is 32% versus 21% with cyclosporine use [9]. Whereas cyclosporine neurotoxicity does not directly correlate with blood levels, the risk of tacrolimus-associated headache is significantly correlated with the tacrolimus blood level. Headaches can also be a manifestation of hypertension and, as such, can herald impending cerebrovascular accidents. Meningitis is always a concern in immunosuppressed patients and should be part of the differential diagnosis of headaches.

Pheochromocytomas are catecholamine-secreting tumors that arise from chromaffin cells of the adrenal medulla. They are rare tumors, with an estimated annual incidence of 0.8 per 100,000 person years [10]. The classic triad of symptoms in patients with pheochromocytoma consists of episodic headache, sweating, and tachycardia. About half have paroxysmal hypertension. The symptoms are caused by tumoral hypersecretion of norepinephrine, epinephrine, and dopamine. Approximately 95% of pheochromocytomas are in the abdomen, 85% to 90% of which are intra-adrenal. About 10% are malignant. Malignant pheochromocytomas are histologically and biochemically the same as benign ones. The only diagnostic tool of a malignant pheochromocytoma is local invasion into surrounding tissues and organs or distant metastases, which may occur up to 20 years after resection [11].

In summary, this is the second case report in the literature of a de novo pheochromocytoma after solid organ transplantation. It shows that new onset of common symptoms in transplant recipients is always challenging and deserves a very thorough work-up until the cause of the symptoms is elucidated. A broad differential diagnosis should always be included in the study of any abnormalities in this patient population. The case highlights as well the significant disability that a pheochromocytoma can cause and the complete resolution of the symptoms after removal of the tumor.

References

[1] L. Backman, M. Nicar, M. Levy et al., "FK506 trough levels in whole blood and plasma in liver transplant recipients. Correlation with clinical events and side effects," *Transplantation*, vol. 57, no. 4, pp. 519–525, 1994.

[2] S. Saigal, S. Norris, P. Muiesan, M. Rela, N. Heaton, and J. O'Grady, "Evidence of differential risk for posttransplantation malignancy based on pretransplantation caused in patients undergoing liver transplantation," *Liver Transplantation*, vol. 8, no. 5, pp. 482–487, 2002.

[3] E. J. Gallagher, R. Courgi, S. Heiba, and R. Tamler, "Resolution of insulin-requiring diabetes in a liver transplant recipient after treatment of a pheochromocytoma: case report and review of literature," *Minerva Endocrinologica*, vol. 36, no. 4, pp. 341–345, 2011.

[4] I. Penn, "Occurrence of cancers in immunosuppressed organ transplant recipients," *Clinical Transplants*, pp. 147–158, 1998.

[5] I. Penn, C. G. Halgrimson, and T. E. Starzl, "De novo malignant tumors in organ transplant recipients," *Transplantation Proceedings*, vol. 3, no. 1, pp. 773–778, 1971.

[6] F. Y. Yao, M. Gautam, C. Palese et al., "De novo malignancies following liver transplantation: a case-control study with long-term follow-up," *Clinical Transplantation*, vol. 20, no. 5, pp. 617–623, 2006.

[7] R. Baehner, G. Magrane, R. Balassanian et al., "Donor origin of neuroendocrine carcinoma in 2 transplant patients determined by molecular cytogenetics," *Human Pathology*, vol. 31, no. 11, pp. 1425–1429, 2000.

[8] S. S. Desai, E. Loh, M. L. Kochman, D. Fraker, and D. DeNofrio, "De novo ampullary neuroendocrine tumor in an orthotopic heart transplant recipient," *The American Journal of Gastroenterology*, vol. 94, no. 11, pp. 3382–3383, 1999.

[9] P. Neuhaus, P. McMaster, R. Calne et al., "Neurological complications in the European multicentre study of FK 506 and cyclosporin in primary liver transplantation," *Transplant International*, vol. 7, pp. S27–S31, 1994.

[10] C. M. Beard, S. G. Sheps, L. T. Kurland, J. A. Carney, and J. T. Lie, "Occurrence of pheochromocytoma in Rochester, Minnesota, 1950 through 1979," *Mayo Clinic Proceedings*, vol. 58, no. 12, pp. 802–804, 1983.

[11] R. E. Goldstein, J. A. O'Neill Jr., G. W. Holcomb III et al., "Clinical experience over 48 years with pheochromocytoma," *Annals of Surgery*, vol. 229, no. 6, pp. 755–766, 1999.

30

Ligation of Left Renal Vein for Spontaneous Splenorenal Shunt to Prevent Portal Hypoperfusion after Orthotopic Liver Transplantation

Lampros Kousoulas,[1] Kristina Imeen Ringe,[2] Michael Winkler,[1] Frank Lehner,[1] Nicolas Richter,[1] Juergen Klempnauer,[1] and Fabian Helfritz[1]

[1] *Department of General, Visceral and Transplant Surgery, Hannover Medical School, Carl-Neuberg-Street 1, 30625 Hanover, Germany*
[2] *Institute of Radiology, Hannover Medical School, Carl-Neuberg-Street 1, 30625 Hanover, Germany*

Correspondence should be addressed to Lampros Kousoulas; kousoulas.lampros@mh-hannover.de

Academic Editors: P. Boraschi, S. Faenza, and S. Pinney

We report a case of recovered portal flow by ligation of the left renal vein on the first postoperative day after orthotopic liver transplantation of a 54-year-old female with alcoholic liver cirrhosis, chronic kidney failure, and spontaneous splenorenal shunt. After reperfusion, Doppler ultrasonography showed almost total diversion of the portal flow into the existing splenorenal shunt, but because of severe coagulopathy and diffuse bleeding, ligation of the shunt was not attempted. A programmed relaparotomy was performed on the first postoperative day, and the left renal vein was ligated just to the left of the inferior vena cava. Portal flows subsequently increased to 37 cm/sec, and the patient presented a good and stable liver function. We conclude that patients with known preoperative splenorenal shunts should be closely monitored, and if the portal flow becomes insufficient, ligation of the left renal vein should be attempted in order to optimize the portal perfusion of the liver.

1. Introduction

In cirrhotic patients with portal hypertension, collateral vessels into systemic circulation are well known. The amount of collateral flow depends on the stage of portal hypertension. In advanced stages, the development of a reversal hepatofugal portal flow may lead to a portal steal syndrome [1]. After orthotopic liver transplantation, usually the portal flow and pressure normalize and, providing that there is an adequate-sized graft, collateral vessels collapse and obliterate [2–4].

Low portal vein flows after orthotopic liver transplantation, due to persisting splenorenal shunt, are associated with hepatic hypoperfusion and poor allograft survival [2]. Splenorenal shunts are present in cirrhotic patients from nearly 14% up to 21%, and several studies have suggested that spontaneous portosystemic shunts should be treated in order to recover the portal flow of the liver graft [5, 6]. Beside direct division of the shunt vessels with or without splenectomy, the ligation of the left renal vein is described to be an effective technique and has been reported to be safe in adult liver transplant patients with large splenorenal shunts [7–9].

2. Case Report

The patient is a 54-year-old female with alcoholic liver cirrhosis and chronic kidney failure, listed for liver and sequential renal transplantation. The patient underwent a percutaneous ethanol injection therapy for a solitary hepatocellular carcinoma in 2009. At the timepoint of transplantation the MELD score was 37.

The preoperatively conducted abdominal computed tomographic (CT) scan showed severe portal-systemic collateral vessels of the abdomen, including a splenorenal shunt (Figure 1).

The patient underwent an orthotopic liver transplantation using a full-size organ. Donor age was 56 years, and the organ quality was rated as "acceptable" by the explant surgeon. Histopathological rating of steatosis was 25–30%.

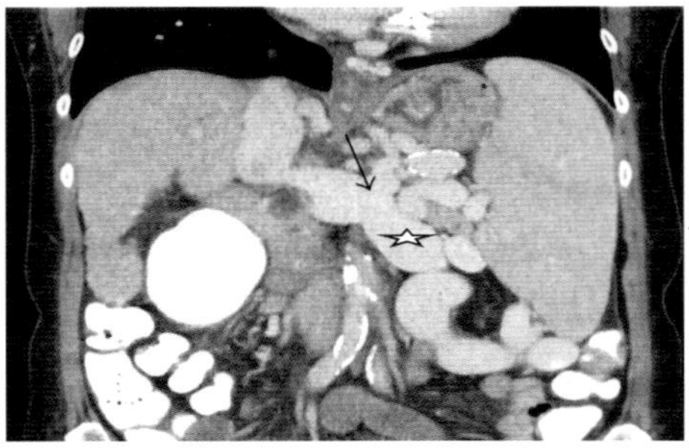

FIGURE 1: Preoperative CT imaging showing the splenorenal shunt (arrow) and a splenomegaly (left renal vein = star).

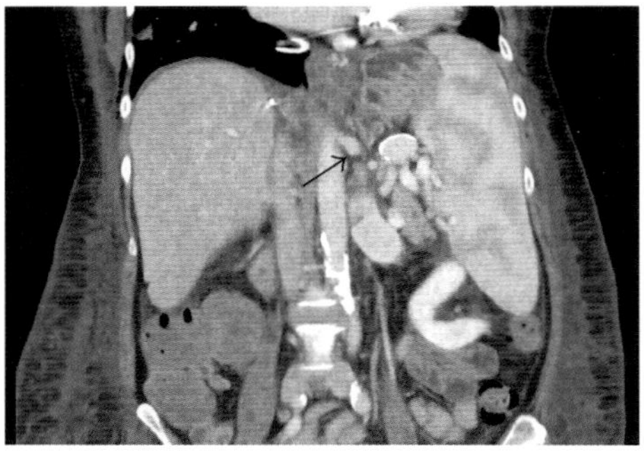

FIGURE 2: Postoperative CT imaging (day 5) after the ligation of the left renal vein. The arrow shows the point of ligation.

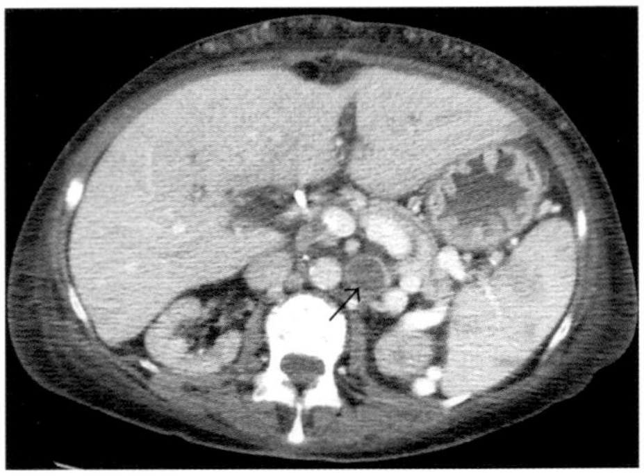

FIGURE 3: Postoperative CT imaging (day 47) showing the thrombosis of the left renal vein at the point of ligation (arrow).

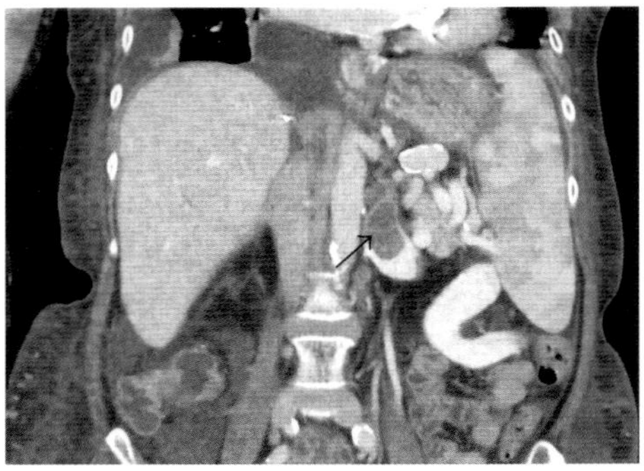

FIGURE 4: Postoperative CT imaging (day 47) showing in axial form the thrombosis of the left renal vein (arrow).

The center standardised transplant procedure was performed with replacement of the retrohepatic inferior vena cava and without any bypass procedure. Anastomosis time was 43 min, incision to suture time was 3 hours 09 min, and cold ischemic time was 8 hours 47 min.

After reperfusion, Doppler ultrasonography showed total diversion of the portal flow into the existing splenorenal shunt, but because of severe coagulopathy and diffuse bleeding, ligation of the shunt was not attempted. A programmed relaparotomy was performed on the first postoperative day, and the left renal vein was ligated at its confluence to the inferior vena cava (Figure 2).

Portal flows subsequently increased to 37 cm/sec. The postoperative graft function was excellent and substitution of plasma or coagulation factors was not necessary. The postoperative Doppler ultrasound examination showed normal flows for both the hepatic artery and portal vein. The further postoperative course was uncomplicated.

About two months after the liver transplantation, another CT scan of the abdomen was performed, and progredient thrombosis of the left renal vein was observed (Figures 3 and 4). Due to the preexisting chronic renal failure, this fact was without any consequence for our patient, but it demonstrates that the procedure of renal vein ligation bears the potential risk of renal impairment. The patient currently enjoys good allograft function with normal liver function tests.

3. Discussion

Preexisting splenorenal shunts may lead to insufficient portal flow after orthotopic liver transplantation, which is associated with hepatic hypoperfusion and poor allograft survival [10, 11]. As an adequate portal venous inflow is critical for graft function and survival, spontaneous or surgically created portosystemic shunts have to be treated after the liver transplantation in order to improve the portal flow to the allograft [12]. Direct ligation of a splenorenal shunt, with or without splenectomy, is technically challenging and is associated with a high risk of bleeding or of infection [13, 14]. Furthermore, the ligation of the shunt may not always significantly improve the portal flow. Therefore, the ligation of the left renal vein at the inferior vena cava has been proposed as an alternative therapeutic approach. Given the fact that the venous renal blood flow accelerates the portal flow after the ligation of the renal vein, this procedure can lead to sufficient portal flow.

Our case report shows that the ligation of the left renal vein can be performed safely in order to optimize the flow of the portal vein after the liver transplantation, but this procedure could also lead to renal impairment due to outflow problems and thrombosis of the left renal vein [2, 7, 8]. In our case, because of the chronic kidney failure of the patient, the decision to ligate the left renal vein was easily made, but in patients with normal kidney function, this aspect should be taken into consideration.

Thus, we conclude that patients with known preoperative splenorenal shunt should be closely monitored after orthotopic liver transplantation, and if the portal flow becomes insufficient, direct ligation of the splenorenal shunt or ligation of the left renal vein at the inferior vena cava should be attempted in order to prevent portal flow steal and optimize the portal perfusion of the liver. The selection of the method performed should be based not only on the ability to identify and ligate the shunt vessels, but also on the special characteristics of the patient and on the experience of the surgeon.

References

[1] A. von Herbay, T. Frieling, and D. Haussinger, "Color Doppler sonographic evaluation of spontaneous portosystemic shunts and inversion of portal venous flow in patients with cirrhosis," *Journal of Clinical Ultrasound*, vol. 28, pp. 332–339, 2000.

[2] F. Castillo-Suescun, G. C. Oniscu, and E. Hidalgo, "Hemodynamic consequences of spontaneous splenorenal shunts in deceased donor liver transplantation," *Liver Transplantation*, vol. 17, no. 8, pp. 891–895, 2011.

[3] Y. Kita, Y. Harihara, K. Sano et al., "Reversible hepatofugal portal flow after liver transplantation using a small-for-size graft from a living donor," *Transplant International*, vol. 14, no. 4, pp. 217–222, 2001.

[4] L. De Carlis, E. Del Favero, G. Rondinara et al., "The role of spontaneous portosystemic shunts in the course of orthotopic liver transplantation," *Transplant International*, vol. 5, no. 1, pp. 9–14, 1992.

[5] G. Tarantino, V. Citro, P. Conca et al., "What are the implications of the spontaneous spleno-renal shunts in liver cirrhosis?" *BMC Gastroenterology*, vol. 9, article 89, 2009.

[6] E. M. Zardi, V. Uwechie, D. Caccavo et al., "Portosystemic shunts in a large cohort of patients with liver cirrhosis: detection rate and clinical relevance," *Journal of Gastroenterology*, vol. 44, no. 1, pp. 76–83, 2009.

[7] S. G. Lee, D. B. Moon, C. S. Ahn et al., "Ligation of left renal vein for large spontaneous splenorenal shunt to prevent portal flow steal in adult living donor liver transplantation," *Transplant International*, vol. 20, no. 1, pp. 45–50, 2007.

[8] R. R. Slater, N. Jabbour, A. A. Abbass et al., "Left renal vein ligation: a technique to mitigate low portal flow from splenic vein siphon during liver transplantation," *American Journal of Transplantation*, vol. 11, no. 8, pp. 1743–1747, 2011.

[9] S. Y. Cho, S. H. Kim, K. W. Lee, S. J. Park, S. S. Han, and Y. K. Kim, "Ligation of left renal vein as a salvage procedure for splenorenal shunt after living donor liver transplantation: a case report," *Transplantation Proceedings*, vol. 41, no. 10, pp. 4243–4245, 2009.

[10] H. Sadamori, T. Yagi, H. Matsukawa et al., "The outcome of living donor liver transplantation with prior spontaneous large portasystemic shunts," *Transplant International*, vol. 21, no. 2, pp. 156–162, 2008.

[11] R. S. Shapiro, C. V. R. Varma, M. E. Schwartz, and C. M. Miller, "Splenorenal shunt closure after liver transplantation: intraoperative Doppler assessment of portal hemodynamics," *Liver Transplantation and Surgery*, vol. 3, no. 6, pp. 641–642, 1997.

[12] H. Sadamori, T. Yagi, S. Shinoura et al., "New surgical approach to large splenorenal shunt in living donor liver transplantation: diversion of SMV and SPV blood flow," *Journal of Gastrointestinal Surgery*, vol. 17, no. 2, pp. 403–407.

[13] U. Settmacher, N. C. Nüssler, M. Glanemann et al., "Venous complications after orthotopic liver transplantation," *Clinical Transplantation*, vol. 14, no. 3, pp. 235–241, 2000.

[14] R. Troisi, U. J. Hesse, J. Decruyenaere et al., "Functional, life-threatening disorders and splenectomy following liver transplantation," *Clinical Transplantation*, vol. 13, no. 5, pp. 380–388, 1999.

Rapid Resolution of Cholangitic Abscess and Biliary Sepsis in a Liver Transplant Recipient after Hepatic Artery Revascularization

Sushrut Trakroo[1] and Kamran Qureshi[2]

[1]*Department of Surgery, Temple University Hospital, Philadelphia, PA 19140, USA*
[2]*Section of Gastroenterology and Hepatology, Temple University Lewis Katz School of Medicine, Philadelphia, PA 19140, USA*

Correspondence should be addressed to Kamran Qureshi; kamran.qureshi@temple.edu

Academic Editor: Carl Classen

Hepatic arterial flow is paramount in preserving biliary integrity. We present an interesting clinical scenario of a liver transplant recipient with biliary anastomotic stricture who developed biliary abscess and sepsis after Endoscopic Retrograde Cholangiopancreatography. The abscess did not respond to maximal medical management, percutaneous drainage, and adequate endoscopic biliary drainage. Clinically, patient continued to deteriorate and imaging identified hepatic artery stenosis which was treated with percutaneous intra-arterial stenting. Revascularization and perfusion of infected area led to rapid resolution of abscess and sepsis. This case emphasizes the anatomic basis of biliary ductal pathology. An important educational point is to understand that interrupted hepatic arterial supply can lead to biliary complications in liver transplant recipients and early correction of perfusion deficit should be pursued in such cases. In nonresolving hepatobiliary infections after liver transplantation, hepatic arterial compromise should be looked for and if present promptly treated. Reperfusion of biliary system in our patient led to improved antibiotics penetration, resolution of abscess and sepsis, and healing of biliary stricture.

1. Introduction

Branches of hepatic artery and arterioles supply the arterial blood to whole of biliary tree via peribiliary plexus of capillaries and then drain into hepatic sinusoids. Incidence of hepatic artery stenosis (HAS) after liver transplant (LT) is considered to be 4 to 10% after deceased donor LT [1, 2]. Presentation of delayed HAS is less clear, ranging from asymptomatic to progressive biliary disease in the form of strictures [3]. Studies have shown decreased incidence of biliary pathology with early intervention [4].

2. Case Report

This sixty-year-old male with a history of deceased donor LT done for cryptogenic liver cirrhosis over 3 years ago presented to the emergency department with 3 days of high grade fevers and chills. He was found to be tachycardiac and hypotensive and thus was admitted to the Intensive Care Unit (ICU) for management of septic shock. Review of his past history revealed uneventful 2.5 years after LT course and a diagnosis of late onset biliary anastomotic stricture, which was recognized during the work-up of new onset cholestatic hepatitis 6 months prior to this admission. During the original LT operation, surgeons had to perform hepatic arterial reconstruction because of donor to recipient arterial size mismatch. For the treatment of biliary anastomotic stricture he underwent Endoscopic Retrograde Cholangiopancreatography (ERCP) with biliary stent placement 3 times during the course of subsequent 6 months. His last ERCP procedure was performed 7 days prior to this ICU admission; during which a severe localized biliary stricture was found and was treated with balloon dilation and exchange of biliary stents. Four days after the ERCP he started mounting high

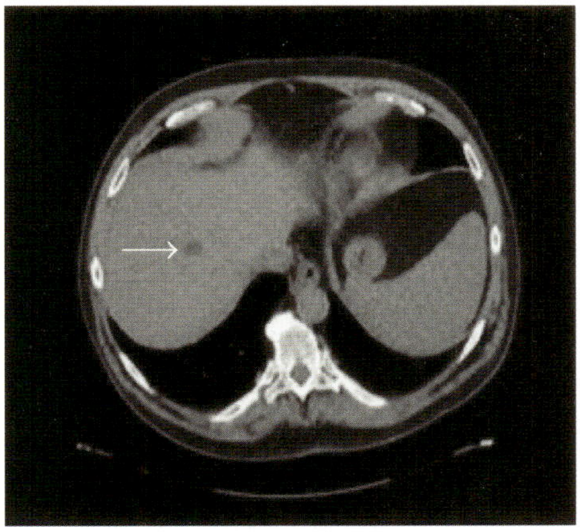

FIGURE 1: Multidetector CT of the abdomen on the day of admission showed a new ill-defined hypodense lesion in the right hepatic lobe.

grade fevers with chills, which brought him to the hospital. Clinical presentation on admission (day 0) suggested presence of septic shock with right upper abdominal pain and new onset jaundice. After initial fluid resuscitation, an abdominal computerized tomography (CT) scan was done which showed a new liver lesion (Figure 1) thought to be abscess in this clinical scenario. He was managed for septic shock secondary to a working diagnosis of ascending cholangitis/hepatic abscess and was started on broad-spectrum antibiotics (vancomycin with piperacillin/tazobactam), along with vasopressor support. Blood cultures (BC) from admission eventually grew extended spectrum beta-lactamase producing (ESBL) *Klebsiella pneumoniae* and antibiotic coverage was accordingly modified to imipenem/cilastatin. With an adequate antibacterial coverage and following initial response to imipenem/cliastatin regimen (and negative BC), he started to develop fevers again. Repeat BC (day 8) showed the same bacterial growth of ESBL *Klebsiella pneumonia* (Figure 2). Subsequently antibiotic coverage was broadened with double carbapenem regimen (ertapenem with meropenem) for presumed carbapenemase producing pandrug resistant *Klebsiella pneumonia*. Repeat CT scan showed enlarging liver abscess (Figure 3), as he continued to have fever and bacteremia despite the addition of doxycycline in the antimicrobial regimen. Thus, CT guided percutaneous drainage of abscess was performed (day 16) and aspirate grew the same ESBL *Klebsiella pneumonia*, which was persistently seen in the blood stream. Despite aggressive medical management for total of 3 weeks, he remained febrile with bacteremia and sepsis. HAS been suspected and was identified on ultrasound arterial Doppler study. Subsequently, he underwent hepatic artery angiogram (day 21), which showed critical anastomotic stenosis of the replaced common hepatic artery that arose directly off the aorta. Nitroglycerin (200 mcg) was administered for vasodilatation and mechanical dilatation of the stricture was performed with a 4 mm balloon dilatation catheter across the stenotic segment. A 5 mm × 15 mm express SD stent was then deployed across the stenotic segment. Completion angiogram demonstrated excellent perfusion to

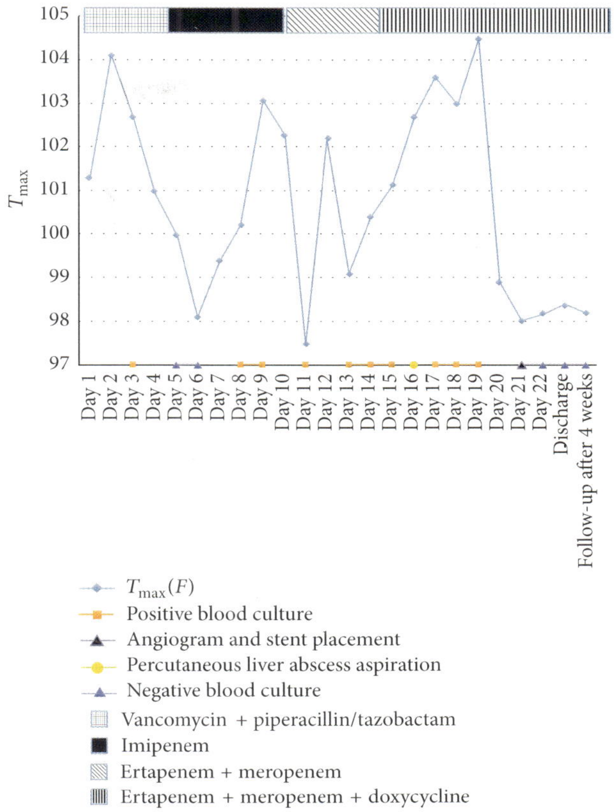

FIGURE 2: Timeline graph to depict various clinical parameters during the admission and after discharge from hospital.

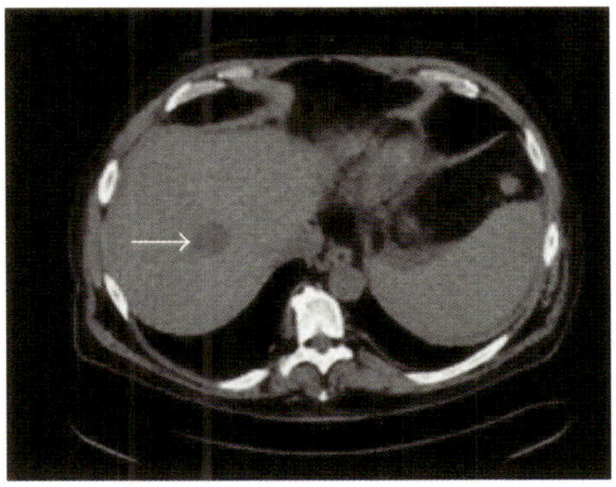

FIGURE 3: CT image on day 14 redemonstrated enlarged ill-defined hypodensity within the right hepatic lobe.

the liver (Figure 4). The revascularization resulted in reperfusion of the biliary system and better access and penetration of antibiotics to the infected area and abscess. He showed dramatic clinical and hemodynamic improvement over the subsequent 24 hours. Blood cultures drawn the day after the arterial stenting showed no growth and he was discharged 3 days after revascularization along with the confirmation of sterile BC. 3 months follow-up CT scan (Figure 5) showed resolution of liver abscess and ERCP done afterwards showed a resolved biliary anastomotic stricture.

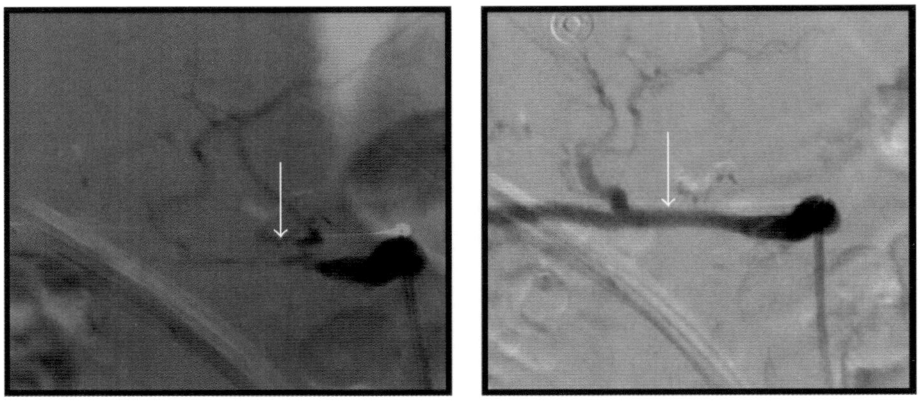

FIGURE 4: Angiogram with hepatic artery stent placement on day 21 showed critical stenosis of the anastomotic segment of replaced hepatic artery. Subsequent balloon dilatation and stenting with 2–5 mm stents was completed.

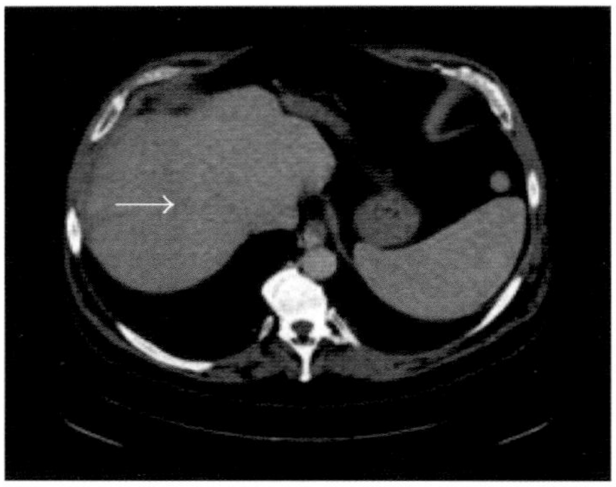

FIGURE 5: Follow-up CT image at 3 months after hepatic artery revascularization with stent placement showed resolution of liver abscess.

3. Discussion

Hepatic arterial flow is paramount in preserving biliary integrity [5, 6]. Delayed presentation of HAS after LT is rare and can lead to potential graft loss and mortality [7]. Pathophysiology of delayed HAS includes transplant associated arteriosclerosis, vascular intimal thickening, medial attenuation, and vasoconstriction [8, 9]. Our patient's clinical condition deteriorated despite maximal medical management and percutaneous abscess drainage. This can be explained on the basis of impaired perfusion of the affected/infected area which limited antibiotic penetration. Recognition and stenting of HAS led not only to immediate resolution of sepsis and abscess but also to the resolution of biliary stricture. He did not require any further interventions for biliary stricture on the follow-up ERCP done 3 months later.

Competing Interests

The authors declare that there are no competing interests regarding the publication of this paper.

References

[1] J. P. Duffy, J. C. Hong, D. G. Farmer et al., "Vascular complications of orthotopic liver transplantation: experience in more than 4,200 patients," *Journal of the American College of Surgeons*, vol. 208, no. 5, pp. 896–903, 2009.

[2] R. F. Da Silva, R. Raphe, H. C. Felício et al., "Prevalence, treatment, and outcomes of the hepatic artery stenosis after liver transplantation," *Transplantation Proceedings*, vol. 40, no. 3, pp. 805–807, 2008.

[3] P. M. Porrett, J. Hsu, and A. Shaked, "Late surgical complications following liver transplantation," *Liver Transplantation*, vol. 15, supplement 2, pp. S12–S18, 2009.

[4] O. Abbasoglu, M. F. Levy, M. S. Vodapally et al., "Hepatic artery stenosis after liver transplantation—incidence, presentation, treatment, and long term outcome," *Transplantation*, vol. 63, no. 2, pp. 250–255, 1997.

[5] J. M. A. Northover and J. Terblanche, "A new look at the arterial supply of the bile duct in man and its surgical implications," *British Journal of Surgery*, vol. 66, no. 6, pp. 379–384, 1979.

[6] D. Castaing, "Surgical anatomy of the biliary tract," *HPB*, vol. 10, no. 2, pp. 72–76, 2008.

[7] C. Pulitano, D. Joseph, C. Sroussi et al., "Hepatic artery stenosis after liver transplantation: is endovascular treatment always necessary?" *Liver Transplantation*, vol. 21, no. 2, pp. 162–168, 2015.

[8] R. N. Mitchell and P. Libby, "Vascular remodeling in transplant vasculopathy," *Circulation Research*, vol. 100, no. 7, pp. 967–978, 2007.

[9] O. S. Plekhanova, E. V. Parfenova, and V. A. Tkachuk, "Mechanisms of vascular remodeling following arterial injury," *Kardiologiya*, vol. 55, no. 7, pp. 63–77, 2015.

Methicillin-Resistant *Staphylococcus aureus* Prostatic Abscess in a Liver Transplant Recipient

Tanima Jana,[1] Jorge D. Machicado,[1] Giovanni E. Davogustto,[1] and Jen-Jung Pan[2]

[1] *Department of Internal Medicine, University of Texas Medical School at Houston, Houston, TX 77030, USA*
[2] *Division of Gastroenterology, Hepatology and Nutrition, Department of Internal Medicine, University of Texas Medical School at Houston, Houston, TX 77030, USA*

Correspondence should be addressed to Tanima Jana; tanima.jana@uth.tmc.edu

Academic Editor: David Conti

Prostatic abscesses are usually related to gram-negative bacilli. However, methicillin-resistant *Staphylococcus aureus* (MRSA) has emerged as a substantial cause of prostatic abscesses in recent years. Herein, we report the case of a 31-year-old man with a history of orthotopic liver transplantation 10 years ago who presented with acute onset dysuria and abdominal pain and was diagnosed with a MRSA prostatic abscess. To our knowledge, this is the first case describing a prostatic abscess in a liver transplant recipient and the first reporting MRSA as the causative organism of a prostatic abscess in a solid organ transplant recipient.

1. Introduction

A prostatic abscess is a rare entity, usually caused by organisms from the family Enterobacteriaceae or genus *Enterococcus*. Although *Staphylococcus aureus* infection is typically associated with skin diseases, it has emerged as a substantial cause of prostatic abscesses in recent years [1]. *S. aureus*, a major cause of infection among solid organ transplant recipients, occurs most commonly within the first 2 months following liver transplantation and is associated with a high morbidity and mortality [2]. Herein, we report the case of a 31-year-old man with a history of orthotopic liver transplantation 10 years ago, chronic immunosuppression, and ulcerative colitis, who presented with acute onset dysuria and abdominal pain. He was ultimately found to have a prostatic abscess and bacteremia caused by methicillin-resistant *Staphylococcus aureus* (MRSA). To the best of our knowledge, this is the first case describing a prostatic abscess in a liver transplant recipient and the first reporting MRSA as the causative organism of a prostatic abscess in a solid organ transplant recipient.

2. Case Presentation

A 31-year-old African-American man underwent orthotopic liver transplantation 10 years ago for primary sclerosing cholangitis (PSC). He had moderate acute cellular rejection five months after the transplant but had no history of any transplant-related infections. He presented to the emergency department with a one-week history of lower abdominal pain and dysuria. His past medical history was pertinent for ulcerative colitis and type 2 diabetes mellitus. He had been hospitalized multiple times in the past year for abdominal pain. Extensive investigation had shown partial small bowel obstruction caused by intussusception that was treated conservatively, in addition to chronic elevation of total bilirubin, alkaline phosphatase, and transaminases attributed to possible recurrence of PSC in the hepatic graft. At the time of suspicion of possible PSC recurrence, his prednisone dosage had been increased and later tapered when liver function studies improved. He had last been admitted to the hospital 2 weeks earlier for diarrhea and fever, diagnosed with *Clostridium difficile* infection (CDI), and discharged

10 days prior with oral vancomycin. At the time of current presentation, his immunosuppression regimen included tacrolimus 1 mg twice daily, mycophenolate mofetil 500 mg twice daily, and prednisone 5 mg daily. He reported temporal insertion of indwelling urinary catheters during some of his previous hospital admissions for management of small bowel obstruction. Otherwise, he denied any intravenous (IV) drug use, history of urethral instrumentation, or chronic indwelling urinary catheters. His vital signs on admission revealed blood pressure 134/68 mmHg, heart rate 80 beats per minute, 20 respirations per minute, and temperature 98.5°F. On physical exam, his abdomen was soft with mild tenderness to palpation in the left lower quadrant. Rectal exam revealed a normal-sized, painless prostate with fluctuation at the right base. Laboratory investigation showed white blood cell count of 22,600/μL (94% neutrophils, 2% lymphocytes, 1% bands), hemoglobin 12.3 g/dL, and platelet count 309,000/μL. Biochemistry tests revealed creatinine 1.2 mg/dL, alanine aminotransferase 199 U/L, aspartate aminotransferase 157 U/L, alkaline phosphatase 719 U/L, and total bilirubin 18.3 mg/dL (direct bilirubin 15.6 mg/dL), which were unchanged compared to previous laboratory results. Human immunodeficiency virus (HIV) antibody was negative. Urinalysis showed 11–20 white blood cells/high power field (HPF), 0–2 red blood cells/HPF, few bacteria, and no casts. Contrast-enhanced computed tomography (CT) of the abdomen and pelvis revealed multiple stable areas of intussusception and a 3.0 cm × 1.9 cm prostatic abscess (Figures 1(a) and 1(b)). We empirically treated for infection with IV ceftriaxone and vancomycin. MRSA was isolated from both urine (<10,000 CFU/mL) and 2 sets of blood cultures (aerobic and anaerobic bottles) obtained upon admission. Cultures were sensitive to daptomycin, clindamycin, gentamycin, rifampin, tetracycline, levofloxacin, trimethoprim-sulfamethoxazole, and vancomycin (MIC < 0.5). Both transthoracic and transesophageal echocardiography were negative for vegetations. Based on his recent hospitalizations, he was diagnosed with health-care associated MRSA bacteremia. Detailed review of his hospital records revealed that colonization with MRSA had been detected 2 weeks prior in a nasal swab sample and treated accordingly with topical chlorhexidine and mupirocin. A final diagnosis of MRSA prostatic abscess with bacteremia was made. Due to his immunosuppression and bacteremia, it was decided that he was not a candidate for oral antibiotics. IV vancomycin was continued while ceftriaxone was stopped. We opted for conservative management in this case, which showed rapid improvement of symptoms and inflammatory response. Therefore, abscess aspiration was not deemed necessary. We also continued oral vancomycin to complete 14 days of treatment for CDI. The same dosage of immunosuppressant medications was continued, with the exception of tacrolimus, which was held due to acute kidney injury. Leukocytosis resolved at day 3 while symptoms started to improve at day 5. Repeat blood cultures at day 4 were negative. Urine cultures failed to grow any organism at day 11 of active therapy. His creatinine rose to 1.6 mg/dL and IV vancomycin was switched to daptomycin on day 12 of treatment. He was discharged from the hospital at day 22, with instructions to continue daptomycin for a total of 6 weeks of antibiotics. During a follow-up clinic appointment at 8 weeks after completion of antibiotics, his symptoms were resolved, cultures were negative, and repeat CT of the abdomen and pelvis showed complete resolution of the prostatic abscess (Figures 2(a) and 2(b)).

3. Discussion

Prostatic abscess is most commonly caused by gram-negative bacilli, primarily *Escherichia coli*, (60–80% of cases), although *Neisseria gonorrhoeae* was the most common pathogen in the past (75% of cases in the preantibiotic era) [3, 4]. *Staphylococcus aureus* is an uncommon cause of prostatic abscess but it has been reported more commonly in recent years. We searched the literature from inception through August 2014 on PubMed and Ovid MEDLINE to identify the cases of prostatic abscess caused by *S. aureus*. The databases were searched using the keywords "*Staphylococcus aureus*" OR "methicillin-resistant *Staphylococcus aureus*" OR "MRSA" AND "prostatic abscess" OR "prostate abscess" OR "prostatic infection" OR "prostate infection." We found 33 documented cases of *S. aureus* prostatic abscess (Table 1), 21 of which were found to be MRSA, 3 methicillin-sensitive *Staphylococcus aureus* (MSSA), and 9 in which susceptibilities were not available. Of the 21 MRSA cases, 20 (95%) involved patients with predisposing conditions, 18 (86%) fell within the 40–60-year-old age group, and 16 (76%) had associated bacteremia. Predisposing history included immunocompromised conditions (e.g., diabetes mellitus, HIV, immunosuppressive drugs), IV drug use, recent genitourinary infection, chronic or recent indwelling urinary catheter, and preexisting prostatic disease, such as benign prostatic hypertrophy. Additional risk factors for prostatic abscess described in the literature include chronic dialysis, prostate biopsy, chronic bacterial prostatitis, and obstructive uropathy [4–7]. In the case of our patient, he was colonized by MRSA most likely due to his multiple hospital admissions and was receiving immunosuppressant agents for liver allograft protection. In addition, he had been admitted multiple times for partial small bowel obstruction during the last year and undergone temporal indwelling urinary catheter insertions.

Common symptoms of a prostatic abscess include fever, dysuria, increased urinary frequency, acute urinary retention, perineal pain, back pain, and hematuria [3, 7]. Many of these symptoms might be absent in immunosuppressed subjects, and thus a prostatic abscess should be suspected in these patients if found with MRSA bacteriuria or MRSA bacteremia of unknown source. MRSA bacteriuria is rare, with a study from a single institution in Rochester, Minnesota, describing it in 0.5% of 17,085 urine cultures obtained over two years [8]. Risk factors associated with MRSA bacteriuria in this study included recent urinary catheter use, recent healthcare exposure, history of genitourinary surgery, presence of comorbidities, and increasing patient age. Identification of the source of bacteriuria was not described in the study, but it was effectively treated as a urinary tract infection [8]. Clinicians should be reminded that the

TABLE 1: Reported cases of *Staphylococcus aureus* prostatic abscess.

	Age (years)	Comorbidities/risk factors	Treatment	Microbiology
Our patient	31	DM, OLT	Vancomycin + daptomycin	HA-MRSA (urine, blood)
Deshpande et al., 2013 [19]	49	BPH	Vancomycin + doxycycline, TURP	CA-MRSA (N/A)
Docekal et al., 2013 [5]	56	DM	Vancomycin, IR-guided abscess drainage ×2, pigtail drain placement, TURP	CA-MRSA (prostate abscess)
Krishnamohan et al., 2013 [1]	47	Recent *Trichomonas* infection	Vancomycin + linezolid, TURP, percutaneous and transperineal abscess drainage	CA-MRSA (urine, prostate abscess)
	20	Hepatitis C	Vancomycin + linezolid, TURP	CA-MRSA (prostate abscess)
Lachant et al., 2013 [7]	47	Recent penile furuncle, history of hypospadias with urethral stricture	Vancomycin, TURP	CA-MRSA (urine, blood, lung, heart valve vegetation, kidney, prostate abscess)
	31	None	Vancomycin + daptomycin + TMP-SMX, TURP, transrectal abscess drainage	CA-MRSA (blood, prostate abscess)
Naboush et al., 2013 [4]	52	DM	Vancomycin + TMP-SMX + rifampin, TURP, transurethral unroofing of abscess	CA-MRSA (urine, blood, prostate abscess)
Sukhal et al., 2013 [20]	57	DM	Vancomycin	CA-MRSA (urine, blood, nares)
Flannery and Humphrey 2012 [6]	49	DM	Vancomycin + doxycycline, TURP	CA-MRSA (urine, blood, prostate tissue)
Javeed et al., 2012 [21]	50	DM	Vancomycin + daptomycin, CT-guided abscess drainage	CA-MRSA (urine, blood, prostate abscess)
Matsumoto et al., 2012 [22]	65	DM, indwelling urethral catheter	Antibiotics, transrectal abscess drainage	MSSA (blood, prostate abscess, heart valve vegetation)
Abreu et al., 2011 [23]	59	DM, suppurative lesions in nasal cavity	TMP-SMX + ciprofloxacin + vancomycin, percutaneous abscess drainage	CA-MRSA (blood, prostate abscess)
Park et al., 2011 [24]	45	DM	Vancomycin, percutaneous abscess drainage, TURP	CA-MRSA (blood, prostate abscess)
Tiwari et al., 2011 [25]	N/A	N/A	Intravenous and oral antibiotics, surgical treatment	*S. aureus*[#]
	N/A	N/A	Intravenous and oral antibiotics, surgical treatment	*S. aureus*[#]
Chao et al., 2009 [26]	40	N/A	Vancomycin + gentamicin, transperineal abscess drainage	CA-MRSA (blood, prostate abscess)
Baradkar et al., 2008 [27]	50	DM	Ciprofloxacin	MSSA
Gautam et al., 2008 [28]	51	HIV	Ciprofloxacin + TMP-SMX + vancomycin, transurethral abscess drainage	CA-MRSA (blood, prostate abscess)
Lin et al., 2008 [29]	55	BPH	Vancomycin	CA-MRSA (blood)
Pierce et al., 2008 [30]	64	DM	Vancomycin, percutaneous abscess drainage	CA-MRSA (urine, blood, prostate abscess)
Beckman and Edson 2007 [31]	53	DM	Vancomycin + TMP-SMX + rifampin	CA-MRSA (blood, prostate tissue, nares)
Cabrera Meirás et al., 2007 [32]	51	N/A	Antibiotics, transrectal abscess drainage, urinary diversion	*S. aureus*[#] (prostate abscess)
Tobian and Ober 2007 [33]	56	DM, BPH, history of self-digital rectal examinations	Vancomycin + rifampin, cystoscopy, percutaneous abscess drainage, transurethral unroofing of abscess	MRSA (urine, blood)[*]
Shindel et al., 2006 [34]	29	Straddle injury to urethra, hepatitis C	Vancomycin, Cope loop catheter placement, urethroplasty	CA-MRSA (prostate abscess)
Baker et al., 2004 [35]	43	Hepatitis C, intravenous drug abuse	Vancomycin + nafcillin + TMP-SMX, TURP	CA-MRSA (blood, prostate abscess)

Table 1: Continued.

	Age (years)	Comorbidities/risk factors	Treatment	Microbiology
Fraser et al., 2003 [36]	63	DM, recent scrotal abscess drainage	Vancomycin, percutaneous abscess drainage, TURP	HA-MRSA (urine, blood, prostate abscess)
Oliveira et al., 2003 [37]	38	HIV	Intravenous antibiotics, surgical procedure unclear	*S. aureus*#
	41	None	Intravenous antibiotics, surgical procedure unclear	*S. aureus*#
	50	DM	Intravenous antibiotics, surgical procedure unclear	*S. aureus*#
	50	None	Intravenous antibiotics, surgical procedure unclear	*S. aureus*#
Trauzzi et al., 1994 [38]	35	HIV	Intravenous antibiotics	*S. aureus*#
Savarirayan et al., 1995 [39]	50	Recent salivary gland abscess treated with antibiotics	Ciprofloxacin + erythromycin, transperineal abscess drainage, perineal unroofing of abscess	*S. aureus*#
Gill et al., 1991 [40]	42	Recent fall with closed arm fracture	Oxytetracycline, transperineal abscess drainage	MSSA (prostate abscess)

BPH, benign prostate hypertrophy; CA, community-acquired; DM, diabetes mellitus; HA, hospital-acquired; HIV, human immunodeficiency virus; IR, interventional radiology; OLT, orthotopic liver transplant; TURP, transurethral resection of prostate; TMP-SMX, trimethoprim-sulfamethoxazole; MRSA, methicillin-resistant *Staphylococcus aureus*; MSSA, methicillin-sensitive *Staphylococcus aureus*; N/A, not available.

*Community versus hospital-acquired MRSA status not given.

#Susceptibility to methicillin was not reported.

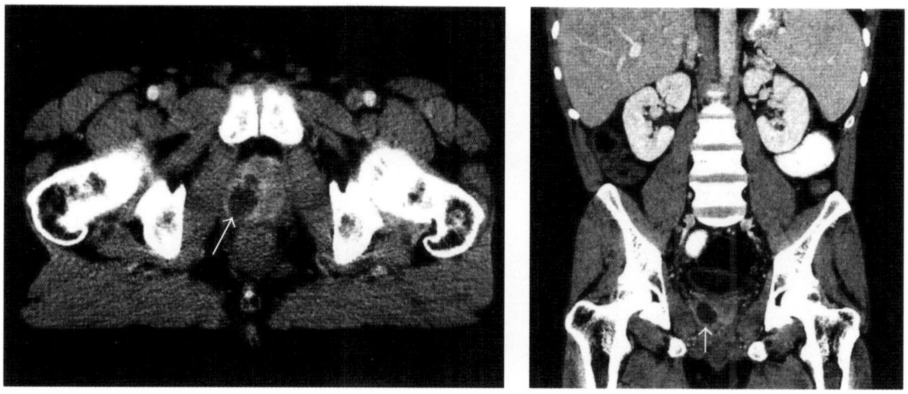

(a) (b)

FIGURE 1: Axial (a) and coronal (b) views of CT abdomen and pelvis revealing a 3.0 cm × 1.9 cm prostatic abscess (arrow).

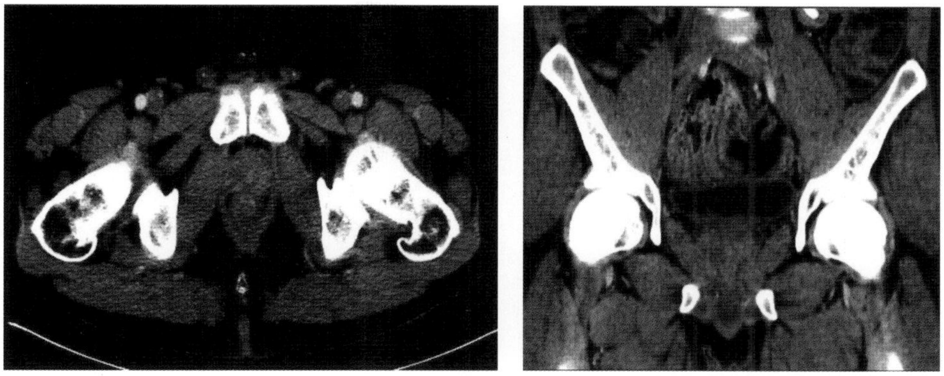

(a) (b)

FIGURE 2: Axial (a) and coronal (b) views of CT abdomen and pelvis with contrast after completion of 6 weeks of intravenous antibiotic therapy showing resolution of prostatic abscess.

differential diagnosis after detecting MRSA in the urine should include pyelonephritis, renal abscess, prostate abscess, endocarditis, skin infection, or staphylococcal bacteremia originating from another site [3, 7, 9]. MRSA bacteremia can be the origin or the consequence of a prostatic abscess. In our case, further investigation to identify the origin of the bacteremia, including careful history, physical examination, and echocardiogram, was negative except for the presence of the prostatic abscess.

Imaging studies obtained by CT and transrectal ultrasound (TRUS) are useful in the diagnosis of prostatic abscesses. There are no studies that have described superiority of any of these techniques over the others. TRUS is often used initially and can show one or more hypoechoic areas with well-defined and thick walls containing fluid. However, it may be inconclusive in the initial stages of abscess formation [3, 10]. Additionally, it may cause pain to patients and abscess size may be altered based on the angle of TRUS. CT is not painful, has less operator dependence, and can detect spread of infection to nearby organs [3]. In addition, CT offers better characterization of the lesion and can differentiate an abscess from a cyst, granuloma, or malignancy [4]. There is no consensus regarding which imaging modality to use, and some authors advocate starting with TRUS, as one study showed 100% accuracy in diagnosis of prostate abscesses [11].

While it is widely agreed that prompt treatment is crucial to prevent morbidity and mortality, there are no randomized clinical trials or expert consensus statements that recommend conservative management, percutaneous aspiration, or surgical incision and drainage as the particular treatment strategy of choice [3, 4, 7]. Conservative management is limited to antibiotics targeted against the organism found in the cultures. If an additional intervention is decided, it depends on local experience to decide between transurethral resection of prostate (TURP) and transperineal percutaneous drainage. A 2012 retrospective study from Korea [3] described 52 patients with prostatic abscess of any etiology, where 11 received conservative treatment, 23 underwent TURP, and 18 had transperineal aspiration. The average length of hospital stay was 17.5 days. Of the 18 who underwent needle aspiration, hospital stay was longer (23 days) and 4 suffered recurrence within one month of discharge. Two patients died after conservative treatment, but it is unclear if this strategy was chosen due to poor general functional status. It was concluded that patients treated with TURP have a shorter length of stay than patients treated with needle aspiration, but the former is a more invasive procedure and carries the risk of greater complications [3]. Another retrospective study examined 48 patients with a prostatic abscess and devised an algorithm for treatment recommendations. For patients with an abscess size <2 cm, minimal symptoms, and no leukocytosis, antibiotics for 2 weeks were suggested. If these criteria were not fulfilled or if there was a persistent abscess, transperineal aspiration was recommended [11].

Of the 21 cases of MRSA prostatic abscess found in the literature, 4 were treated with antibiotics alone and 17 with the combination of antibiotics and at least one additional intervention (TURP, abscess drainage). Two patients died, one who was treated conservatively, and the other with transurethral abscess drainage. The choice of antibiotics, duration, and route of administration have not been well-defined for the treatment of MRSA prostatic abscess. One author has suggested one week of IV vancomycin followed by 4 weeks of trimethoprim and/or rifampin [4]. In our case, vancomycin was given initially and then switched to daptomycin due to ongoing renal injury. We decided to complete 6 weeks of therapy with IV daptomycin for the treatment of MRSA prostatic abscess and bacteremia and had symptomatic, microbiologic, and radiologic resolution. Daptomycin was considered sufficient therapy, as research has shown that it is highly excreted in the urine, has good penetration into biofilms, and is not affected by alkaline pH, which is often seen in prostate tissue [12, 13]. Our case is an example that, even in immunosuppressed patients, a conservative approach can be opted for if adequate follow-up is reassured.

We found 5 case reports of patients with prostatic abscess of any etiology following solid organ transplantation: 4 cases described after kidney transplant and 1 case following heart transplantation. The associated organisms were *Histoplasma capsulatum* [14, 15], *Cladophialophora carrionii* [16], *Pseudomonas aeruginosa* [17], and *Cryptococcus neoformans* [18]. In the cases of the renal transplant patients, the prostatic abscess was found at 2.5 and 3 years (*Histoplasma*), 10 months (*Cladophialophora*), and 6 days (*Pseudomonas*) after transplant. In the heart transplant patient, the abscess was found after 7 years (*Cryptococcus*). To our knowledge, this is the first case describing a prostatic abscess in a liver transplant recipient and the first case of MRSA prostatic abscess described in a solid organ transplant recipient.

4. Conclusion

In summary, we present a unique case of a patient with a MRSA prostatic abscess and bacteremia. Abnormal fluctuation of the prostate during rectal examination together with MRSA bacteriuria or MRSA bacteremia of unknown origin should raise the suspicion for this diagnosis. While *S. aureus* is not a common cause of a prostatic abscess, the growing number of these cases in the literature emphasizes the importance of early recognition in susceptible individuals, such as solid organ transplant recipients. Treatment should be individualized based on each patient's clinical condition.

Authors' Contribution

Tanima Jana, Jorge D. Machicado, and Giovanni E. Davogustto were involved with data collection and initial drafting of the paper. Jorge D. Machicado and Jen-Jung Pan were involved in critical revision of the paper.

References

[1] P. Krishnamohan, T. Schaninger, L. M. Baddour, and M. N. Al-Hasan, "Community-acquired methicillin-resistant Staphylococcus aureus prostatic abscesses," *American Journal of the Medical Sciences*, vol. 346, no. 4, pp. 341–344, 2013.

[2] S.-O. Lee, S. H. Kang, R. C. Abdel-Massih, R. A. Brown, and R. R. Razonable, "Spectrum of early-onset and late-onset bacteremias after liver transplantation: implications for management," *Liver Transplantation*, vol. 17, no. 6, pp. 733–741, 2011.

[3] K. Jang, D. H. Lee, S. H. Lee, and B. H. Chung, "Treatment of prostatic abscess: case collection and comparison of treatment methods," *Korean Journal of Urology*, vol. 53, no. 12, pp. 860–864, 2012.

[4] A. Naboush, A. A. Yassine, M. Yasmin, and N. Mobarakai, "Community-acquired methicillin-resistant *Staphylococcus aureus* prostatic abscess presenting as acute urinary retention: a case report and review of the literature," *Case Reports in Infectious Diseases*, vol. 2013, Article ID 761793, 5 pages, 2013.

[5] J. Docekal, J. Hall, B. Reese, J. Jones, and T. Ferguson, "A rare presentation of community acquired methicillin resistant *Staphylococcus aureus*," *Case Reports*, vol. 2013, Article ID 543762, 3 pages, 2013.

[6] M. T. Flannery and D. Humphrey, "Case report of a prostatic abscess with a review of the literature," *Case Reports in Medicine*, vol. 2012, Article ID 430657, 2 pages, 2012.

[7] D. J. Lachant, M. Apostolakos, and A. Pietropaoli, "Methicillin resistant *Staphylococcus aureus* prostatic abscess with bacteremia," *Case Reports in Infections Diseases*, vol. 2013, Article ID 613961, 5 pages, 2013.

[8] J. C. Routh, A. L. Alt, R. A. Ashley, S. A. Kramer, and T. G. Boyce, "Increasing prevalence and associated risk factors for methicillin resistant Staphylococcus aureus bacteriuria," *Journal of Urology*, vol. 181, no. 4, pp. 1694–1698, 2009.

[9] R. R. Muder, C. Brennen, J. D. Ribs et al., "Isolation of Staphylococcus aureus from the urinary tract: Association of isolation with symptomatic urinary tract infection and subsequent staphylococcal bacteremia," *Clinical Infectious Diseases*, vol. 42, no. 1, pp. 46–50, 2006.

[10] P. Singh, M. K. Yadav, S. K. Singh, A. Lal, and N. Khandelwal, "Case series: diffusion weighted MRI appearance in prostatic abscess," *Indian Journal of Radiology and Imaging*, vol. 21, no. 1, pp. 46–48, 2011.

[11] J. Vyas, S. Ganpule, A. Ganpule, R. Sabnis, and M. Desai, "Transrectal ultrasound-guided aspiration in the management

of prostatic abscess: a single-center experience," *Indian Journal of Radiology and Imaging*, vol. 23, no. 3, pp. 253–257, 2013.

[12] R. Cantón, P. Ruiz-Garbajosa, R. L. Chaves, and A. P. Johnson, "A potential role for daptomycin in enterococcal infections: what is the evidence?" *Journal of Antimicrobial Chemotherapy*, vol. 65, no. 6, pp. 1126–1136, 2010.

[13] K. C. Lamp, M. J. Rybak, E. M. Bailey, and G. W. Kaatz, "In vitro pharmacodynamic effects of concentration, pH, and growth phase on serum bactericidal activities of daptomycin and vancomycin," *Antimicrobial Agents and Chemotherapy*, vol. 36, no. 12, pp. 2709–2714, 1992.

[14] W. W. Baig, R. P. Attur, A. Chawla et al., "Epididymal and prostatic histoplasmosis in a renal transplant recipient from southern India," *Transplant Infectious Disease*, vol. 13, no. 5, pp. 489–491, 2011.

[15] A. Chawla, K. Chawla, and J. Thomas, "Genitourinary histoplasmosis in post-renal transplant patient: diagnostic dilemma," *Indian Journal of Urology*, vol. 28, no. 3, pp. 359–361, 2012.

[16] A. J. Kindo, S. Ramalakshmi, S. Giri, and G. Abraham, "A fatal case of prostatic abscess in a post-renal transplant recipient caused by Cladophialophora carrionii," *Saudi Journal of Kidney Diseases and Transplantation*, vol. 24, no. 1, pp. 76–79, 2013.

[17] B. S. Zeidan, W. C. Waltzer, Z. Frischer, F. Miller, and F. T. Rapaport, "Prostatic abscess in a renal transplant recipient—a case report," *Transplantation Proceedings*, vol. 24, no. 2, pp. 755–756, 1992.

[18] P. E. Sax and A. R. Mattia, "Case records of the Massachusetts General Hospital. Weekly clinicopathological exercises. Case 7-1994, A 55-year-old heart transplant recipient with a tender, enlarged prostate gland," *The New England Journal of Medicine*, vol. 330, no. 7, pp. 490–496, 1994.

[19] A. Deshpande, G. Haleblian, and A. Rapose, "Prostate abscess: MRSA spreading its influence into Gram-negative territory: case report and literature review," *BMJ Case Reports*, 2013.

[20] S. Sukhal, J. G. Zamora, and P. Herrera, "An unusual cause of prostatic abscess: a case report and review of literature," *Infectious Diseases in Clinical Practice*, vol. 21, no. 5, pp. 289–291, 2013.

[21] I. Javeed, P. Kaushik, M. Chowdhury, B. Palermo, and C. L. Emery, "Community acquired methicillin resistant *Staphylococcus aureus* (CA-MRSA) prostatic abscess in a diabetic patient," *International Journal of Case Reports and Images*, vol. 3, no. 2, pp. 20–23, 2012.

[22] M. Matsumoto, K. Shigemura, F. Yamamichi et al., "A case of prostate abscess with sepsis, infectious endocarditis and pyogenic spondylitis," *Hinyokika Kiyo*, vol. 58, no. 10, pp. 565–568, 2012.

[23] D. Abreu, C. Arroyo, R. Suarez et al., "Community-acquired methicillin resistant Staphylococcus aureus: a new aetiological agent of prostatic abscess," *British Medical Journal Case Reports*, vol. 2011, 4 pages, 2011.

[24] S. C. Park, J. W. Lee, and J. S. Rim, "Prostatic abscess caused by community-acquired methicillin-resistant Staphylococcus aureus," *International Journal of Urology*, vol. 18, no. 7, pp. 536–538, 2011.

[25] P. Tiwari, D. K. Pal, A. Tripathi et al., "Prostatic abscess: diagnosis and management in the modern antibiotic era," *Saudi Journal of Kidney Diseases and Transplantation*, vol. 22, no. 2, pp. 298–301, 2011.

[26] B. H. Chao, J. M. Kidd, and A. W. Dow, "Methicillin-resistant Staphylococcus aureus bacteremia due to prostatic abscess," *Journal of Hospital Medicine*, vol. 4, no. 1, pp. E9–E11, 2009.

[27] V. Baradkar, M. Mathur, and S. Kumar, "Prostatic abscess by *Staphylococcus aureus* in a diabetic patient," *Indian Journal of Medical Microbiology*, vol. 26, no. 4, pp. 395–397, 2008.

[28] M. Gautam, A. Gandhi, and F. Rose, "Methicillin-resistant Staphylococcus aureus: fatal prostatic abscess in an AIDS patient," *Southern Medical Journal*, vol. 101, no. 4, article 449, 2008.

[29] M. Y. Lin, K. Rezai, and D. N. Schwartz, "Septic pulmonary emboli and bacteremia associated with deep tissue infections caused by community-acquired methicillin-resistant *Staphylococcus aureus*," *Journal of Clinical Microbiology*, vol. 46, no. 4, pp. 1553–1555, 2008.

[30] J. R. Pierce Jr., Q. Saeed, and W. R. Davis, "Prostatic abscess due to community-acquired methicillin-resistant Staphylococcus aureus," *American Journal of the Medical Sciences*, vol. 335, no. 2, pp. 154–156, 2008.

[31] T. J. Beckman and R. S. Edson, "Methicillin-resistant *Staphylococcus aureus* prostatitis," *Urology*, vol. 69, no. 4, pp. 771.e1–779.e3, 2007.

[32] F. Cabrera Meirás, A. Sanchís Bonet, O. Blanco Carballo, A. Martín Parada, G. Duque Ruiz, and O. Leiva Galvis, "Sthapylococcus aureus prostatic abscess and subdural empyema: a case report," *Actas Urólogicas Españolas*, vol. 31, no. 5, pp. 548–552, 2007.

[33] A. A. R. Tobian and S. K. Ober, "Dual perinephric and prostatic abscesses from methacillin-resistant *Staphylococcus aureus*," *Southern Medical Journal*, vol. 100, no. 5, pp. 515–516, 2007.

[34] A. W. Shindel, M. D. Darcy, and S. B. Brandes, "Management of prostatic abscess with community-acquired methicillin-resistant Staphylococcus aureus after straddle injury to the urethra," *Journal of Trauma—Injury, Infection and Critical Care*, vol. 61, no. 1, pp. 219–221, 2006.

[35] S. D. Baker, D. C. Horger, and T. E. Keane, "Community-acquired methicillin-resistant *Staphylococcus aureus* prostatic abscess," *Urology*, vol. 64, no. 4, pp. 808–810, 2004.

[36] T. G. Fraser, N. D. Smith, and G. A. Noskin, "Persistent methicillin-resistant Staphylococcus aureus bacteremia due to a prostatic abscess," *Scandinavian Journal of Infectious Diseases*, vol. 35, no. 4, pp. 273–274, 2003.

[37] P. Oliveira, J. A. Andrade, H. C. Porto, J. E. P. Filho, and A. F. J. Vinhaes, "Diagnosis and treatment of prostatic abscess," *International Brazilian Journal of Urology*, vol. 29, no. 1, pp. 30–34, 2003.

[38] S. J. Trauzzi, C. J. Kay, D. G. Kaufman, and F. C. Lowe, "Management of prostatic abscess in patients with human immunodeficiency syndrome," *Urology*, vol. 43, no. 5, pp. 629–633, 1994.

[39] S. Savarirayan, Y. Shenykin, R. Gerard, and G. J. Wise, "Staphylococcus periprostatic abscess: an unusual cause of acute urinary retention," *Urology*, vol. 46, no. 4, pp. 573–574, 1995.

[40] S. K. Gill, R. J. C. Gilson, and D. Rickards, "Multiple prostatic abscesses presenting with urethral discharge," *Genitourinary Medicine*, vol. 67, no. 5, pp. 411–412, 1991.

33

Liver Transplant for Unusually Large Polycystic Liver Disease: Challenges and Pitfalls

Pablo Serrano Rodriguez,[1] **Alfred Sidney Barritt IV**,[2] **David Allen Gerber**,[1] **and Chirag Sureshchandra Desai**[1]

[1]*Department of Surgery, Division of Abdominal Transplant Surgery, The University of North Carolina at Chapel Hill, Chapel Hill, NC 27599, USA*
[2]*Division of Gastroenterology and Hepatology, The University of North Carolina at Chapel Hill, Chapel Hill, NC 27599, USA*

Correspondence should be addressed to Chirag Sureshchandra Desai; chirag_desai@med.unc.edu

Academic Editor: Ryszard Grenda

Patients with polycystic liver disease are described in the literature as both recipient and donor for liver transplant. Due to well-preserved liver function, it is often difficult for these patients to receive an organ. Livers of these patients are often large and heavier than a normal organ. We describe two cases who had exceedingly large livers, weighing 14 and 19 kg. To the best of our knowledge and search, these are some of the heaviest explanted livers, and one of the patients incidentally received a liver from a donor with ADPKD. The aim of this report is to discuss the challenges and pitfalls of evaluating and listing, technical aspect of the transplant, possibility of transplanting a liver from a donor with a genetic cystic disease to a cystic disease recipient, and the related literature with some highlights on the facts from UNOS/OPTN data.

1. Introduction

Polycystic liver disease (PLD) can be associated with autosomal dominant polycystic kidney disease (ADPKD) and autosomal dominant polycystic liver disease (ADPLD) [1–3]. These are progressive diseases that can have an increase in liver size of up to 3.7% annually [4]. Patients can have cysts at an early age but normally do not have renal and/or hepatic manifestations until the 5th-6th decades of life. With large cysts, quality of life is affected due to either compressive symptoms or end organ damage that can progress to death [5, 6]. The medical management includes avoiding exogenous estrogen, medications like somatostatin analogues like octreotide, and mTOR inhibitors with variable success [3, 7, 8]. Invasive options include aspiration sclerotherapy, laparoscopic fenestration, and liver resection [9–14].

Of all patients diagnosed with PLD, 60% present with symptoms, 42% of the patients require at least one treatment of any kind, 23% require more than 1 intervention, 17% present with complications, and 8% of the patients fail to respond to any of these therapies. Patients with progressive disease with failed therapies either become overtly decompensated due to comorbidities or progress to end stage liver disease requiring orthotopic liver transplant (OLT) [15]. In most patients, model for end stage liver disease (MELD) score remains low. As MELD is the metric for liver graft allocation in the United States, these patients rarely receive priority for transplant. Since 2013, after the establishment of the share 35 rule, regional sharing of donor organs has increased, making it much harder for lower MELD score patients to have an opportunity for transplant. Some patients with PLD have associated renal impairment making their MELD score more competitive, but in the large majority, their score is still lower than other cirrhotic patients [16]. For that reason in 2015 the Organ Procurement and Transplantation Network (OPTN) published guidelines to standardize the allocation of exception points for patients with PLD. In order to be eligible for exception points, the patient needs to demonstrate hepatic decompensation, hemodialysis, or "compensated comorbidities" [17], rather than quality of life issue [18]. Patients transplanted for PCLD have 30-day morbidity of 41% and mortality of 5%. The 1- and 5-year survival of liver transplant alone are 93 and 91%. In patients receiving a simultaneous liver-kidney transplant, 1- and 5-year survival are lower, 86 and 80%, respectively [19], and 6% of patients required retransplantation. A majority of patients experience improvement in quality of life [20].

The large livers increase the technical difficulty of these procedures. We describe two cases of 51 and 98 kg women who had unusually large livers, weighing 14 and 19 kg, respectively. To the best of our knowledge and literature search, these are some of the heaviest explanted livers. Incidentally, one of our patients received a liver from a donor with ADPKD with multiple small liver cysts. The aim of reporting this series is to discuss the challenges and pitfalls of evaluating and listing this complex patient, the technical aspect of the transplant, and utility of transplanting a liver from one cystic disease donor to a cystic disease recipient while discussing the related literature.

2. Case Reports

A 57-year-old female [177 cm (5′10) 51 kg (113)] with ADPKD had an extensive history of comorbidities, including ascites with multiple paracenteses, repeated spontaneous bacterial peritonitis, pyrosis, hyporexia, early satiety, abdominal pain, severe weight loss, and malnutrition. In the year prior to the transplant, she clinically deteriorated and was unable to perform basic chores. She had portal hypertension with esophageal varices and thrombocytopenia. She was listed at that point with MELD score of 18. Since MRI failed to detail vascular patency and anatomy, because of large cysts, CT venogram was done as a preoperative workup, which showed displacement of the inferior vena cava pushing it to the left side of the aorta due to large caudate lobe cyst (Figure 1). Portal vein was stretched and patent and hepatic artery was normal. While listed, she developed a right common iliac deep venous thrombosis (DVT) due to external compression from her hepatic cysts requiring her to be on anticoagulation pushing MELD score to 25. A suitable organ was offered to her from the local organ procurement organization. Donor details are described in Table 1.

Of note, during the donor evaluation, ADPKD was diagnosed with multiple kidney cysts and with liver involvement including small-disseminated cysts but with almost normal size. During the transplant hepatectomy, the extremely enlarged liver was difficult to mobilize, and multiple cysts had to be transected in order to mobilize the organ from the abdominal cavity and obtain vascular control. Anatomy was distorted making the dissection of the portal vain and the inferior vena cava more complicated. We kept all vessels as long as possible. After explant the liver weighed 14 kg. A standard technique was followed with caval replacement without venovenous bypass (VVB). After the procedure, the patient was extubated on postoperative day one with downtrending LFTs. She was started on tacrolimus, mycofenolic acid, and a steroid taper. She was discharged home 10 days after the procedure without any complications. At 6-month follow-up, she has significant improvement in quality of life, increased appetite, and improved nutritional status.

The second case was a 53-year-old female [177 cm (5′10) 93 kg (205)] with history of ADPKD with similar symptoms as the first case; she had a hepatic hydrothorax that required monthly tapping to improve her shortness of breath. She had a native MELD of 10 with severe malnutrition. Exception points were obtained to increase to a MELD of 23. Donor details are in Table 1.

During the transplant, 21 liters of ascites was removed. Transplant surgery was performed similar to the first case and the patient received the same immunosuppression as the previous one. Explant in this case weighed 19.4 kg (Figure 2). Of note, during the explant, when we started cutting the suprahepatic cava, after clamping vessels, and cutting PV and infrahepatic IVC, due to the weight of the liver, RHV area tore and got retracted in the clamp. We applied another clamp above after dissecting the diaphragm to get adequate cuff for the anastomosis. Postoperative course was significant for ascites and hydrothorax requiring prolonged weaning and tracheostomy. She had an episode of rejection, which was successfully treated. After a month long stay, she has been discharged to rehab.

3. Discussion

Data from OPTN/UNOS from February 2002 to December 2015 show that from 117,427 patients listed, 620 (0.5%) were PLD cases. Of these cases, 351 (56.6%) had transplants and 81 (13.1%) died on the waitlist or became too sick to transplant. The average wait time was 196 days, that is, longer than the wait time of patients with HCC (130 days) and patients with chronic liver failure (58 days). Of all PLD patients listed, 269 (43.4%) received exception points, making them more likely to have transplant compared with those who were listed without exception points (78.8% versus 39.6%). Their waitlist mortality and removal from the list were significantly higher than those of HCC though lower than those of CLF (21.4% versus 5.2% versus 26.9%, resp.) [21]. Looking at these numbers, it is highly intuitive that exception petitions should be filed for these patients and listing be considered very early on.

The sheer size of the liver can make it difficult to evaluate patency of the portal vein and vena cava. As many centers perform MRI for pretransplant evaluation of liver disease, it is noteworthy that the multiple cysts make it difficult to assess vascular patency and anatomy. In contrast, a triple-phase CT scan and reconstructed venogram were very useful in both of our cases. Nutritional status of these patients is also a concern, thereby requiring these patients to be on either enteral or parenteral nutritional support preoperatively.

During the surgery, the typical cirrhotic liver is small and can be easily manipulated. Enlarged polycystic livers make mobilization and dissection of the hilum more complicated. The typical liver volume is 1.1 kg, and the average polycystic liver increases to 6.695 kg [22]. Mobilization and visualization improves with fenestration of select cysts, and this has to be performed carefully to avoid injuring the displaced vessels and collaterals. Most of the vessels are under tension making them susceptible to tearing and rupture. The IVC

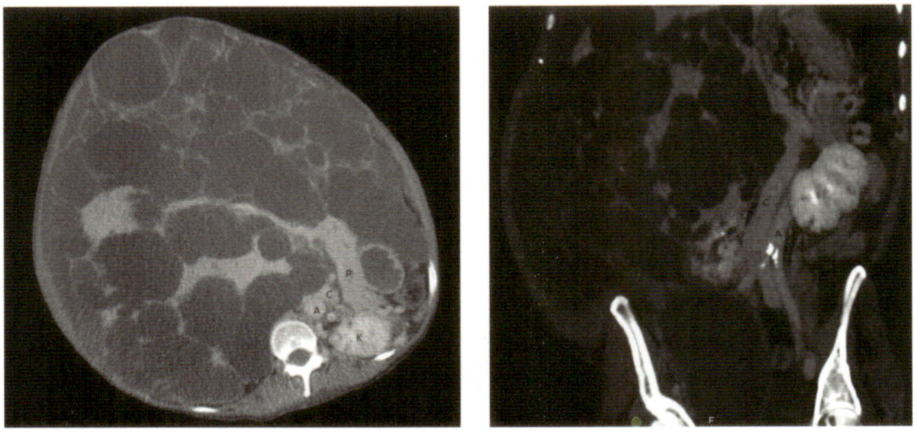

(a) (b)

FIGURE 1: (a) Axial section CT showing abdominal anatomy with kidney (K) and pancreas (P) in relation to liver. (b) Coronal plane CT venogram showing vena cava (C) pushed on the left side of the aorta (A).

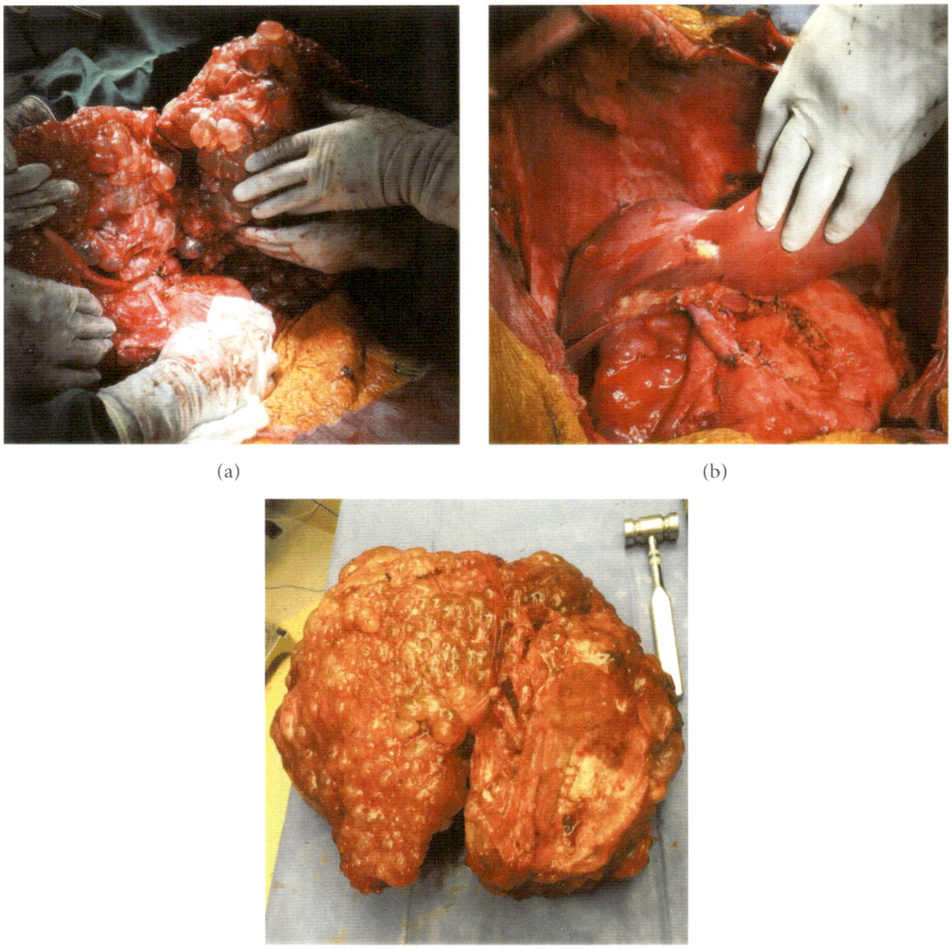

(a) (b)

(c)

FIGURE 2: (a) Intraop. imaging of native liver. (b) Liver after reperfusion. (c) Explanted recipient liver.

TABLE 1: Demographics and lab work for both donors showing terminal value and peak value in parenthesis.

	Donor 1	Donor 2
Age (years)	32	21
Race	African American	Caucasian
Gender	Male	Female
AST	25 (83)	48 (84)
ALT	20 (58)	17 (25)
Alkaline phosphatase	53 (60)	35 (49)
Bilirubin	0.3 (0.4)	4 (4)
Creatinine	0.74 (1.65)	0.9 (1.7)
INR	0.9 (1.1)	1.4 (1.6)
Albumin	3.6 (2.1)	3.1 (3.8)
Sodium	155 (158)	134 (155)
Potassium	4 (5.1)	4 (4.1)
Hemoglobin	7.7 (13.3)	10.5 (10.5)
Platelet	246 (383)	88 (164)
Vasopressors	No	No

is frequently displaced and compressed in 60% of patients [22]. During the hepatectomy, it is imperative to preserve vascular length to compensate for the size mismatch of the donor graft and avoid tension during implantation. Due to such a large size, it is preferable to do standard bicaval replacement technique over the piggyback technique for the transplant. These patients have portal hypertension, and with modern anesthetic management, they usually do not require venovenous bypass (VVB). One problem we had encountered as mentioned earlier is weight dragging the suprahepatic cava and causing retraction. In hindsight, maybe in such a heavy liver, to prevent this drag, we should cut the suprahepatic cava before the infrahepatic, so that natural tendency while cutting top cava to pull on the liver is avoided.

Due to the lack of availability of suitable donor liver grafts, there is increasing pressure to accept more unconventional donors for the purpose of transplantation [23]. Patients with PLD have been described in the literature as donors, for both living and cadaveric donation [24, 25]. Following Gigot's classification, type 1 includes the presence of less than 10 large hepatic cysts measuring no more than 10 cm in maximum diameter [24] and can be suitable for transplantation as a donor. It would be interesting to evaluate strategies to prevent enlargement of cyst from donor, but current literature does not support any evidence-based measure. PLD patients can undergo transplant from living donors, but this may be suitable only in few cases. Development of postsurgical ascites is a challenge after any form of surgery for PLD. However, with good graft function, improved nutrition, and gentle diuretics, most can be controlled.

In conclusion, patients with PLD are more complicated and disadvantaged. They often require exception point petition and the utilization of innovative donors. It is essential to avoid undue tension on small vessels during the hepatectomy and be aware of the distorted anatomy preoperatively. Size and weight of the liver are the most challenging parts of this surgery, but with appropriate precautions, good outcomes can be obtained.

Abbreviations

ADPKD: Autosomal dominant polycystic kidney disease
ADPLD: Autosomal dominant polycystic liver disease
CLF: Chronic liver failure
HA: Hepatic artery
IVC: Inferior vena cava
MELD: Model for end stage liver disease
OLT: Orthotopic liver transplant
PLD: Polycystic liver disease
PV: Portal vein
RHV: Right hepatic vein.

References

[1] T. Roskams and V. Desmet, "Embryology of extra- and intrahepatic bile ducts, the ductal plate," *Anatomical Record*, vol. 291, no. 6, pp. 628–635, 2008.

[2] D. M. Reynolds, C. T. Falk, A. Li et al., "Identification of a locus for autosomal dominant polycystic liver disease, on chromosome 19p13.2-13.1," *American Journal of Human Genetics*, vol. 67, no. 6, pp. 1598–1604, 2000.

[3] G. T. Everson and M. R. G. Taylor, "Management of polycystic liver disease," *Current Fungal Infection Reports*, vol. 7, no. 1, pp. 19–25, 2005.

[4] M. C. Hogan, T. V. Masyuk, L. J. Page et al., "Randomized clinical trial of long-acting somatostatin for autosomal dominant polycystic kidney and liver disease," *Journal of the American Society of Nephrology*, vol. 21, no. 6, pp. 1052–1061, 2010.

[5] G. I. Kirchner, K. Rifai, T. Cantz et al., "Outcome and quality of life in patients with polycystic liver disease after liver or combined liver-kidney transplantation," *Liver Transplantation*, vol. 12, no. 8, pp. 1268–1277, 2006.

[6] W. Uddin, J. K. Ramage, B. Portmann et al., "Hepatic venous outflow obstruction in patients with polycystic liver disease:

pathogenesis and treatment," *Gut*, vol. 36, no. 1, pp. 142–145, 1995.

[7] Q. Qian, H. Du, B. F. King et al., "Sirolimus reduces polycystic liver volume in ADPKD patients," *Journal of the American Society of Nephrology*, vol. 19, no. 3, pp. 631–638, 2008.

[8] M. Chrispijn, T. J. G. Gevers, J. C. Hol, R. Monshouwer, H. M. Dekker, and J. P. H. Drenth, "Everolimus does not further reduce polycystic liver volume when added to long acting octreotide: Results from a randomized controlled trial," *Journal of Hepatology*, vol. 59, no. 1, pp. 153–159, 2013.

[9] E. VanSonnenberg, J. T. Wroblicka, H. B. D'Agostino et al., "Symptomatic hepatic cysts: Percutaneous drainage and sclerosis," *Radiology*, vol. 190, no. 2, pp. 387–392, 1994.

[10] T. Iijima, T. Suwabe, K. Sumida et al., "Prediction of hepatic cyst recurrence after minocycline hydrochloride aspiration sclerotherapy using cyst computed tomography values," *Hepatology Research*, vol. 47, no. 5, pp. 419–424, 2017.

[11] M. Kabbej, A. Sauvanet, D. Chauveau, O. Farges, and J. Belghiti, "Laparoscopic fenestration in polycystic liver disease," *British Journal of Surgery*, vol. 83, no. 12, pp. 1697–1701, 1996.

[12] T. Koperna, S. Vogl, U. Satzinger, and F. Schulz, "Nonparasitic cysts of the liver: results and options of surgical treatment," *World Journal of Surgery*, vol. 21, no. 8, pp. 850–855, 1997.

[13] C. Vons, D. Chauveau, E. Martinod, C. Smadja, F. Capron, J. P. Grunfeld et al., "Liver resection in patients with polycystic liver disease," *Gastroenterologie clinique et biologique*, vol. 22, pp. 50–54, 1998.

[14] F. Que, D. M. Nagorney, J. B. Gross Jr., and V. E. Torres, "Liver resection and cyst fenestration in the treatment of severe polycystic liver disease," *Gastroenterology*, vol. 108, no. 2, pp. 487–494, 1995.

[15] L. Van Keimpema, D. B. De Koning, B. Van Hoek et al., "Patients with isolated polycystic liver disease referred to liver centres: Clinical characterization of 137 cases," *Liver International*, vol. 31, no. 1, pp. 92–98, 2011.

[16] L. Arrazola, D. Moonka, R. G. Gish, and G. T. Everson, "Model for End-Stage Liver Disease (MELD) exception for polycystic liver disease," *Liver Transplantation*, vol. 12, no. 12, pp. S110–S111, 2006.

[17] U. S. Department of, U.S. Department of Health & Human Services. Guidance on MELD PELD exception review. Organ Procure Transplant Network, US Dep Heal Hum Serv 2015. https://optn.transplant.hrsa.gov/resources/by-organ/liver-intestine/guidance-on-meld-peld-exception-review/.

[18] C. M. Flavin, Guidance to Liver Transplant Programs and the National Liver Review Board for Adult MELD Exception Review OPTN/UNOS Liver and Intestinal Organ Transplantation Committee. OPTN/UNOS Liver Intest Organ Transplant Comm 2016. https://optn.transplant.hrsa.gov/governance/public-comment/adult-meld-exception-review-guidance/.

[19] E. S. Orman, M. E. Mayorga, S. B. Wheeler et al., "Declining liver graft quality threatens the future of liver transplantation in the United States," *Liver Transplantation*, vol. 21, no. 8, pp. 1040–1050, 2015.

[20] J. P. H. Drenth, M. Chrispijn, D. M. Nagorney, P. S. Kamath, and V. E. Torres, "Medical and surgical treatment options for polycystic liver disease1," *Hepatology*, vol. 52, no. 6, pp. 2223–2230, 2010.

[21] G. T. Everson, M. R. G. Taylor, and R. B. Doctor, "Polycystic disease of the liver," *Hepatology*, vol. 40, no. 4, pp. 774–782, 2004.

[22] S. D. Doshi, T. Bittermann, T. D. Schiano, and D. S. Goldberg, "Waitlisted Candidates with Polycystic Liver Disease Are More Likely to be Transplanted Than Those with Chronic Liver Failure," *Transplantation*, vol. 101, no. 8, pp. 1838–1844, 2017.

[23] T. Schnelldorfer, V. E. Torres, S. Zakaria, C. B. Rosen, and D. M. Nagorney, "Polycystic liver disease: a critical appraisal of hepatic resection, cyst fenestration, and liver transplantation," *Annals Surgery*, vol. 250, pp. 112–118, 2009.

[24] E. S. Orman, A. S. Barritt, S. B. Wheeler, and P. H. Hayashi, "Declining liver utilization for transplantation in the United States and the impact of donation after cardiac death," *Liver Transplantation*, vol. 19, no. 1, pp. 59–68, 2013.

[25] B. Abu-Wasel, C. Walsh, V. Keough, and M. Molinari, "Pathophysiology, epidemiology, classification and treatment options for polycystic liver diseases," *World Journal of Gastroenterology*, vol. 19, no. 35, pp. 5775–5786, 2013.

34

Tacrolimus Aggravated Tube Feeding Syndrome with Acute Renal Failure in a Pediatric Liver Transplant Recipient

R. Kula, M. Melter, J. Kunkel, C. Dörfler, S. Alikadic, B. Knoppke, and R. Zant

KUNO University Children's Hospital, Regensburg, Germany

Correspondence should be addressed to R. Zant; robert.zant@ukr.de

Academic Editor: Federica Meloni

Acute renal failure can be caused by calcineurin inhibitors (CNIs), due to arteriolopathy and altered tubular function. Within this context, we present the case of a 14-month-old liver transplant recipient who suffered an acute polyuric renal failure during a short episode of hypercaloric feeding. In our case, CNI-induced distal RTA led to nephrocalcinosis and therefore to secondary nephrogenic diabetes insipidus. The diet with high renal solute load consequently resulted in an acute polyuric renal failure with severe hypernatremic dehydration. In conclusion, a hypercaloric diet in children with potentially impaired renal function due to therapy with CNIs requires precise calculation of the potential renal solute load and the associated fluid requirements.

1. Introduction

Tacrolimus and cyclosporine are widely used calcineurin inhibitors (CNIs) with a narrow therapeutic window and multiple drug-drug interactions [1]. They have the potency to induce renal failure due to acute arteriolopathy. Moreover, CNIs lead to altered tubular function, resulting in an impaired renal concentrating ability [2].

Within this context, we report the case of a pediatric liver transplant recipient who suffered acute polyuric renal failure leading to severe dehydration during a diet with high renal solute load.

Informed consent was obtained from the parents for publication of this report.

2. Case Presentation

A 14-month-old girl with a body weight of 7.7 kg was admitted to our pediatric intensive care unit (PICU) in acute polyuric renal failure including severe hypernatremia, hyperchloremia, hyperkalemia, hyperuricemia, and metabolic acidosis. Clinically she was irritable and appeared only mildly dehydrated. Her heart rate on admission was 150 beats per minute with an arterial blood pressure of 83/43 (63) mmHg. Renal ultrasound on admission revealed bilateral nephrocalcinosis type IIa. Her laboratory findings on admission are summarized in Table 1. The girl was treated with tacrolimus after liver transplantation 7 months prior to admission for extrahepatic biliary atresia. Renal ultrasound before liver transplantation showed a normal finding. She was discharged home from a former hospital stay 8 days prior to this admission with the recommendation for 800 ml Nutrini Energy MultiFibre® (Table 2) a day in addition to complementary feeding. Against medical advice she drank no additional water. Therefore, her calculated water deficit over the last 8 days was 23.6% of her body weight (Table 3). In PICU the high protein diet was interrupted and the girl was intravenously rehydrated. The average diuresis in the first 12 hours after admission was 8.1 ml/kg/hour. Additionally, bicarbonate was administered and the antihypertensive therapy with enalapril was paused for 2 days. Under these therapeutic measures the renal function recovered and the serum electrolytes returned to normal values. After reinstating feeding with Nutrini MultiFibre plus oral bicarbonate instead of Nutrini Energy MultiFibre the child was transferred to the normal ward. On day 9 after admission she was discharged home. At the time of discharge the patient's serum urea and creatinine values were within the normal range, her glomerular filtration rate assessed by serum cystatin C was 76 ml/min/1.73 sqm. In the later course immunosuppression was changed from tacrolimus monotherapy to low-dose tacrolimus plus mycophenolate mofetil.

Table 1: Laboratory findings on admission to the pediatric intensive care unit.

Laboratory findings on admission	
Serum pH	7.19
Serum bicarbonate	11.8 mmol/L
Serum base excess	−15 mmol/L
Serum sodium	170 mmol/L
Serum potassium	7.4 mmol/L
Serum chloride	143 mmol/L
Serum calcium	1.9 mmol/L
Serum phosphate	2.85 mmol/L
Serum creatinine	1.6 mg/dL
Serum urea	364 mg/dL
Serum osmolality (measured)	425 mmol/kg
Tacrolimus level	7.7 mcg/L
Urine pH	5.6
Urine osmolality	465 mmol/kg
Urine sodium/creatinine ratio	86 (mM based reference: <58)
Urine potassium/creatinine ratio	25 (mM based reference: <68)
Urine phosphate/creatinine ratio	18 (mM based reference: <14)

Table 2: Nutrini Energy MultiFibre.

Nutrini Energy MultiFibre	
Energy	1.5 kcal/ml
Protein	40 g/L
Sodium	39,1 mmol/L
Chloride	40.3 mmol/L
Potassium	42.2 mmol/L
Calcium	22.4 mmo/L
Phosphorus	24.2 mmol/L
Nitrogen	6400 mg/L
Osmolarity	315 mosmol/L
Potential renal solute load	374 mosmol/L

3. Discussion

The etiology of calcineurin inhibitor induced nephrotoxicity has not been clearly established yet. It is thought to be multifactorial, resulting from a combination of an increase in vasoconstrictive factors (endothelin and thromboxane), activation of the renin-angiotensin-aldosterone system, reduction of vasodilator factors (nitric oxide and prostacyclin), and formation of free radicals. CNIs also lead to tubular functional alterations and ion homeostasis disturbances like hyperkalemia, hypomagnesemia and magnesium wasting, distal tubular acidosis, and hyperuricemia. Some of the effects of CNIs on tubular function can be explained by reduced expression of the Na^+-K^+-$2Cl^-$-cotransporter (NKCC2) on the apical membrane of tubular epithelial cells. Decreased expression of NKCC2 would lead to polyuria, nephrocalcinosis, magnesium wasting, and hyperreninemic hyperaldosteronism [5]. As mentioned above, distal RTA is one of several features of nephrotoxicity induced by tacrolimus treatment [2]. Patients with distal RTA have a metabolic acidosis with an inability to acidify the urine appropriately. This type of RTA is caused by impaired distal acidification and is characterized by the inability to lower urinary pH maximally (<5.5) under the stimulus of systemic acidemia [6]. Hypercalciuria and nephrocalcinosis are typically present. The mainstay of therapy in all forms of RTA is bicarbonate replacement. The base requirement for distal RTAs is generally in the range of 2–4 mEq/kg/24 hours. Patients with distal RTA should be monitored for the development of hypercalciuria [7]. The defining characteristic of nephrocalcinosis is generalized calcium deposition in the kidney. Nephrocalcinosis can involve the renal medulla or, much less often, the cortex. The most common cause of nephrocalcinosis is increased urinary calcium excretion with or without hypercalcemia. Distal RTA is the most common cause of nephrocalcinosis (particularly in children) due to hypercalciuria without hypercalcemia. The reported prevalence of nephrocalcinosis in patients with distal RTA ranges from 60 to 80 percent. However, it is clinically difficult to differentiate since nephrocalcinosis itself frequently causes defects in distal acidification. Nocturia, polyuria, and polydipsia due to an impaired urinary concentrating ability (nephrogenic diabetes insipidus) may occur in patients with hypercalcemia or medullary nephrocalcinosis of any cause [8]. Recent data support the hypothesis that in vivo external calcium, through activation of calcium-sensing receptors, modulates the expression/trafficking of aquaporin 2 (AQP2). Short-term control of water permeability occurs via vesicular trafficking of AQP2 and long-term control through changes in the abundance of AQP2 and AQP3 water channels. Defective AQP2 trafficking causes nephrogenic diabetes insipidus, a condition characterized by the kidney's inability to produce concentrated urine because of the insensitivity of the distal nephron to vasopressin [9]. The underlying cause of nephrocalcinosis should be determined and treated if possible. No specific treatment has been shown to prevent progression of nephrocalcinosis. Increased fluid intake may be beneficial for all patients with nephrocalcinosis. Among patients with hypercalciuria, urinary calcium excretion may be reduced by dietary modifications that include restriction of animal protein and sodium intake [10]. Infant formulas have a lower protein content and therefore a lower renal solute load compared to products designed for patients aged over 1 year. Children with increased metabolic needs (e.g., after liver transplantation) and/or decreased fluid tolerance may not be able to consume an adequate volume of standard formulas to promote growth. In this instance, a more concentrated formula may be needed. However, a protein intake which accounts for more than 16% of calories could contribute to azotemia and negative water balance if associated fluid intakes are low. In these cases the caloric density can be increased by utilizing modular additives of carbohydrate or fat because both do not increase the renal solute load. The potential renal solute load does not need to be calculated routinely, but it is important with patients who have medical problems [11]. If healthy infants consume a predominantly liquid diet ad libitum, their ability to excrete unneeded solutes and to maintain water balance is more than adequate [3]. But the renal solute load and fluid balance should be closely monitored if children have a low fluid

TABLE 3: The patient's calculated water deficit over the last 8 days prior to admission to the pediatric intensive care unit.

Equations
Water intake = food intake × water content
Water requirement = (food intake × potential renal solute load/age dependent estimated maximal renal concentration capacity) + (insensible water losses × patient's body surface area)
Water deficit = water intake − water requirement
Case specific calculations
Water intake per day = 0.8 L/day × 0.77 L/L = 0.616 L/day
Water requirement per day = (0.8 L/day × 374 mOsmol/L/465 mOsmol/L) + (0.5 L/day/sqm × 0.4 sqm) = 0.843 L/day
Water deficit per day = 0.616 L/day − 0.843 L/day = −0.227 L/day
Water deficit within 8 days = 1.820 L
Percent of body weight = 1.820 L/7.7 kg~23.6%

Potential renal solute load (PRSL) refers to solutes of dietary origin that would need to be excreted in the urine if none were diverted into synthesis of new tissue or lost through nonrenal routes. It is calculated by the following equation: PRSL = nitrogen/28 + sodium + chloride + potassium + phosphorus. The units are in milliosmoles, except for nitrogen, which is total nitrogen in milligrams. Available phosphorus is assumed to be total phosphorus of milk-based formulas and two-thirds of the phosphorus of soy-based formulas. PRSL is expressed as milliosmoles per liter [3]. The renal concentration capacity on admission was 465 mOsmol/L. The insensible fluid losses under normal condition are 0.5 L/sqm/day [4].

intake, if they are receiving calorically dense feedings, or if they have increased extrarenal fluid losses and/or an impaired renal concentrating ability. In these children additional water may be required [12].

In summary, renal dysfunction in pediatric liver transplant recipients treated with CNIs like tacrolimus is well known and well documented in the existing literature [13]. The overall prevalence of chronic kidney disease in this population ranges up to 32% [14]. Renal failure due to nephrocalcinosis in pediatric liver transplantation is usually described in the context of hyperoxaluria; however, information on tacrolimus induced acute renal failure associated with nephrocalcinosis is scarce and to the best of our knowledge this is the first describing report [15]. Previously published reports include early graft failure in an adult kidney transplanted recipient with severe renal calcifications under tacrolimus treatment [16]. A likely pathophysiologic scenario in our case may have been that tacrolimus induced distal RTA led to nephrocalcinosis and therefore to secondary nephrogenic diabetes insipidus. Insufficient water intake in a diet with high renal solute load and further renal impairment due to enalapril treatment consequently resulted in an acute polyuric renal failure with severe hypernatremic dehydration.

4. Conclusion

A hypercaloric diet in children with potentially impaired renal function due to therapy with CNIs requires precise determination of the potential renal solute load and the associated fluid requirements. Pediatric liver transplant recipients treated with CNIs should be assessed for nephrocalcinosis and associated impaired renal function at regular intervals.

Abbreviations

AQP2: Aquaporin 2
CNIs: Calcineurin inhibitors
NKCC2: Na^+-K^+-$2Cl^-$-cotransporter
PICU: Pediatric intensive care unit
PRSL: Potential renal solute load
RTA: Renal tubular acidosis.

References

[1] Hesselink D. A., van Schaik R. H., van der Heiden I. P. et al., "Genetic polymorphisms of the CYP3A4, CYP3A5, and MDR-1 genes and pharmacokinetics of the calcineurin inhibitors cyclosporine and tacrolimus," *Clinical Pharmacology & Therapeutics*, vol. 74, pp. 245–254, 2003.

[2] M. Riveiro-Barciela, I. Campos-Varela, J. L. Tovar et al., "Hyperkalemic distal renal tubular acidosis caused by immunosuppressant treatment with tacrolimus in a liver transplant patient: case report," *Transplantation Proceedings*, vol. 43, no. 10, pp. 4016–4018, 2011.

[3] S. J. Fomon and E. E. Ziegler, "Renal solute load and potential renal solute load in infancy," *Journal of Pediatrics*, vol. 134, no. 1, pp. 11–14, 1999.

[4] J. S. Dallas and T. P. Foly Jr., "Foly TPJr. Thyromegaly," in *Pediatric Endocrinology*, F. Lifshitz, Ed., p. 663, Marcel Decker, Inc, New York, NY, USA, 5th edition, 2009.

[5] M. Naesens, D. R. J. Kuypers, and M. Sarwal, "Calcineurin inhibitor nephrotoxicity," *Clinical Journal of the American Society of Nephrology*, vol. 4, no. 2, pp. 481–508, 2009.

[6] J. R. Soriano, "Renal tubular acidosis: the clinical entity," *Journal of the American Society of Nephrology*, vol. 13, no. 8, pp. 2160–2170, 2002.

[7] R. W. Chesney, "Rickets associated with renal tubular acidosis," in *Nelson textbook of pediatrics*, R. M. Kliegman, B. F. Stanton, J. W. Geme, N. F. Schor, and R. E. Behrman, Eds., p. 1811, Elsevier Saunders, Philadelphia, PA, USA, 19th edition, 2011.

[8] G. Procino, L. Mastrofrancesco, A. Mira et al., "Aquaporin 2 and apical calcium-sensing receptor: new players in polyuric disorders associated with hypercalciuria," *Seminars in Nephrology*, vol. 28, no. 3, pp. 297–305, 2008.

[9] G. Valenti, G. Procino, G. Tamma, M. Carmosino, and M. Svelto, "Minireview: aquaporin 2 trafficking," *Endocrinology*, vol. 146, no. 12, pp. 5063–5070, 2005.

[10] L. Borghi, T. Schianchi, T. Meschi et al., "Comparison of two diets for the prevention of recurrent stones in idiopathic hypercalciuria," *The New England Journal of Medicine*, vol. 346, no. 2, pp. 77–84, 2002.

[11] S. J. Fomon, "Nutrition of normal infants," in *Mosby-Year Book*, M. O. St. Louis, Ed., vol. 100, Mosby-Year Book, St. Louis, MO, 1993.

[12] N. Nevin-Folino and T. Mayes, "Enteral nutrition," in *Handbook of pediatric nutrition*, P. Q. Samour and K. King, Eds., pp. 499–524, 2005.

[13] R. N. Fine, "Renal function following liver transplantation in children," *Pediatric Transplantation*, vol. 9, no. 5, pp. 680–684, 2005.

[14] K. M. Campbell, N. Yazigi, F. C. Ryckman et al., "High prevalence of renal dysfunction in long-term survivors after pediatric liver transplantation," *Journal of Pediatrics*, vol. 148, no. 4, pp. 475–480, 2006.

[15] M. Galanti and A. Contreras, "Excellent renal function and reversal of nephrocalcinosis 8 years after isolated liver transplantation in an infant with primary hyperoxaluria type 1," *Pediatric Nephrology*, vol. 25, no. 11, pp. 2359–2362, 2010.

[16] P. Esposito, G. Bedino, A. Gallotti, M. Gregorini, T. Rampino, and A. Dal Canton, "Early allograft calcifications after kidney transplantation," *Urology*, vol. 79, no. 3, p. e44, 2012.

35

Gallstone Pancreatitis: A Common but Often Overlooked Cause of Abdominal Pain in Post-Liver-Transplant Patients

Napatt Kanjanahattakij,[1] Kamolyut Lapumnuaypol,[1] Sanna Fatima,[1] and Eyob Feyssa[2]

[1] *Department of Internal Medicine, Einstein Medical Center, Philadelphia, PA, USA*
[2] *Department of Transplantation, Einstein Medical Center, Philadelphia, PA, USA*

Correspondence should be addressed to Napatt Kanjanahattakij; napattkj@gmail.com

Academic Editor: Piero Boraschi

Introduction. In general population, gallstone pancreatitis is the most common cause of pancreatitis. However, there are very few literatures that address this topic in post-liver-transplant patients. *Clinical Case.* A 69-year-old female who had a liver transplant in 2015 due to hepatocellular carcinoma and nonalcoholic steatohepatitis (NASH) cirrhosis. She had a recent episode of acute cellular rejection that was treated with high dose methylprednisolone 1 week prior to admission. She presented with severe epigastric abdominal pain associated with nausea and vomiting. Her laboratory studies showed significantly elevated serum lipase, AST, and ALT from her baseline. She underwent urgent Endoscopic Ultrasound (EUS) with Endoscopic Retrograde Cholangiopancreatography (ERCP) that showed common bile duct stone that was extracted. *Discussion.* Biliary sludge and stones accounted for 22% of late onset acute pancreatitis after liver transplant. Corticosteroids have been identified as one of the potential causes of drug-induced pancreatitis. However, she is more likely to have gall stone pancreatitis since she also had dilated common bile duct and intrahepatic duct. In addition, there was CBD stone noted on ERCP. *Conclusion.* Acute gallstone associated pancreatitis after liver transplant is not uncommon. Patients generally have good outcomes. Further prospective studies are warranted.

1. Introduction

Over the past decade, there has been an increase in the number of liver transplants in the United States. Over 70,000 adults are living with the liver allograft [1]. Biliary complication is one of the most common complications after liver transplant. The most common biliary complication after transplant is biliary stricture and bile leak [2]. Posttransplant bile ducts stone can also occur in 5–10% of liver-transplant recipients and it is associated with serious complication such as cholangitis and pancreatitis [3]. Acute pancreatitis can occur in 3–8% of post-liver-transplant patients [4]. However, there are very few case reports that specifically address this topic. We hereby report a case of a post-liver-transplant patient who presented to our center with abdominal pain and elevated serum lipase.

2. Case Presentation

We present a case of a 69-year-old female who had a liver transplant in 2015 due to hepatocellular carcinoma and nonalcoholic steatohepatitis (NASH) cirrhosis. Her posttransplant course was complicated by multiple episodes of acute cellular rejection. She had a recent episode of acute cellular rejection that was treated with high dose methylprednisolone 1 week prior to admission. Her immunosuppressive regimen included prednisone, mycophenolate mofetil, and tacrolimus.

She presented to the emergency department with severe epigastric abdominal pain associated with nausea and vomiting. She reported no recent alcohol or drug abuse. On abdominal examination, she had tenderness to palpation at epigastrium and right upper quadrant area without rigidity or rebound tenderness. Her laboratory studies showed

TABLE 1: Summary of laboratory results.

	Day 2	Day 1	Baseline
BUN (8–27 mg/dL)	32	38	33
Creatinine (0.6–1 mg/dL)	0.9	1.0	1.1
ALT (0–55 IU/L)	303	101	141
AST (5–34 IU/L)	246	42	33
Total bilirubin (0.2–1.2 mg/dL)	0.8	0.5	0.5
Direct bilirubin (0.1–1.5 mg/dL)	0.4	n/a	0.3
ALP (40–150 IU/L)	152	94	95
INR (0.9–1.1)	1.0	n/a	1.0
Lipase (8–78 IU/L)	530	186	n/a
Albumin (3.4–4.8 g/dL)	3.6	4.1	3.5

BUN = blood urea nitrogen, ALT = alanine aminotransferase, AST = aspartate aminotransferase, INR = international normalized ratio, and ALP = alkaline phosphatase.

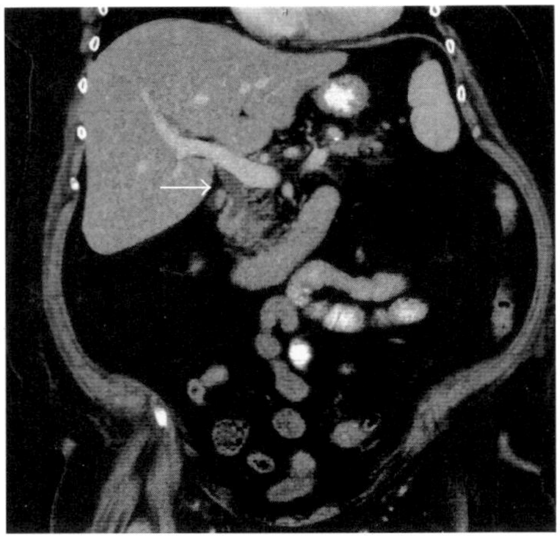

FIGURE 1: Dilated common bile duct (arrow).

significantly elevated serum lipase, AST, and ALT from her baseline (Table 1).

Her abdominal Computed Tomography (CT) scans with contrast showed acute edematous interstitial pancreatitis with enlarged common bile duct and intrahepatic duct without any calculus or discrete obstruction (Figure 1).

Our differential diagnosis included gall stone pancreatitis and drug-induced pancreatitis secondary to high dose steroid. Her prednisone was stopped. She underwent urgent Endoscopic Ultrasound (EUS) with Endoscopic Retrograde Cholangiopancreatography (ERCP) that showed dilated common bile duct with 4 mm hyperechoic stone that was extracted. She was diagnosed with gall stone pancreatitis.

Her pain significantly improved after the stone extraction.

3. Discussion

Acute pancreatitis is one of the serious complications after liver transplant, which can occur in up to 8% of patients after liver transplant. Our patient presented with signs and symptoms of pancreatitis caused by CBD stone.

3.1. Diagnosis. The criteria for diagnosis of pancreatitis are similar in normal population and posttransplant patients. To establish the diagnosis, it requires two out of the three of the following criteria: (1) abdominal pain that is consistent with the disease, (2) serum amylase and/or lipase greater than 3 times of the upper normal limit, and (3) abnormal imaging that is consistent with the disease [5]. Isolated elevation of lipase or amylase is nondiagnostic without signs and symptoms of pancreatitis.

3.2. Etiology. Multiple studies reported various identified etiology of acute pancreatitis after liver transplant. In one study of 1832 patients undergoing liver transplant, postoperative acute pancreatitis occurred in 3% of the patients [6]. The etiology is believed to be from intraoperative manipulation and ischemia [4].

Infection has also been linked to post-liver-transplant acute pancreatitis. CMV and varicella-zoster viruses have been reported as rare causes of posttransplant acute pancreatitis [7–9].

Posttransplant ERCP is also common after liver transplant. The ERCP is commonly performed in posttransplant period to rule out biliary complications, such as biliary stricture that can occur in 5–15% after deceased donor liver transplant [2]. ERCP is usually required to correct these complications resulting in high incidence of post-ERCP pancreatitis up to 11% of post-liver-transplant pancreatitis [4, 10, 11].

Biliary sludge and stones accounted for 22% of late onset acute pancreatitis after liver transplant [11]. Corticosteroids are the first-line treatment for acute rejection in post-liver-transplant population. Corticosteroids have been identified as one of the potential causes of drug-induced pancreatitis [12].

Our patient received steroid for the treatment of her acute rejection. However, she is more likely to have gall stone pancreatitis since she also had dilated common bile duct and intrahepatic duct. In addition there was CBD stone noted on ERCP.

3.3. Biliary Stone after Liver Transplant. A large study of 1650 subjects showed that bile duct filling defects can occur in 5.7% of patients after liver transplant. 56% percent of bile duct filling defects are from biliary sludge or cast, and 32% are from stone [13].

In a case control study, patients with bile duct stone were more likely to have underlying bile duct pathology after transplant and higher triglyceride and cholesterol.

3.4. Management. Management of acute pancreatitis in post-liver-transplant patient is generally the same as in normal population. There is no specific guideline for this specific population. Management of pancreatitis involves intravenous hydration, bowel rest, and etiology specific management [4, 5].

Our patient underwent ERCP and the stone was removed and she had significant symptom improvement. ERCP in the period after liver transplant is generally a safe procedure. A retrospective study, which included 157 post-liver-transplant patients who underwent ERCP, showed that complication occurred in 15% of the patients. The most common complication of ERCP is pancreatitis followed by bleeding [14].

3.5. Prognosis. Late post-liver-transplant pancreatitis has similar prognosis with general population. Mortality rate could be up to 11% of the patients [4].

4. Conclusion

Acute gallstone associated pancreatitis in post-liver-transplant patient generally has good outcomes. There is a paucity of data regarding the understanding of disease and specific risk factors associated with it. Further prospective studies are warranted for better understanding of the disease.

References

[1] S. A. Fayek, C. Quintini, K. D. Chavin, and C. L. Marsh, "The Current State of Liver Transplantation in the United States: Perspective From American Society of Transplant Surgeons (ASTS) Scientific Studies Committee and Endorsed by ASTS Council," *American Journal of Transplantation*, vol. 16, no. 11, pp. 3093–3104, 2016.

[2] W. S. Ayoub, C. O. Esquivel, and P. Martin, "Biliary complications following liver transplantation," *Digestive Diseases and Sciences*, vol. 55, no. 6, pp. 1540–1546, 2010.

[3] B. J. Spier, P. R. Pfau, K. R. Lorenze, S. J. Knechtle, and A. Said, "Risk factors and outcomes in post-liver transplantation bile duct stones and casts: A case-control study," *Liver Transplantation*, vol. 14, no. 10, pp. 1461–1465, 2008.

[4] A. Danalioğlu, O. J. Mitchell, V. K. Singh et al., "Acute pancreatitis following adult liver transplantation: A systematic review," *The Turkish Journal of Gastroenterology*, vol. 26, no. 6, pp. 450–455, 2015.

[5] S. Tenner, J. Baillie, J. Dewitt, and S. S. Vege, "American college of gastroenterology guideline: management of acute pancreatitis," *American Journal of Gastroenterology*, vol. 108, no. 9, pp. 1400–1415, 2013.

[6] N. V. Krokos, D. Karavias, A. Tzakis et al., "Acute pancreatitis after liver transplantation: incidence and contributing factors," *Transplant International*, vol. 8, no. 1, pp. 1–7, 1995.

[7] J. C. Coelho, J. C. Wiederkehr, A. C. Campos, C. Zeni Neto, and V. Oliva, "Acute pancreatitis caused by varicella-zoster virus after liver transplantation," *Journal de Chirurgie*, vol. 131, no. 2, pp. 96–98, 1994.

[8] J. C. U. Coelho, J. C. Wiederkehr, M. B. Parolin, E. Balbi, and A. E. Nassif, "Isolated tuberculosis of the pancreas after orthotopic liver transplantation," *Liver Transplantation and Surgery*, vol. 5, no. 2, pp. 153–155, 1999.

[9] A. Pascher and P. Neuhaus, "Bile duct complications after liver transplantation," *Transplant International*, vol. 18, no. 6, pp. 627–642, 2005.

[10] L. Lupo, J. Pirenne, B. Gunson et al., "Acute pancreatitis after orthotopic liver transplantation," *Transplantation Proceedings*, vol. 29, no. 1-2, p. 473, 1997.

[11] D. J. Verran, A. Gurkan, A. K. Chui et al., "Pancreatitis in adult orthotopic liver allograft recipients: Risk factors and outcome," *Liver Transplantation*, vol. 6, no. 3, pp. 362–366, 2000.

[12] N. Badalov, R. Baradarian, K. Iswara, J. Li, W. Steinberg, and S. Tenner, "Drug-Induced Acute Pancreatitis: An Evidence-Based Review," *Clinical Gastroenterology and Hepatology*, vol. 5, no. 6, pp. 648–e3, 2007.

[13] R. Sheng, C. B. Ramirez, A. B. Zajko, and W. L. Campbell, "Biliary stones and sludge in liver transplant patients: A 13-year experience," *Radiology*, vol. 198, no. 1, pp. 243–247, 1996.

[14] A. Hüsing, V. R. Cicinnati, M. Maschmeier et al., "Complications after endoscopic sphincterotomy in liver transplant recipients: A retrospective single-centre study," *Arab Journal of Gastroenterology*, vol. 16, no. 2, pp. 46–49, 2015.

Emergent Management of Intracardiac Thrombosis during Liver Transplantation

Caroline Protin,[1] Dmitri Bezinover,[1] Zakiyah Kadry,[2] and Thomas Verbeek[1]

[1]Department of Anesthesia and Perioperative Medicine, Penn State Health Milton S. Hershey Medical Center, Hershey, PA, USA
[2]Department of Surgery, Penn State Health Milton S. Hershey Medical Center, Hershey, PA, USA

Correspondence should be addressed to Dmitri Bezinover; dbezinover@hmc.psu.edu

Academic Editor: Luca Cicalese

Intraoperative thromboembolism is a well-documented complication associated with orthotopic liver transplantation (OLT) but its identification and intraoperative treatment are still an emerging topic in anesthesia. Intracardiac thrombus during OLT is associated with a high mortality rate. There are only a few reports describing the successful management of thromboembolism during OLT. We describe a case where routine intraoperative transesophageal echocardiography during a live donor liver transplantation enabled early detection of an intracardiac thrombus with subsequent successful heparin treatment. Our case suggests that if an intracardiac thrombus is identified early (before hemodynamic instability occurs), the use of IV heparin may be a safe therapeutic option.

1. Introduction

End-stage liver disease (ESLD) is associated with an increased risk for both hypo- and hypercoagulopathy [1]. Hypocoagulability is relatively easy to detect and treat. Hypercoagulability, on the other hand, is frequently unexpected and difficult to diagnose before hemodynamic instability occurs. Once diagnosed, treatment is challenging and outcomes vary. Intracardiac thrombus (ICT) formation during orthotopic liver transplantation (OLT) is associated with a mortality rate as high as 68% [2]. A small number of published reports describe the successful use of recombinant tissue plasminogen activator (rTPA) as well as thrombectomy in the treatment of both intracardiac and pulmonary thrombi [3]. There are some reports of the use of intravenous heparin for the treatment of ICT during OLT in hemodynamically unstable patients [3]. All of these attempts failed. In this report, we describe a case where an intraoperative ICT was detected early in a hemodynamically stable patient and treated successfully with IV heparin.

2. Case Description

A 42-year-old female with a history of extrahepatic cholangiocarcinoma presented for a Living Donor Liver Transplant (LDLT). She was status post en bloc extrahepatic bile duct resection with right hepatectomy three years earlier with subsequent neoadjuvant chemotherapy and had developed high-grade recurrence. The patient's other pertinent past medical history included depression, asthma, and an episode of acute renal failure secondary to dehydration. The patient's only medications at the time of surgery were albuterol/ipratropium, cetirizine, and sertraline. Model for End-Stage Liver Disease (MELD) score was 25.

Anesthesia was administered according to institutional protocol. In addition to standard American Society of Anesthesiologists monitoring, a transesophageal echocardiography (TEE) probe was placed after anesthesia induction. Coagulation was monitored using thromboelastography (TEG) and standard laboratory tests included International Normalized Ratio (INR), activated Partial Thromboplastin Time (aPTT), Prothrombin Time (PT), and fibrinogen concentration. The patient received 5000 units of subcutaneous heparin prior to anesthesia induction as routine deep venous thrombosis prophylaxis. Initial TEE exam performed after induction did not reveal any abnormalities. Standard midesophageal 4-chamber view was used for intraoperative monitoring. During the case, cardiac evaluation was performed every 20–30 minutes using midesophageal bicaval and midesophageal right ventricular inflow-outflow views,

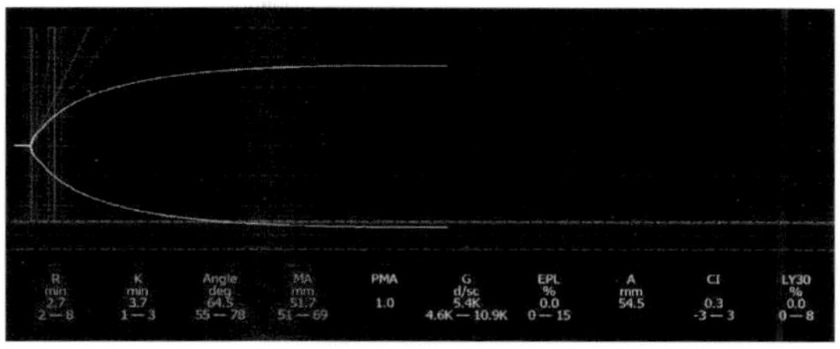

FIGURE 1: Thromboelastogram during preanhepatic phase after surgical incision.

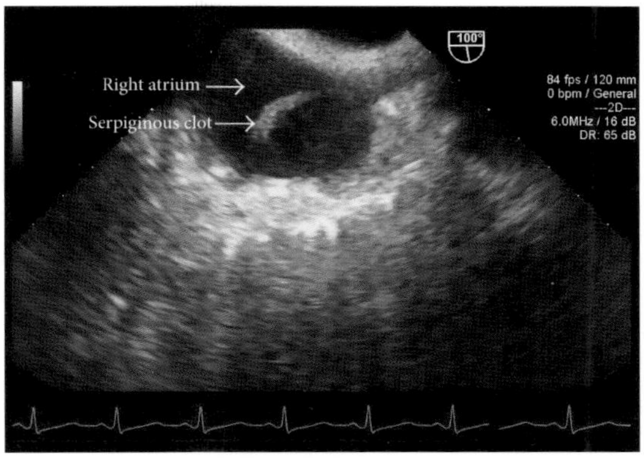

FIGURE 2: Preanhepatic phase. TEE midesophageal bicaval view: fibrous clot in right atrium.

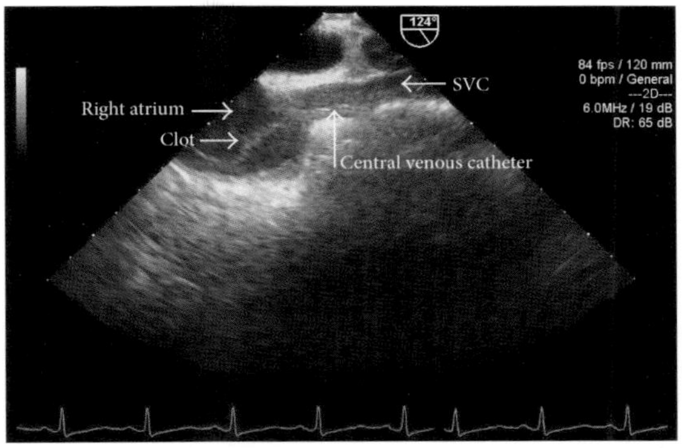

FIGURE 3: Preanhepatic phase. TEE midesophageal view: clot in the right atrium appears to be attached to 9 French catheter.

according to institutional protocol. All baseline standard laboratory tests including coagulation studies were obtained after induction and were within normal reference ranges. A TEG obtained during the preanhepatic phase was also within normal limits, with the exception of a k value that was mildly elevated (Figure 1).

Six hours after induction, during dissection of the liver, the midesophageal bicaval TEE view demonstrated a mobile serpiginous fibrous clot, 2.5 cm × 1 cm, in the right atrium (Figure 2) which appeared to be attached to the 9 French catheter placed in the right internal jugular vein (Figure 3).

We confirmed the presence of the clot using different TEE views (Figure 4). A discussion ensued between the surgical and anesthesia teams as to how to best proceed with the case. Options included the use of rTPA, cardiopulmonary bypass, thrombectomy, and IV heparin administration. Until this point, the patient had been hemodynamically stable. Point of care blood gas analysis did not reveal any abnormalities. Repeat TEE evaluation revealed a slight increase in clot size but the patient's hemodynamic status remained stable. Right and left ventricular function was not affected. The patient did not have any signs of increased pulmonary arterial pressure. Ultimately, it was decided to administer an initial bolus of 5000 units of IV heparin followed by a continuous infusion with a target aPTT of >60 seconds.

After graft reperfusion, TEE demonstrated a decrease in size of the clot and normal right and left ventricular function (Figure 5).

The patient remained stable throughout the case, requiring transfusion of two units of packed red blood cells (PRBC). The patient was transferred to the surgical intensive care unit postoperatively in stable condition and was successfully

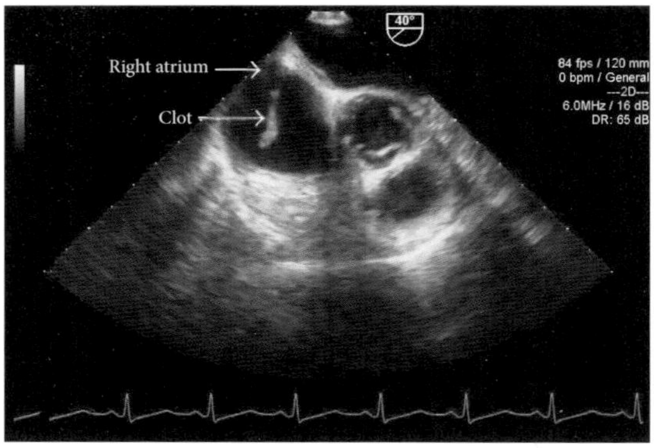

FIGURE 4: Preanhepatic phase. Modified TEE midesophageal right verticular inflow-outflow view: serpiginous clot in the right atrium.

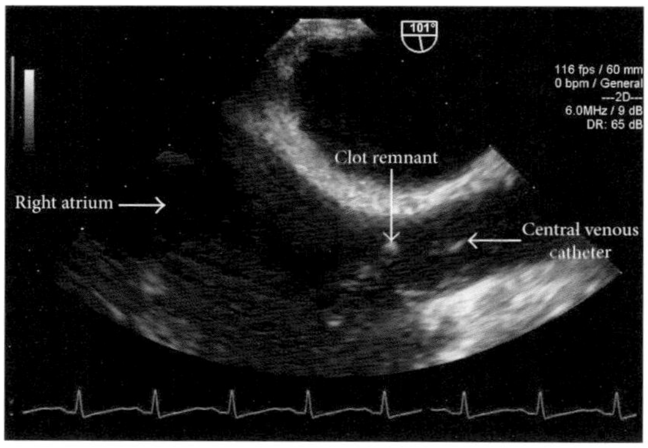

FIGURE 5: Neohepatic phase. TEE midesophageal bicaval view (depth decreased to 6 cm): significant reduction in clot size.

extubated on postoperative day (POD) 4. Graft function at that time was normal and there was no evidence of bleeding. The heparin infusion was continued postoperatively for 5 days after which anticoagulation therapy was transitioned to warfarin as soon as the patient was extubated and her surgical drains were removed.

A transthoracic echocardiogram (TTE) performed on POD 1 demonstrated a mobile, shaggy mass suggestive of a right atrial thrombus but was otherwise normal. There was no evidence of right heart strain. A repeat TTE on POD 9 was unable to demonstrate the presence of a clot in the right atrium and was also negative for any right heart strain.

3. Discussion

The incidence of intraoperative thrombosis in adult patients undergoing OLT ranges from 1.2% to 6.25% [4–6]. Eighty-five percent of thromboses occurred during the neohepatic phase of OLT and can pose a significant threat to both patient and graft survival [5, 7]. This hypercoagulability is related to complex changes in the coagulation profile seen in patients with ESLD. While there is a decrease in the synthesis and concentration of procoagulation factors by the liver, there is also a decrease in the synthesis and concentration of anticoagulation factors as well as a pronounced increase in production of liver-independent factors such as factor VIII, von Willebrand factor (vWF), and Plasminogen Activator Inhibitor 1 (PAI-1) [8–11]. Additionally, serum concentration of ADAMTS13, the protein responsible for splitting vWF, is decreased during OLT and its concentration does not immediately return to normal reference values after transplantation [11]. This results in a fragile coagulation/anticoagulation equilibrium that can easily be tipped towards bleeding or clotting.

Considering that our patient had a low MELD score but an oncologic etiology of her ESLD, she was predisposed to hypercoagulability. Vigilant monitoring is warranted in this patient population. The routine use of TEE during OLT can help detect clotting early; it also allows monitoring of cardiac function and guides management of hemodynamic instability should it occur. Shillcutt et al. demonstrated, in a retrospective study, that pulmonary microemboli were found in 44% of OLT patents. Twenty-seven percent of patients had thromboembolic events (24% intracardiac thrombus and 5% pulmonary thrombus) and the majority of these events occurred after graft reperfusion. ICT was associated with likelihood of early (30 days) and late (1 year) major postoperative adverse events and decreased survival (OR = 4.7, OR = 3.15, and OR = 3.46, resp.) [12].

The timely diagnosis of clotting events is crucial for intraoperative management. Several different methods to treat intracardiac thrombus formation and pulmonary thromboembolism previously have been described: IV heparin, rTPA, thrombectomy, and extracorporeal membrane oxygenation (ECMO). Heik et al. have demonstrated the effectiveness of high dose heparin administration for treatment of echocardiographically documented left ventricle thrombi but not in the OLT setting. In their report, the clots were significantly reduced in size or disappeared within 1 to 3 weeks without complications [13]. Boone et al. reported a case series of four patients where they used low dose rTPA (0.5 mg–4 mg) to treat intracardiac and pulmonary thrombosis during OLT [3]. In each of these cases, patients were hemodynamically unstable and in different stages of surgery. In two of the cases, a bolus of IV heparin was given with no change in hemodynamics. The administration of low dose rTPA in each of the four cases resulted in rapid hemodynamic improvement. In all of these cases, TEE was performed routinely allowing for rapid evaluation and treatment of thromboembolic events. All four patients had favorable postoperative outcomes.

Thrombectomy is another treatment option for intraoperative ICT and pulmonary embolus. However, while this method of intervention is more aggressive, it has not been demonstrated to improve patient outcome [2, 3, 14]. Other acute rescue therapeutic modalities such as ECMO or the Angiovac system (AngioDynamics, Latham, NY) have been used [15].

The use of TEE for routine monitoring during OLT is becoming commonplace in the USA. Considering that OLT is often associated with significant hemodynamic instability, intraoperative TEE is an important diagnostic tool for this patient population. It has been demonstrated that echocardiography used as a rescue modality can significantly improve

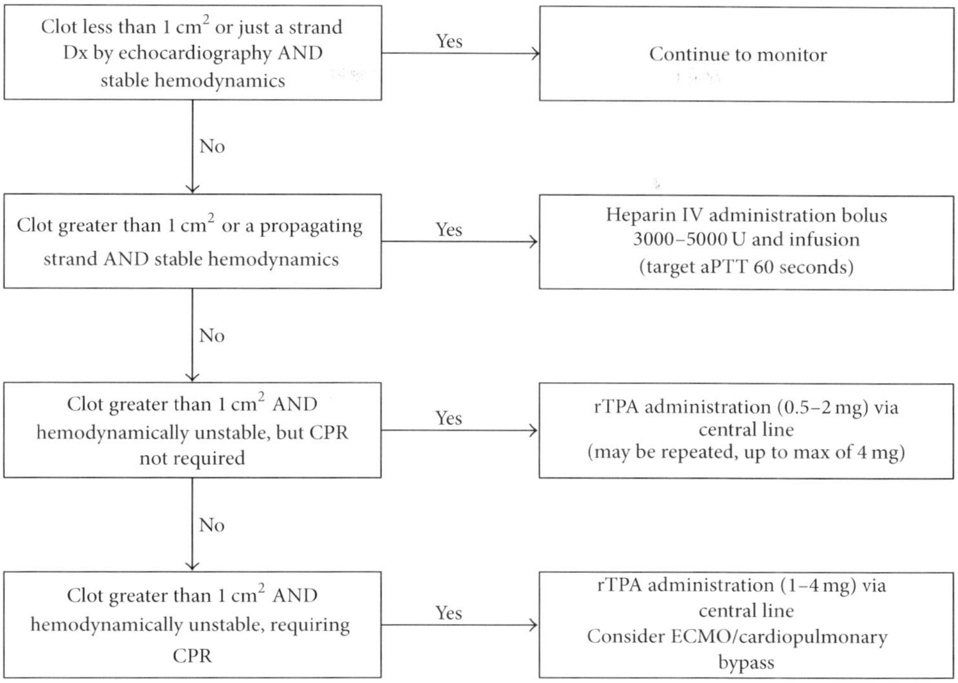

Figure 6: Management of an intraoperative intracardiac clotting event.

outcome of patients with hemodynamic instability during noncardiac surgery [16]. Once a clot is detected, therapeutic options should be considered and immediately implemented. Based on our experience and current literature we established an algorithm in our institution for the management of ICT during OLT (Figure 6). The risk of bleeding complications may be reduced when low dose rTPA is used instead of the previously recommended dose of 100 mg for thrombolysis [3].

Our case suggests that the use of TEE may allow early detection of ICT prior to the development of hemodynamic instability. When identified early, intravenous heparin administration should be considered as a treatment option in this patient population as this approach may mitigate the need for more aggressive therapy.

Competing Interests

The authors declare that they have no competing interests.

References

[1] A. Tripodi and P. M. Mannucci, "The coagulopathy of chronic liver disease," *The New England Journal of Medicine*, vol. 365, no. 2, pp. 147–156, 2011.

[2] N. Warnaar, I. Q. Molenaar, S. D. Colquhoun et al., "Intraoperative pulmonary embolism and intracardiac thrombosis complicating liver transplantation: a systematic review," *Journal of Thrombosis and Haemostasis*, vol. 6, no. 2, pp. 297–302, 2008.

[3] J. D. Boone, S. S. Sherwani, J. C. Herborn, K. M. Patel, and A. M. De Wolf, "The successful use of low-dose recombinant tissue plasminogen activator for treatment of intracardiac/pulmonary thrombosis during liver transplantation," *Anesthesia & Analgesia*, vol. 112, no. 2, pp. 319–321, 2011.

[4] E. Gologorsky, A. M. De Wolf, V. Scott, S. Aggarwal, M. Dishart, and Y. Kang, "Intracardiac thrombus formation and pulmonary thromboembolism immediately after graft reperfusion in 7 patients undergoing liver transplantation," *Liver Transplantation*, vol. 7, no. 9, pp. 783–789, 2001.

[5] T. Sakai, T. Matsusaki, F. Dai et al., "Pulmonary thromboembolism during adult liver transplantation: incidence, clinical presentation, outcome, risk factors, and diagnostic predictors," *British Journal of Anaesthesia*, vol. 108, no. 3, pp. 469–477, 2012.

[6] A. B. Lerner, E. Sundar, F. Mahmood, T. Sarge, D. W. Hanto, and P. J. Panzica, "Four cases of cardiopulmonary thromboembolism during liver transplantation without the use of antifibrinolytic drugs," *Anesthesia and Analgesia*, vol. 101, no. 6, pp. 1608–1612, 2005.

[7] F. Arshad, T. Lisman, and R. J. Porte, "Hypercoagulability as a contributor to thrombotic complications in the liver transplant recipient," *Liver International*, vol. 33, no. 6, pp. 820–827, 2013.

[8] B. Agarwal, G. Wright, A. Gatt et al., "Evaluation of coagulation abnormalities in acute liver failure," *Journal of Hepatology*, vol. 57, no. 4, pp. 780–786, 2012.

[9] M. Habib, L. N. Roberts, R. K. Patel, J. Wendon, W. Bernal, and R. Arya, "Evidence of rebalanced coagulation in acute liver injury and acute liver failure as measured by thrombin generation," *Liver International*, vol. 34, no. 5, pp. 672–678, 2014.

[10] L. Q. Huang, J. A. Whitworth, and C. N. Chesterman, "Effects of cyclosporin A and dexamethasone on haemostatic and vasoactive functions of vascular endothelial cells," *Blood Coagulation and Fibrinolysis*, vol. 6, no. 5, pp. 438–445, 1995.

[11] I. T. A. Pereboom, J. Adelmeijer, Y. van Leeuwen, H. G. D. Hendriks, R. J. Porte, and T. Lisman, "Development of a severe von Willebrand factor/ADAMTS13 dysbalance during orthotopic liver transplantation," *American Journal of Transplantation*, vol. 9, no. 5, pp. 1189–1196, 2009.

[12] S. K. Shillcutt, K. J. Ringenberg, M. M. Chacon et al., "Liver transplantation: intraoperative transesophageal echocardiography findings and relationship to major postoperative adverse cardiac events," *Journal of Cardiothoracic and Vascular Anesthesia*, vol. 30, no. 1, pp. 107–114, 2016.

[13] S. C. W. Heik, W. Kupper, C. Hamm et al., "Efficacy of high dose intravenous heparin for treatment of left ventricular thrombi with high embolic risk," *Journal of the American College of Cardiology*, vol. 24, no. 5, pp. 1305–1309, 1994.

[14] M. Manji, J. L. Isaac, and J. Bion, "Survival from massive intraoperative pulmonary thromboembolism during orthotopic liver transplantation," *British Journal of Anaesthesia*, vol. 80, no. 5, pp. 685–687, 1998.

[15] J. Szocik, S. Rudich, and M. Csete, "ECMO resuscitation after massive pulmonary embolism during liver transplantation," *Anesthesiology*, vol. 97, no. 3, pp. 763–764, 2002.

[16] S. K. Shillcutt, N. W. Markin, C. R. Montzingo, and T. R. Brakke, "Use of rapid 'rescue' perioperative echocardiography to improve outcomes after hemodynamic instability in noncardiac surgical patients," *Journal of Cardiothoracic and Vascular Anesthesia*, vol. 26, no. 3, pp. 362–370, 2012.

Application of the Liver Maximum Function Capacity Test in Acute Liver Failure: A Helpful Tool for Decision-Making in Liver Transplantation?

Florian Wolfgang Rudolf Vondran,[1] Carsten Schumacher,[2] Kai Johanning,[2] Björn Hartleben,[3] Wolfgang Knitsch,[1] Olaf Wiesner,[4] Elmar Jaeckel,[5] Michael Peter Manns,[5] Juergen Klempnauer,[1] Hueseyin Bektas,[1] and Frank Lehner[1]

[1] *Department of General, Visceral and Transplant Surgery, Hannover Medical School, 30625 Hannover, Germany*
[2] *Department of Anaesthesiology and Intensive Care Medicine, Hannover Medical School, 30625 Hannover, Germany*
[3] *Institute of Pathology, Hannover Medical School, 30625 Hannover, Germany*
[4] *Department of Respiratory Medicine, Hannover Medical School, 30625 Hannover, Germany*
[5] *Department of Gastroenterology, Hepatology and Endocrinology, Hannover Medical School, 30625 Hannover, Germany*

Correspondence should be addressed to Florian Wolfgang Rudolf Vondran; vondran.florian@mh-hannover.de

Academic Editor: Sandeep Mukherjee

Background. Despite aggressive intensive medical management acute liver failure (ALF) may require high-urgency liver transplantation (LTx). Available prognostic scores do not apply for all patients; reliable tools to identify individuals in need of LTx are highly required. The liver maximum function capacity test (LiMAx) might represent an appropriate option. Referring to a case of ALF after *Amanita phalloides*-intoxication the potential of the LiMAx-test in this setting is discussed. *Presentation of Case.* LiMAx was performed in a 27-year-old patient prior to and after high-urgency LTx. In accordance with clinical appearance of hepatic encephalopathy, coagulopathy, and acute kidney failure, the LiMAx-test constituted a fulminant course of ALF with hardly any detectable metabolic activity. Following LTx with a marginal donor organ (95% hepatosteatosis), uptake of liver function was demonstrated by postoperative increase of the LiMAx-value. The patient was discharged from hospital on postoperative day 26. *Discussion.* ALF often is associated with a critical state of the patient that requires almost immediate decision-making regarding further therapy. Application of a noninvasive liver function test might help to determine the prognosis of ALF and support decision-making for or against LTx as well as acceptance of a critical donor organ in case of a critically ill patient.

1. Introduction

Acute liver failure (ALF) represents a potentially fatal complication of severe hepatic illness due to various reasons. Many patients suffering from ALF profit from aggressive intensive medical management; nonetheless, salvage of a substantial proportion of affected individuals still relies on orthotopic liver transplantation (LTx) [1, 2]. Since the clinical state of patients suffering from ALF can be most critical, short-term decision-making regarding further treatment might be vital [3]. In this setting, not only determination for or against LTx but also decision-making regarding acceptance of a critical donor organ in case of high-urgency- (HU-) LTx might be necessary. Since the available prognostic clinical scores do not apply for all patients [3], reliable tools to allow for identification of those individuals who need a liver transplant and those who can be managed with medical treatment to achieve full recovery after ALF thus are highly desired. The liver maximum function capacity test (LiMAx) is known to predict postoperative outcomes in liver surgery [4]. Regarding non-acetaminophen and non-*Amanita phalloides* toxin induced ALF first promising data has been reported using the LiMAx-test [5]. As this noninvasive measurement allows for rapid quantification of liver function selectively looking at the

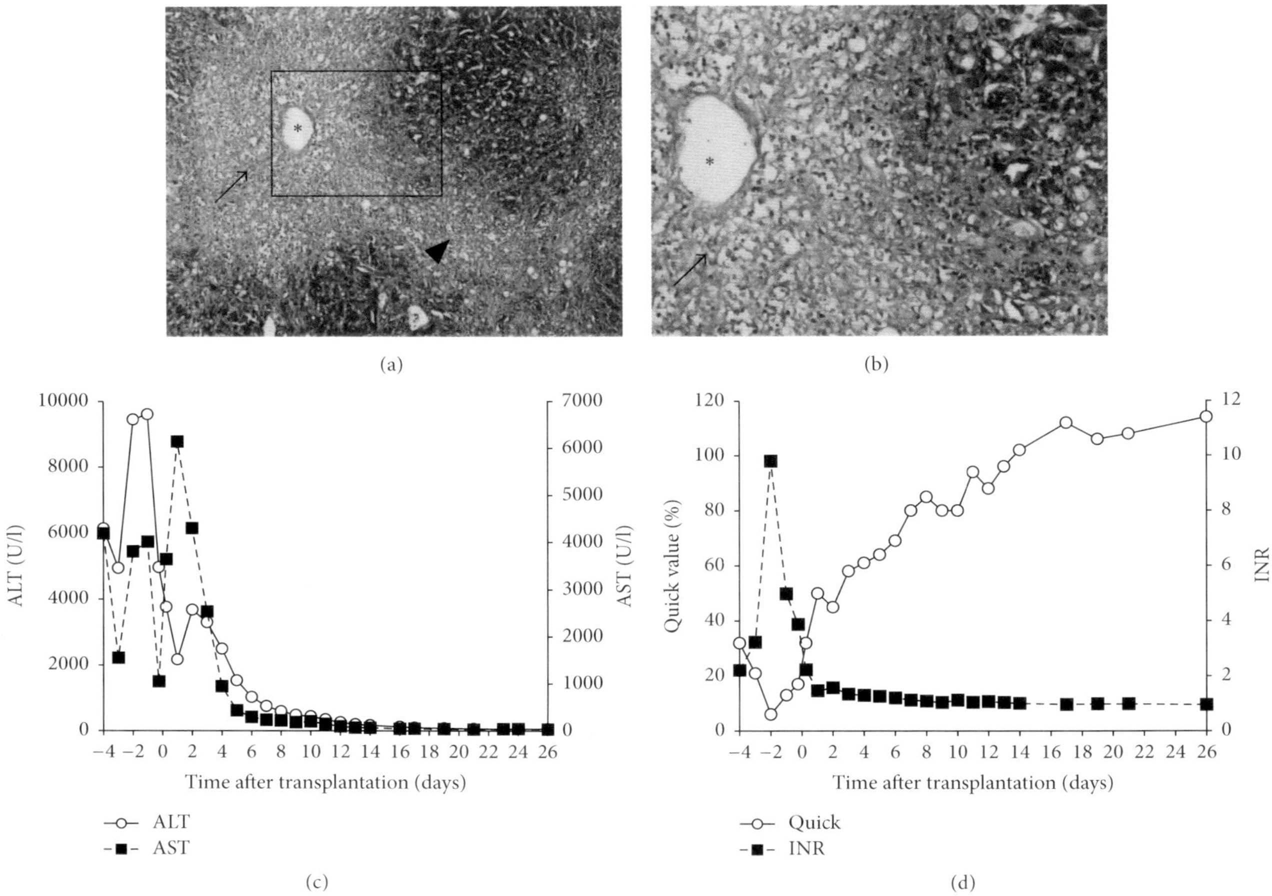

FIGURE 1: *Amanita phalloides* toxin can cause severe liver damage as observed in the explanted liver of our patient in terms of severe centrilobular necrosis (arrow) and bridging necrosis (arrowhead) of the liver epithelial cells. Asterisk marks central vein (HE staining; magnification: 40x and 100x, resp.) (a, b). This toxin-induced acute liver failure was associated with an appropriate increase of the liver transaminases (AST, ALT) (c) as well as coagulopathy depicted by decrease of the Quick value and increase of the INR (d).

Cytochrome P450 1A2 metabolism, liver function also can be determined when conventional laboratory parameters are not meaningful as during coagulopathy requiring blood product substitution and toxin-induced release of liver enzymes.

Amanita phalloides is a wild mushroom that can cause severe liver damage in man (Figures 1(a) and 1(b)) clinically ranging from diarrhea to ALF. If not treated, mortality is as high as 80% [6]. Despite treatment (i.e., supportive measures, inactivation of the toxin) mortality still is 10–20% [7]. If ALF occurs, LTx so far seems to be the only therapeutic option, since the effectiveness of therapeutic concepts based on artificial liver devices is still suboptimal [8, 9]. Nevertheless, the criteria for LTx in ALF due to *Amanita phalloides*-intoxication are not consensual [10], and conventional laboratory parameters were not of any prognostic value [11].

Referring to a case of ALF after *Amanita phalloides*-intoxication the potential of the LiMAx-test in this setting will be discussed. Furthermore, the possible implication for the management of HU-LTx candidates in respect to the increasing number of critical donor organs will be pointed out.

2. Presentation of Case

We report on a healthy 27-year-old male patient who received HU-LTx due to ALF following *Amanita phalloides*-intoxication eating mushrooms collected by his girlfriend. Approximately 11 h after poisoning he suffered from diarrhea, vomiting, and abdominal pain. He was admitted to a local hospital where therapy with orally applied charcoal (25 g/d) and intravenous silibinin (20 mg/kg/body weight) was initiated immediately. Due to significant rise of transaminases (at norm on admission) and development of coagulopathy (Figures 1(c) and 1(d)) therapy was extended by acetylcysteine (5 g/d) as well as thiamine (300 mg/d) followed by transfer to our liver center the day after. Upon admission the patient presented with further aggravation of toxin-induced ALF (Figures 1(c) and 1(d)) but still no signs of hepatic encephalopathy. Therapy with charcoal, silibinin, acetylcysteine, and thiamine was continued. Urine screening 50 h after mushroom-ingestion still revealed positive *Amanita phalloides* toxin levels (1.6 μg/L).

Despite continuation of the aforementioned therapy the patient's condition worsened continuously with requirement for intensive care treatment: transaminases further increased, coagulopathy worsened dramatically (Figures 1(c) and 1(d)), and relevant lactate levels (up to 14.9 mmol/L) were recorded; clinically he still suffered from diarrhea, whereas nausea, vomiting, and abdominal pain persisted; he developed hepatic encephalopathy grade II. Since the patient's medical history was free of further diseases, he thus was listed at Eurotransplant for HU-LTx with a MELD-score of 36 on day 4 after intoxication. He now received daily substitution with fresh frozen plasma (FFP) (4 units/d) and fibrinogen (2 g/d), but apart from mild hemorrhagic defecation no further bleeding events were observed. Due to development of acute kidney failure hemodialysis was begun.

On day 6 after toxin ingestion the patient received the first offer for LTx. The sighted deceased donor was a 59-year-old obese (body mass index of 28) female who suffered from a subarachnoidal bleeding due to a ruptured cerebral aneurysm. The donor liver was deemed steatotic by macroscopic appearance with confirmation by histology (60% micro- and 35% macrosteatosis). Since no other organ was available and the patient's condition was most critical, the organ eventually was accepted for transplantation following extensive interdisciplinary discussion.

Waiting for the organ to arrive, the patient's liver maximum function capacity was determined applying the LiMAx-test (Humedics GmbH, Germany) by intravenously injecting a body weight-adapted dose of methacetin (2 mg/kg body weight) followed by detection of the exhaled ^{13}C-labeled CO_2 using the "Fast Liver Investigation Package" (FLIP) according to the manufacturer's instructions. By this means, onset of fulminant ALF was confirmed, as hardly any liver metabolism could be detected (Figure 2).

In accordance with this finding severe derangement of blood coagulation was found performing rotational thromboelastometry (ROTEM) according to the manufacturer's instructions (Tem Innovations GmbH, Germany) and interpreted referring to published reference ranges [12] (Figure 3).

The patient was transplanted with the large (2422 g) steatotic organ of the aforementioned donor and a cold ischemic time of 7 h 37 min. LTx was performed with end-to-end vascular and biliary anastomoses. The warm ischemic time was 47 min. Due to diffuse bleeding the liver was packed and a planned second look was performed after 36 h. Triple immunosuppression (tacrolimus/mycophenolate mofetil/steroids) with anti-CD25 induction-therapy was provided. Histopathological work-up of the recipient's own liver demonstrated the severe liver damage caused by *Amanita phalloides* toxin (Figures 1(a) and 1(b)).

Despite known hepatosteatosis of 95% the graft showed an acceptable initial function. Only on postoperative day (POD) 1 mass substitution of blood products was performed (i.e., 18x FFPs, 12x packed red blood cells, 3x thrombocyte concentrates, 6 g Fibrinogen, and 3,000 units Antithrombin III). Thereafter no further substitution of blood products apart from Antithrombin III was necessary. The LiMAx-test and ROTEM analysis were repeated on POD 3 and POD 10, respectively, demonstrating continuous recovery of liver function in the course (Figures 2 and 3).

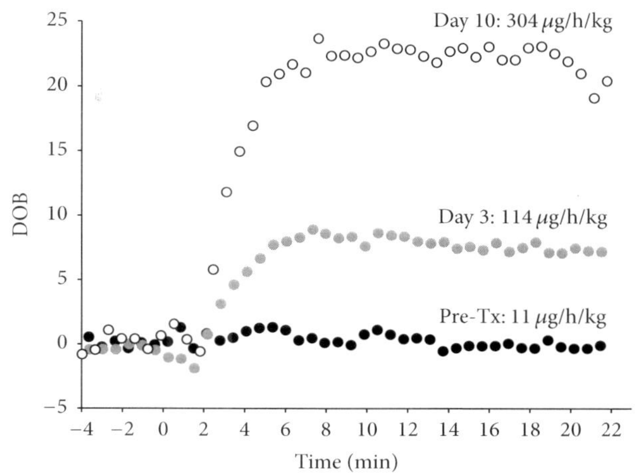

FIGURE 2: Measurement of the liver maximum capacity (LiMAx-test) revealed almost any metabolic activity at the time of transplantation (pre-Tx; black dots) but was seen to normalize in the course thereafter with almost normalized liver function at day 10 (white dots) after LTx (normal liver function = LiMAx value >315 μg/h/kg; DOB: delta over baseline).

Following the second look operation on POD 2, the requirement for catecholamines (initially 0.181 μg/kg/min norepinephrine) decreased continuously and the patient was free of catecholamines on POD 6. He quickly was weaned from the respirator (POD 6). Kidney function likewise rapidly improved following LTx with limited diuresis starting on POD 6 and cessation of hemodialysis on POD 9. Following bacteremia with detection of *Staphylococcus sciuri* but good response to an antibiotic treatment with Vancomycin (in the course switch to Ciprofloxacin), admission to the surgical ward eventually was performed on POD 11. The patient was discharged from hospital in good condition on POD 26.

3. Discussion

At present clinical scores are used for the management of patients suffering from ALF due to various reasons, with their respective limitations [3]. Reliable tools to exclusively monitor the liver function during treatment of ALF that simultaneously allow for valid prediction of prognosis of this condition hence are highly desired. In particular decision-making regarding the need for LTx but also defining the optimal time frame for organ replacement likewise would profit enormously by this means. The latter particularly applies for HU-LTx when critically ill patients receive offers from donors with marginal organs and an almost immediate decision is inevitable.

Primarily, the LiMAx-test has been developed for effective preoperative surgical risk evaluation to prevent major complications or even liver failure-related death. It has proven reliable in the assessment of liver function [13] and determination of postoperative outcomes in liver surgery [4], especially regarding avoidance of postoperative liver failure [14].

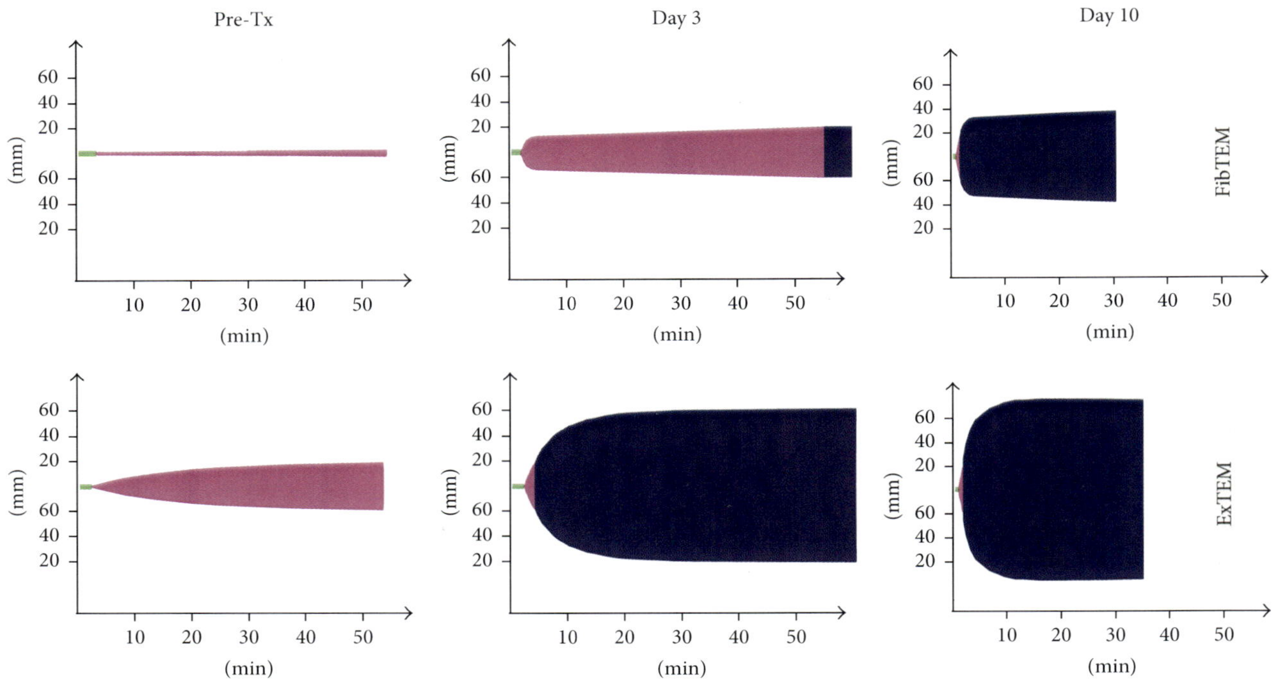

FIGURE 3: ALF also was observed performing pretransplant rotational thromboelastometry (ROTEM): ExTem clotting time (CT-Ex) was significantly prolonged (157 s) and maximum clot firmness in ExTEM (MCF-Ex) and FibTEM (MCF-Fib) reduced (20 and 3 mm, resp.). In line with the LiMAx-test, blood coagulation continuously recovered in the course of transplantation (CT-Ex of 51 s, MCF-Ex of 76 mm, and MCF-Fib of 37 mm at postoperative day 10, resp.).

Impairment of liver recovery in case of nonalcoholic fatty liver disease could be demonstrated [15]. The LiMAx-test further was found to enable early diagnosis of sepsis-related hepatic dysfunction [16] as well as prognosis of early outcome after LTx [17]. Recently, a first small case series on the application of the LiMAx-test in patients suffering from ALF due to viral hepatitis, toxic liver injury (not *Amanita phalloides* induced), or cryptogenic liver failure likewise provided very promising results: whereas all biochemical parameters (i.e., bilirubin, creatinine, AST, ALT, and INR) were statistically indistinct, the liver maximum functional capacity test turned out to be of prognostic relevance with full recovery after ALF for a LiMAx value >38 μg/kg/h [5].

Despite the great potential for the management of ALF and being a noninvasive breath test, the major hypothetical threat of the LiMAx-test in this setting also needs to be discussed: the intravenously applied substrate methacetin is metabolized by the liver to CO_2 and acetaminophen. The latter is a well-known hepatotoxin that may lead to ALF itself when being overdosed [18]. The threshold for induction of ALF in healthy adults has been defined as a single dose of acetaminophen above 10 g or at least 200 mg/kg of bodyweight [19]. Whether the amount of acetaminophen that is set free during metabolism of methacetin may tip the scales regarding full recovery from or definitive development of ALF, or rather aggravate the patient's condition in ALF, remains questionable. It has to be noted though that the average amount of methacetin (applied at 2 mg/kg body weight) required to perform the LiMAx-test is equivalent to an acetaminophen dose of less than 50 mg [4] and thus severe impact on liver function by the LiMAx-test itself seems very unlikely.

Referring to the present case another issue related to transplantation can be discussed: following listing of a patient for HU-LTx it might be of great benefit to further define the time frame in which transplantation should be performed or, in other words, providing further evidence whether there is a need to accept a suboptimal organ to save the patient's life is highly desirable. In case of the young man listed for HU-LTx, we confirmed that ALF has taken a fulminant course applying the LiMAx-test (hardly any metabolic activity detectable). Within 48 h after listing of the patient a first offer for transplantation was obtained, which is in the usual range [20]. Nevertheless, due to the known shortage of donor organs [21] and the current strategy to at least partially counter the gap of supply by use of extended criteria donors (ECD) [22], only a marginal organ was available and the patient in most critical state. In line with data published by others [23], use of this ECD-organ in a good patient still resulted in an acceptable outcome. If the patient's liver maximum function capacity would have demonstrated a better residual liver function or longitudinal measurements would have indicated stable kinetics for the decrease of the liver function, one might have considered waiting for another and possibly better organ offer.

In conclusion, ALF—especially following *Amanita phalloides*-intoxication—often is associated with a critical state of the patient that requires almost immediate decision-making regarding further therapy. Application of a noninvasive liver function test might help to define the prognosis of ALF [5, 24], supporting not only determination for or against LTx but also decision-making regarding acceptance of a critical donor organ in case of a critically ill patient as demonstrated by the presented case.

Competing Interests

The authors declare that there are no competing interests regarding the publication of this paper.

Acknowledgments

The authors thank Kathrin Reinsch for her excellent technical support performing the LiMAx-test.

References

[1] Shalimar and S. K. Acharya, "Management in acute liver failure," *Journal of Clinical and Experimental Hepatology*, vol. 5, supplement 1, pp. S104–S115, 2015.

[2] C. Willars, "Update in intensive care medicine: acute liver failure. Initial management, supportive treatment and who to transplant," *Current Opinion in Critical Care*, vol. 20, no. 2, pp. 202–209, 2014.

[3] M. J. McPhail, H. Farne, N. Senvar, J. A. Wendon, and W. Bernal, "Ability of King's college criteria and model for end-stage liver disease scores to predict mortality of patients with acute liver failure: a meta-analysis," *Clinical Gastroenterology and Hepatology*, vol. 4, no. 4, pp. 516–525.e5, 2015.

[4] M. Stockmann, J. F. Lock, M. Malinowski, S. M. Niehues, D. Seehofer, and P. Neuhaus, "The LiMAx test: a new liver function test for predicting postoperative outcome in liver surgery," *HPB*, vol. 12, no. 2, pp. 139–146, 2010.

[5] J. F. Lock, A. N. Kotobi, M. Malinowski et al., "Predicting the prognosis in acute liver failure: results from a retrospective pilot study using the LiMAx test," *Annals of hepatology*, vol. 12, no. 4, pp. 556–562, 2013.

[6] B. D. Yildiz, O. Abbasoglu, A. Saglam, and C. Sökmensüer, "Urgent liver transplantation for Amanita phalloides poisoning," *Pediatric Transplantation*, vol. 12, no. 1, pp. 105–108, 2008.

[7] L. Santi, C. Maggioli, M. Mastroroberto, M. Tufoni, L. Napoli, and P. Caraceni, "Acute liver failure caused by amanita phalloides poisoning," *International Journal of Hepatology*, vol. 2012, Article ID 487480, 6 pages, 2012.

[8] F. Panaro, E. Andorno, N. Morelli et al., "Liver transplantation represents the optimal treatment for fulminant hepatic failure from amanita phalloides poisoning," *Transplant International*, vol. 19, no. 4, pp. 344–345, 2006.

[9] F. Saliba and D. Samuel, "Artificial liver support: a real step forward," *Minerva Medica*, vol. 106, no. 1, pp. 35–43, 2015.

[10] R. Ferreira, J. M. Romãozinho, P. Amaro, M. Ferreira, and C. Sofia, "Assessment of emergency liver transplantation criteria in acute liver failure due to *Amanita phalloides*," *European Journal of Gastroenterology & Hepatology*, vol. 23, no. 12, pp. 1226–1232, 2011.

[11] H. Bektas, H. J. Schlitt, K. Böker, R. Brunkhorst, K. J. Oldhafer, and R. Pichlmayr, "Indications for liver transplantation in severe amanita phalloides mushroom poisoning," *Der Chirurg—Zeitschrift für alle Gebiete der Operativen Medizin*, vol. 67, no. 10, pp. 996–1001, 1996.

[12] T. Lang, A. Bauters, S. L. Braun et al., "Multi-centre investigation on reference ranges for ROTEM thromboelastometry," *Blood Coagulation & Fibrinolysis*, vol. 16, no. 4, pp. 301–310, 2005.

[13] M. Jara, J. Bednarsch, J. F. Lock et al., "Reliable assessment of liver function using LiMAx," *Journal of Surgical Research*, vol. 193, no. 1, pp. 184–189, 2015.

[14] M. Jara, T. Reese, M. Malinowski et al., "Reductions in post-hepatectomy liver failure and related mortality after implementation of the LiMAx algorithm in preoperative work-up: a single-centre analysis of 1170 hepatectomies of one or more segments," *HPB*, vol. 17, no. 7, pp. 651–658, 2015.

[15] S. Hoppe, C. von Loeffelholz, J. F. Lock et al., "Nonalcoholic steatohepatits and liver steatosis modify partial hepatectomy recovery," *Journal of Investigative Surgery*, vol. 28, no. 1, pp. 24–31, 2015.

[16] M. F. Kaffarnik, J. F. Lock, H. Vetter et al., "Early diagnosis of sepsis-related hepatic dysfunction and its prognostic impact on survival: a prospective study with the LiMAx test," *Critical Care*, vol. 17, no. 5, article R259, 2013.

[17] M. Jara, M. Malinowski, K. Lüttgert, E. Schott, P. Neuhaus, and M. Stockmann, "Prognostic value of enzymatic liver function for the estimation of short-term survival of liver transplant candidates: a prospective study with the LiMAx test," *Transplant International*, vol. 28, no. 1, pp. 52–58, 2015.

[18] E. M. Lancaster, J. R. Hiatt, and A. Zarrinpar, "Acetaminophen hepatotoxicity: an updated review," *Archives of Toxicology*, vol. 89, no. 2, pp. 193–199, 2014.

[19] R. Dart, A. Erdman, K. Olson et al., "Acetaminophen poisoning: an evidence-based consensus guideline for out-of-hospital management," *Clinical Toxicology*, vol. 44, no. 1, pp. 1–18, 2006.

[20] G. Chan, A. Taqi, P. Marotta et al., "Long-term outcomes of emergency liver transplantation for acute liver failure," *Liver Transplantation*, vol. 15, no. 12, pp. 1696–1702, 2009.

[21] R. F. Saidi and S. K. Hejazii Kenari, "Challenges of organ shortage for transplantation: solutions and opportunities," *International Journal of Organ Transplantation Medicine*, vol. 5, no. 3, pp. 87–96, 2014.

[22] A. Nickkholgh, J. Weitz, J. Encke et al., "Utilization of extended donor criteria in liver transplantation: a comprehensive review of the literature," *Nephrology Dialysis Transplantation*, vol. 22, supplement 8, pp. viii29–viii36, 2007.

[23] D. Routh, S. Sharma, C. S. Naidu, P. P. Rao, A. K. Sharma, and P. Ranjan, "Comparison of outcomes in ideal donor and extended criteria donor in deceased donor liver transplant: a prospective study," *International Journal of Surgery*, vol. 12, no. 8, pp. 774–777, 2014.

[24] Y. Ilan, "A fourth dimension in decision making in hepatology," *Hepatology Research*, vol. 40, no. 12, pp. 1143–1154, 2010.

38

Successful Liver Transplantation Case Report from a Deceased Donor with Sickle Cell Anemia

Lucas Souto Nacif,[1] Estrella Bianca de Mello,[1] Rafael Soares Pinheiro,[1] Fabiana Roberto Lima,[2] Rodrigo Bronze de Martino,[1] Wellington Andraus,[1] and Luiz Carneiro D'Albuquerque[1]

[1]*Liver and Gastrointestinal Transplant Division, Department of Gastroenterology, 05403-900 São Paulo, Brazil*
[2]*Department of Pathology, University of São Paulo School of Medicine, 05403-900 São Paulo, Brazil*

Correspondence should be addressed to Lucas Souto Nacif; lucasnacif@usp.br

Academic Editor: Ryszard Grenda

There is a worldwide problem of waiting time and mortality rate associated with remaining on the waiting list for a liver transplant. However, some situations have been encouraging in terms of determining appropriate recipients and expanding the donor criteria. We herein report a case of useful liver donor with sickle cell anemia for liver transplantation. Here we described a case of liver transplantation from a donor with sickle cell anemia to a recipient with hepatocellular carcinoma who was deemed to be at risk of tumor growth and at risk of being dropped from the waiting list. The literature reveals the importance of using safe donors, and we describe the benefits of using a safe, deceased liver donor with sickle cell anemia who was an adequate option for liver transplantation.

1. Introduction

Nowadays, due to the great success of liver transplantation (LT) given advances in technologies and the quality of immunosuppressive drugs, the survival and quality of life have improved [1, 2]. However, a major worldwide problem is still the waiting time and mortality rate associated with remaining on waiting lists [3, 4].

This situation has motivated revisions to the recipient-selection process and an expansion of donor criteria [5]. The risks and benefits of remaining on the waiting list for LT should always be evaluated closely when using doubtful grafts or adopting expanded criteria [1, 5]. Absolute contraindications to deceased organ donation include any evidence of a malignant cancer. Furthermore, other important liver grafts refusal was evaluated by histological analysis with severe steatosis, cholestasis, and fibrosis. Nevertheless, controversies in the relevance of these mandates require that the surgeon team decide the best way to allocate organs.

The purpose of this study is to show the possibility of enlarging use of organs. Moreover, we describe the special case report of a LT from a donor with sickle cell anemia (SCA) and hereditary hemoglobinopathy, with an atypical and inherited disorder of hemoglobin called hemoglobin S (HbS), to a hepatitis B virus (HBV) cirrhosis and hepatocellular carcinoma (HCC) patient who was adjudicated dropping out of the liver transplant waiting list.

2. Case Presentation

2.1. Donor Surgery. The liver graft was from a young male patient, 20 years old, who weighed 57 kg, was 1.78 meters tall, and had a body mass index (BMI) of 18 kg/m^2. He was admitted to a general hospital with a subarachnoid hemorrhage and intracranial hematoma on the left side, and he suffered brain death. He had a previous pathological history of SCA and was treated for his anemia with several blood cell therapies and a splenectomy when he was 16 years old. He was receiving ceftriaxone, meropenem, and vancomycin when he was submitted to donor surgery, five days after the neurosurgery. He was under low doses of vasopressors: norepinephrine

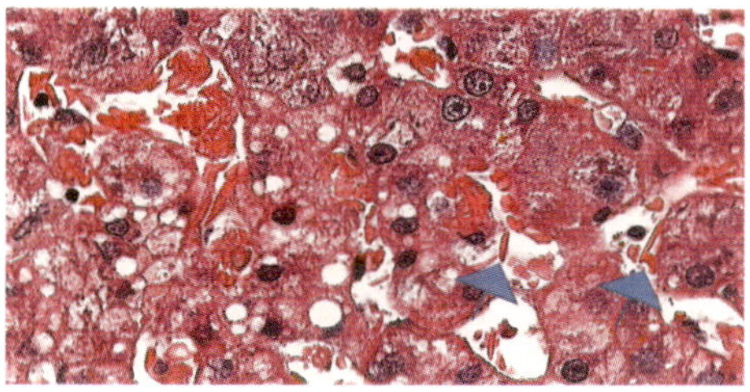

Figure 1: Sinusoidal distension and congestion with many crescent-shaped or needle-shaped red cells and sickle cells (arrowheads) are seen in this field, along with mild steatosis in hepatocytes (H&E, 500x, before reperfusion).

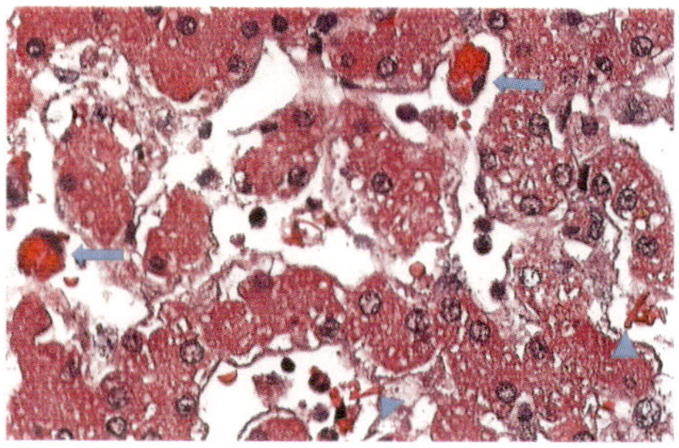

Figure 2: Kupffer cell erythrophagocytosis (arrows) and scarce sickle cells (arrowheads) in sinusoids, as well as some hepatocellular vacuolar degeneration (H&E, 500x).

(0.18 mcg/kg/min) and vasopressin (0.02 mcg/kg/min). The best suitable recipient was chosen by balancing the risk of a hematological disease or thrombotic risk factors associated with the recipient remaining on the waiting list and either dying or dropping out of the list. All laboratory analysis and liver function of the donor were normal. After all analysis and arguments discussed with the transplant team (surgeons, hepatologists, and infectologists), as risk of using SCA graft, probabilities of developing disease, and a few case reports in the literature, on the other hand, the benefits of being an excellent hepatic graft option, the recipient and her family were informed of all risks and probabilities, and a unanimous informed consent decision was made to receive the donor liver and follow with the transplant. The donor surgery was fine and was not associated with any complications. Both of the deceased patient's kidneys and liver were donated to three different recipients in different centers.

2.2. Liver Transplantation. The liver recipient was a 37-year-old woman, and her blood type was the same as that of the donor. She weighed 54 kg and was 1.65 meters tall. Her BMI was 19.8 kg/m^2. She was diagnosed with hepatitis B virus (HBV) cirrhosis and hepatocellular carcinoma (HCC) according to the Milan criteria (2 tumors each with diameter $\leq$ 3 cm, without extrahepatic and major vessel involvement). Model for end-stage liver disease (MELD) score was 18 and Child-Pugh-Turcotte (CPT) classification was B7. The serum alpha-fetoprotein (AFP) value was increasing recently to the transplant (>200 ng/ml). In the waiting list for liver transplant, the patient performed 3 transarterial chemoembolization (TACE) sessions, initially with completely treated areas but afterwards showing partial treatment (progression). The liver allograft weighed 1.495 kg. The cold ischemia time was 8 hours and 30 minutes, and the warm ischemia time was 38 minutes. The transplantation was performed on September 27th, 2016. The patient received four units of red blood cells, three units of platelets, and eight units of plasma during the surgery. The liver biopsy protocol included preclamping and prerevascularization biopsy with mild siderosis and steatosis, hepatocyte ballooning, rare canalicular cholestasis, and moderate sinusoidal congestion with predominance of drepanocytes (Figure 1).

The postrevascularization biopsy revealed mild ischemia reperfusion injury (grade 2), including apoptosis of hepatocytes and a minor neutrophilic sinusoidal infiltrate. Kupffer cell erythrophagocytosis and scarce sickle cells were still seen in a biopsy performed on the following day (Figure 2), along with some ischemic areas. The immunosuppression protocol included corticosteroids every day after the anesthetic induction for 6 months. In terms of the glucocorticoid withdrawal regimen, basiliximab 20 mg was administered on the anesthetic induction and on the fourth postoperative day; mycophenolate mofetil and tacrolimus were administered from the 4th day on (due to the institutional protocol and literature we initiated the onset of tacrolimus later due to acute renal failure and using protocol with corticosteroids and basiliximab). The tacrolimus dose (0.10-0.15 mg/kg/day administered twice a day) was adjusted based on the liver blood tests and the blood level 6-10 ng/ml was maintained during this first year.

2.3. Postoperative Course. The LT recipient also received antibiotics based on the medical profile of the liver donor: vancomycin and meropenem for seven days plus Amicacina for two days. Furthermore, she received hepatitis B immunoglobulin (HBIG) for seven days and then monthly for a year. She still receives entecavir (ETV) daily for preventing hepatitis B recurrence. As part of the LT protocol, she was submitted to a Doppler ultrasound of the vascular graft anastomosis investigation on the first postoperative day, and no abnormalities were noted. The follow-up of the vascular imaging examination will depend on clinical and laboratory data. Despite her good postoperative evolution, she developed acute kidney failure and she required hemodialysis for three weeks. The cause of acute renal failure and hemodialysis was due to liver transplantation procedure and the baseline renal function somewhat altered. Her recovery of renal function was complete, and she did not require renal replacement therapy anymore. She was discharged from hospital on the 37th postoperative day. Postoperative chemotherapy was not necessary due to good evolution and postoperative oncologic control image (CT) with absence of recurrence in the transplanted liver and decrease in the serum tumor marker (AFP <10 ng/ml). A long-term follow-up of 18 months revealed a good evolution, with normal liver blood tests.

2.4. Ethical Aspects. This study was approved by the Institutional Review Board and accomplished the entire requisite for studies in humans according to the guidelines of the 1975 Declaration of Helsinki.

3. Discussion

Sickle cell anemia (SCA) is a hereditary hemoglobinopathy and an atypical inherited disorder of hemoglobin called hemoglobin S (HbS). It is important due to its multifactorial components, diverse clinical manifestations, and impact on patient morbimortality [6]. Sickle cell disease (SCD) presents vascular manifestations leading to complications in multiple organ systems: vasoocclusion of hepatic sinusoids owing to the sickling way, hemosiderosis from chronic transfusions, viral hepatitis, and cholelithiasis in consequence of chronic hemolysis [6].

Some manifestations related to vascular damage have been associated with liver alterations due to acute hepatic crises to chronic liver disease accompanying intrahepatic cholestasis and iron overload. Regardless of this, intrahepatic cholestasis is possibly severe and clinical treatment is often inoperative [7]. SCA or SCD can offer higher morbid-mortality, more hospitalizations, and impaired quality of life [7]. In our case, we observed a nice macroscopic aspect of the liver in the donor harvesting and good donor laboratory tests and hemodynamic controls, so we decided to proceed with the LT. After that we confirm the good microscopic aspect of the liver with the preclamping graft biopsy.

Regarding SCA and SCD liver histology, as one of the limiting factors to use these patients as donors [7], the liver histological analysis is mandatory for a better interpretation of fibrosis, cholestasis, steatosis, and even cirrhosis. So, to maintain the donor's quality of the liver graft we recommend to perform a protocol histological analysis. That was carried out in our case and discarded any problem that reflects this good evolution.

There were few reported published cases of liver transplant in patients with SCD. Furthermore, a recent article review of the literature shows 10 adults and 5 children with SCD that underwent a liver transplant [7]. Orthotopic LT might be included as a treatment choice for SCD patients with end-stage liver disease and with chance to progress the disease with other treatments.

Elsiesy H et al. [8] in 2017 reported in a meeting abstract 7 cases with sickle cell trait patients for liver donation. They conclude that the liver donation is safe from sickle cell trait donors [8]. Nevertheless, we did not find any published articles focusing on donors with SCA.

We have highlighted a literature review and a successful LT case using SCA donor to a HBV cirrhosis and HCC patient with dropout risk from the waiting list for LT. The important objective of this work is to demonstrate this successful recipient and donor match that show that we can expand the donor criteria and share this successful option for liver transplantation. Furthermore, this present report is enhanced to promote to the transplant community this approach with this type of donor.

4. Conclusion

In summary, we have reported that a deceased liver donor with sickle cell anemia is an adequate option for LT. The articles that we found demonstrate the importance of using a safe donor and the real benefits of expanding use of organs.

Abbreviations

LT:	Liver transplantation
HBV:	Hepatitis B virus
HCC:	Hepatocellular carcinoma
BMI:	Body mass index
SCA:	Sickle cell anemia
SCD:	Sickle cell disease
HbS:	Hemoglobin, called hemoglobin S
MELD:	Model for end-stage liver disease
CPT:	Child-Pugh-Turcotte
HBIG:	Hepatitis B immunoglobulin
ETV:	Entecavir.

Authors' Contributions

All authors have approved the final draft of the manuscript submitted. Study conception and design, data collection and analysis, interpretation, and writing the manuscript were the responsibility of Lucas Souto Nacif. Study conception and design, data collection and analysis, interpretation, and critical revision were the responsibility of Estrella Bianca de Mello and Rafael Soares Pinheiro. Data collection and analysis, interpretation, and revision were the responsibility of Fabiana Roberto Lima and Rodrigo Bronze de Martino. Study conception, interpretation, and critical revision were the responsibility of Wellington Andraus and Luiz Carneiro D'Albuquerque.

References

[1] K. J. Halazun, R. C. Quillin, R. Rosenblatt et al., "Expanding the Margins: High Volume Utilization of Marginal Liver Grafts Among >2000 Liver Transplants at a Single Institution," *Annals of Surgery*, vol. 266, no. 3, pp. 441–449, 2017.

[2] L. S. Nacif, A. I. David, R. S. Pinheiro et al., "An analysis of tacrolimus-related complications in the first 30 days after liver transplantation," *Clinics*, vol. 69, no. 11, pp. 745–749, 2014.

[3] L. S. Nacif, R. S. Pinheiro, R. A. De Arruda Pécora et al., "Re-transplantation, higher creatinine levels in hepatitis C virus patients, and donor age are predictors of mortality in long-term analysis of late acute rejection in liver transplantation," *Annals of Transplantation*, vol. 22, pp. 9–16, 2017.

[4] A. J. Kwong, J. C. Lai, J. L. Dodge, and J. P. Roberts, "Outcomes for liver transplant candidates listed with low model for end-stage liver disease score," *Liver Transplantation*, vol. 21, no. 11, pp. 1403–1409, 2015.

[5] J. C. Olson and C. J. Karvellas, "Critical care management of the patient with cirrhosis awaiting liver transplant in the intensive

care unit," *Liver Transplantation*, vol. 23, no. 11, pp. 1465–1476, 2017.

[6] M. H. Steinberg and P. Sebastiani, "Genetic modifiers of sickle cell disease," *American Journal of Hematology*, vol. 87, no. 8, pp. 795–803, 2012.

[7] M. Blinder, B. Geng, M. Lisker-Melman et al., "Successful orthotopic liver transplantation in an adult patient with sickle cell disease and review of the literature," *Case Reports in Hematology*, vol. 5, no. 1, pp. 1–4, 2013.

[8] H. Elsiesy, M. Sturdevant, W. Al-Hamoudi et al., "Safety of Liver Donation from Living Donors with Sickle Cell Trait," *American Journal of Transplantation*, vol. 17, no. Suppl. 3, 2017.

Drug-Induced Liver Injury Associated with the Use of Everolimus in a Liver Transplant Patient

Serena Patel[1], **Michel H. Mendler**[2], **Mark A. Valasek**[3] **and Shirley M. Tsunoda**[1]

[1] *University of California (UC) San Diego, Skaggs School of Pharmacy and Pharmaceutical Sciences, USA*
[2] *UC San Diego, Department of Medicine, Division of Hepatology, USA*
[3] *UC San Diego, Department of Pathology, USA*

Correspondence should be addressed to Shirley M. Tsunoda; smtsunoda@ucsd.edu

Academic Editor: Piero Boraschi

Drug-induced liver injury (DILI) has not been previously reported as a complication of treatment with everolimus. A 56-year-old Caucasian male liver transplant recipient developed DILI after receiving everolimus. Elevations in transaminase levels occurred within a week of starting everolimus and an upward trend in the transaminase levels continued with supporting histopathologic changes confirmed by liver biopsy. Within one week of drug discontinuation, his liver enzymes normalized to baseline. This report includes a brief review of the pharmacokinetic properties of everolimus, a review of the relevant literature, and an analysis using the RUCAM and Naranjo algorithms.

1. Introduction

Everolimus is a mammalian target of rapamycin (mTOR) inhibitor that is FDA approved for use as an immunosuppressive agent in kidney and liver transplantation [1]. In liver transplantation, everolimus is used with low dose tacrolimus and steroids as a kidney-sparing agent to prevent cellular rejection [2]. Everolimus is also approved for advanced cases of breast cancer, pancreatic tumors, and advanced renal cell carcinoma [1]. As a narrow therapeutic index drug, achieving optimal exposure levels (trough concentration ranging from 3 to 8 ng/mL) is critical to its successful use [3].

The mTOR pathway is involved in several physiological pathways including protein, nucleotide, and lipid synthesis. mTOR is a protein kinase that regulates cell growth and cycle progression of B and T lymphocytes from the IL-2 receptor to the nucleus [4]. Consequently, it comes with a diverse range of dose-dependent side effects including hyperlipidemia, edema, wound healing complications, stomatitis, anemia, proteinuria, and interstitial pneumonitis.

In this case, we discuss a patient on everolimus after liver transplant and the histopathologic and laboratory value changes indicative of drug-induced liver injury (DILI).

2. Case Presentation

A 56-year-old Caucasian male with nonalcoholic steatohepatitis (NASH) experienced progression to cirrhosis and its complications including portal hypertension, esophageal varices, and ascites. He had no other significant past medical history. At the time of transplant in July 2015, the patient weighed 228 lbs (BMI 34). He received a liver transplant and was placed on a maintenance immunosuppressive regimen of tacrolimus 9 mg PO BID with a trough goal of 8-10 ng/mL, mycophenolic acid (Myfortic) 720 mg PO BID, and a prednisone taper. The patient remained stable on this regimen and had the following normal laboratory results at the beginning of September (**Figure 1**): ALT 32 IU/L (normal=0-40), AST 23 IU/L (normal= 5-40), alkaline phosphatase (ALP) 83 IU/L (normal= 40-100), gamma-glutamyl transpeptidase (GGT) 36 IU/L (normal=10-64), total bilirubin 0.3 mg/dL (normal=0.3-1.9 mg/dL), BUN 26 (normal 6-20 mg/dL), and Scr 1.18 (normal 0.67-1.17 mg/dL) and INR 1.1.

On September 3, 2015, the patient was switched from mycophenolic acid to everolimus as part of a clinical research study investigating the renal sparing effects of everolimus to target a lower tacrolimus trough concentration of 3-5 ng/mL. At the time of everolimus introduction, the patient's

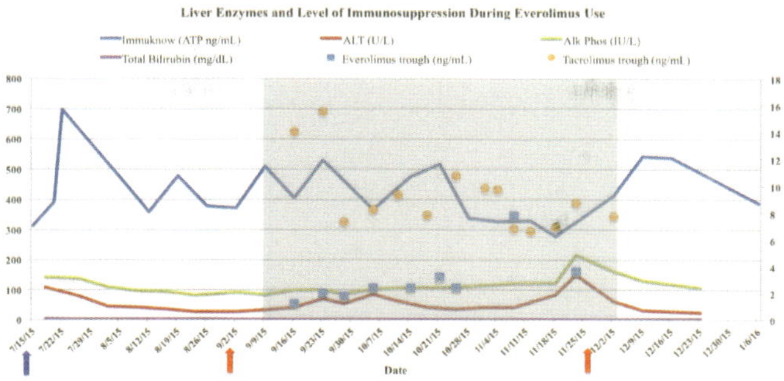

FIGURE 1: Patient's liver enzyme levels and level of immunosuppression after receiving a liver transplant in July 2015. The blue arrow represents the date of the transplant and the shaded area between the red arrows represents the everolimus exposure period (start: 9/3/15; end: 12/1/15).

weight was down to 210 lbs (BMI 31.9) and laboratory values that would impact the pharmacokinetics of everolimus were within a normal range: Hgb 12 mg/dL and albumin 3.7 g/dL. After the patient's first everolimus dose on a starting regimen of 1 mg PO BID, he reported new onset pain to the right flank area. At this time, there was an upward trend in his liver enzymes, ALT (69 IU/L), AST (35 IU/L), ALP (99 IU/L), and GGT (58 IU/L). The everolimus trough was subtherapeutic until late October when a trough of 3.8 ng/mL was achieved on a dose of 3 mg PO qam and 2.5 mg PO qpm (**Figure 1**).

In early October, the patient experienced increasing liver enzymes (ALT=84 IU/L; AST= 42 IU/L; ALP=102 IU/L; GGT=53 IU/L; total bilirubin 0.23 mg/dL) with a tacrolimus trough concentration of 8.2, so a liver biopsy was performed to rule out rejection. The results showed mild portal inflammation with lymphocytes, pericentral sinusoidal dilatation with no hepatic plate atrophy, and inflammation adjacent to the central vein (RAI score = 1 out of 9). The trichrome stain did not have any perisinusoidal staining to indicate chronicity, nor was there duct injury, duct loss, cholestasis, endothelitis, or steatosis. Immunostains for hepatitis B surface antigen (HBsAg) and hepatitis B core antigen (HBcAg) were also negative. There was no report of fever, chills, dark-colored urine, or jaundice or any evidence of an acute hypersensitivity reaction (fever/rash). The immune cell function (ImmuKnow) assay was 338 ng/mL in late October close to the time of the biopsy (10/26/15). It was confirmed that there was no evidence of acute rejection.

By the end of November, two and a half months from the start of everolimus, the patient's serum liver enzymes reached their highest values, ALT (149 IU/L), AST (81 IU/L), and ALP, (215 IU/L) and the ImmuKnow assay done at this time resulted in a level of 412 ng/mL. Tacrolimus doses had not been changed and troughs ranged from 6.9 to 9.8 ng/mL. A second liver biopsy was done on 11/30/15 that showed mild patchy sinusoidal dilatation and focal mild inflammatory infiltrate with lymphocytes, eosinophils, and rare acidophil bodies (**Figure 2**). There was no evidence of acute cellular rejection (RAI score= 1 out of 9), but the presence of eosinophils and focal mild portal inflammation was consistent with the possibility of drug injury. Everolimus was discontinued on December 1, 2015, and the patient went back to a regimen of tacrolimus 5 mg BID and mycophenolic acid 720 mg BID. After one week, the liver enzymes returned to normal: ALT (22 IU/L), AST (20 IU/L), ALP (105 IU/L), and total bilirubin (0.6 mg/dL). Since discontinuation, the patient denied pain and dizziness and reported improved energy.

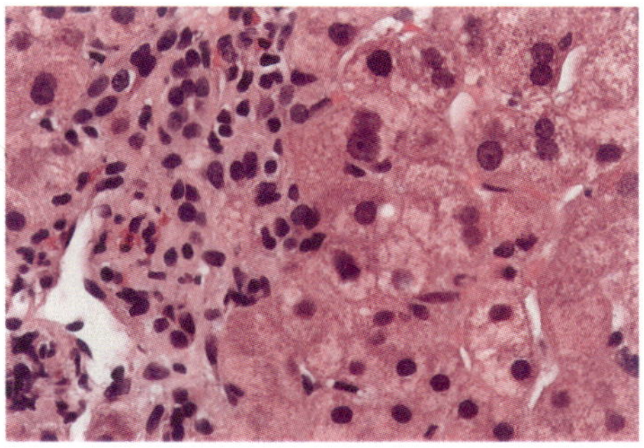

FIGURE 2: Patient's second biopsy done on 11/30/2015 showing features of DILI including portal eosinophils and rare acidophil bodies.

3. Discussion

To our knowledge, this is the first report of everolimus associated DILI. A DILI score model was created to better predict the potential of a drug to cause liver injury and the severity of the injury based on the lipophilicity of the drug (log P $\geq$3), covalent binding of reactive metabolites, and the daily dose of the oral medication ($\geq$ 100 mg) [5]. Everolimus has not been studied in this model directly. However, it does have the property of high lipophilicity with a log P of 5.01, a property associated with greater rates of mitochondrial toxicity and DILI [5, 6]. Secondly, as opposed to sirolimus, it has a stable 2-hydroxy-ethyl substitution at position 40, improving its oral bioavailability [7, 8]. In our patient, the daily dose of everolimus never exceeded 5.5 mg daily, far lower than the 100 mg threshold for the model. The importance of this property for a drug like everolimus may not be significant because there is a poor correlation between the dose and actual systemic exposure of the drug; a stronger correlation is seen between the AUC and trough concentration [7].

Despite the similarity in chemical structures between sirolimus and everolimus, only sirolimus has been included in the FDA's Liver Toxicity Knowledge Base (LTKB) Database as being of "less DILI concern." This is based on both drug-labeling studies of sirolimus and verified causality evidence of hepatotoxicity with elevated trough levels [9–11]. A reference drug list for risk of DILI in humans ranks everolimus as having "ambiguous DILI concern" when taking into account the drug-labeling studies as well as verified causality evidence [9]. Based on the clinical trial studies, everolimus was initially ranked as having "less DILI concern" due to ≤ 10% of patients in each test group having elevations in alkaline phosphatase and liver transaminases [10]. However, the verified DILI concern is still "ambiguous" because there have been no verified causality evidence reports on DILI [9].

In order to rule out other causalities for DILI in this patient, we examined the DILI potential of his concomitant medications. These included tacrolimus, prednisone, sulfamethoxazole/trimethoprim (TMP-SMZ), metformin, glipizide, and propranolol. Tacrolimus, prednisone, and TMP-SMZ are not listed as drugs with a significant risk of DILI in humans based on the reference compiled by Chen et al. [9]. In postmarketing reports, tacrolimus has only been associated with mild to moderate elevations in serum aminotransferases in 5-10% of patients and any elevations are mild, asymptomatic, and self-limiting [12]. Long term and high doses of prednisone and methylprednisolone (500 mg) [13] have been associated with NASH exacerbations, with liver enzyme elevations, and with liver histology showing hepatitis with steatosis, chronic inflammation, and Mallory bodies, which were not consistent with liver biopsy in this patient [11]. Our patient was only on a small oral maintenance dose of 2.5 mg daily. TMP-SMZ can cause mild elevations in ALT that do not proceed to more severe liver injury or jaundice, but in postmarketing reports, the onset is usually within a few days or weeks of starting the medication and resolves within 2-4 weeks [11]. Though idiosyncratic liver injury has been reported with TMP-SMZ with features of drug allergies (eosinophilia), the time course of onset was not consistent with the literature [11]. In our case, TMP-SMZ was started in July 2015 and the patient's liver enzymes (as evident in the graph) were still stable and within normal limits at this time prior to the start of everolimus in September 2015.

Propranolol has been listed as a drug of "ambiguous DILI concern" by Chen et al. and has been rated as an unlikely cause of clinically apparent liver injury. Its rating is based on case reports showing a pattern of serum enzyme elevations that are hepatocellular in nature with typical onset of 2 to 24 weeks [9, 11]. These elevations have been seen in 2% of patients using propranolol and are transient and asymptomatic and tend to resolve even as the patient continues the medication [11]. There are no causal associations because these case reports included patients who were on other well-known hepatotoxic drugs [11]. This patient had started propranolol on 8/28/15, so while the timecourse of propranolol use may be in conjunction with the time for enzyme elevation with its use, the pattern of enzyme elevation was not hepatocellular.

Though metformin was initially listed as a drug with "no-DILI concern," there have been close to twenty case reports in the literature of hepatotoxicity with metformin after 4 to 8 weeks of use [14]. Minor elevations in liver enzymes have been reported to occur during metformin therapy in less than 1% of patients and typically the timing of the injury occurs soon after the agent is started, not during long term therapy [11]. Our patient had been taking metformin for three months, so the likelihood of metformin causing his DILI is low. Glipizide has not been identified as an agent of DILI concern and minor elevations in liver enzymes occur in <1% of patients which is comparable to what can be expected with placebo [9, 11]. Though these medications were started after transplant, the timecourse of transaminase elevations does not correspond to the literature reports.

Additionally, we checked to ensure that elevations in liver enzymes and liver injury were not due to drug interactions. The only major interactions noted were between amlodipine (a CYP3A4 inhibitor) and tacrolimus, leading to increased levels, and prednisone (a CYP3A4 inducer) and tacrolimus leading to decreased levels and potential for transplant rejection [15]. Tacrolimus trough levels were monitored throughout this patient's treatment and were within the trough goal throughout the time of liver injury. Therefore, it is unlikely that drug-drug interactions played a role.

The classification of DILI based on phenotype appears to be mixed [11]. At the peak of the patient's enzyme elevations, the ratio of [ALT/ULN]/[Alk P/ULN] was 2.23. This was based on the patient's enzymes measured on 11/23/15 in which the ALT was 149 U/L (ULN= 40) and the Alk Phos was 215 IU/L (ULN= 129) [11, 16]. Ratios of >5 define hepatocellular, <2 cholestatic, and between 2 and 5 mixed pattern of enzymes [11, 16]. In hepatocellular injury, the ALT is usually >three times the upper limit of normal (ULN), alkaline phosphatase is more than two times the ULN, or total bilirubin is more than twice the ULN [11, 16]. Though elevations to this extent were not evident within the first month, the values did increase and eventually reached levels of ALT or AST that were >3X the ULN and an ALP > 2X the ULN by the end of two months. This indicates that the injury may be mixed hepatocellular and cholestatic.

We suspected everolimus induced DILI based on the chronological association with liver enzyme abnormalities, the pathology findings, and the properties of the drug. We also applied the more standardized causality assessment for drug-induced hepatotoxicity, RUCAM (Roussel Uclaf Causality Assessment Method). This method evaluates drug-induced liver injury based on seven criteria: (1) time to onset of the injury following start of the drug; (2) subsequent course of injury after stopping the drug (time to enzyme normalization after cessation of drug); (3) specific risk factors (age, alcohol use, and pregnancy); (4) use of other medications with a potential for liver injury; (5) exclusion of other causes of liver disease; (6) known potential for hepatotoxicity of the implicated drug; and (7) response to rechallenge [16]. This data is scored and categorized as highly probable, probable, possible, or excluded. RUCAM is specific to liver injury and has been evaluated for accuracy, reproducibility, and intraobserver variability with the advantage of being more

TABLE 1: Adverse drug reaction probability scale (Naranjo) [17].

Question	Yes	No	Do Not Know	Score
1. Are there previous conclusive reports on this reaction?	+1	0	0	0
2. Did the adverse event appear after the suspected drug was administered?	+2	-1	0	+2
3. Did the adverse event improve when the drug was discontinued or a specific antagonist was administered?	+1	0	0	+1
4. Did the adverse event reappear when the drug was readministered?	+2	-1	0	0
5. Are there alternative causes that could on their own have caused the reaction? (alternatives have been excluded =no)	-1	+2	0	+2
6. Did the reaction reappear when a placebo was given?	-1	+1	0	0
7. Was the drug detected in blood or other fluids in concentrations known to be toxic?	+1	0	0	0
8. Was the reaction more severe when the dose was increased or less severe when the dose was decreased? (reaction was less severe when the dose was decreased)	+1	0	0	+1
9. Did the patient have a similar reaction to the same or similar drugs in any previous exposure?	+1	0	0	0
10. Was the adverse event confirmed by any objective evidence?	+1	0	0	+1
			Total Score: 7	

objective [11]. The range of possible RUCAM scores is −9 to +14 with 0 or less indicating that the drug is "excluded" as a cause, 1 to 2 indicating that it is "unlikely," 3 to 5 indicating that it is "possible," 6 to 8 indicating that it is "probable," and greater than 8 indicating that it is "highly probable." In our patient the RUCAM score was 8, which indicates that the link of liver injury as an adverse drug reaction of everolimus is probable (**Figure 3**). While RUCAM is advantageous due to its specificity to liver injury in assessing causality, one drawback is in criterion #6 which asks the observer to consider the known publications of the reaction [16]. The model does not account for differences in type or quantity of publications.

We also applied a second assessment of causality using the Naranjo scale. While the Naranjo scale is not specific for liver injury, it is a widely accepted scale for assessing drug-associated reactions [17]. The assessment takes into consideration ten factors: (1) any previous reports of a reaction; (2) the appearance of the adverse event after starting the drug; (3) improvement in the reaction after drug discontinuation; (4) reappearance of the reaction when the drug is readministered; (5) other possible causes; (6) reappearance of the reaction when placebo is given; (7) detection in the blood or fluids of toxic drug concentrations; (8) worsening or improvement of the reaction with an increase or decrease in dose; (9) previous similar reaction to the drug; and (10) confirmation by objective evidence [17]. The scoring system ranges from −4 to +13 with a score of 0 or less being "doubtful," 1 to 4 being "possible," 5 to 8 being "probable," and 9 or higher being "definite" adverse drug reaction. Based on the Naranjo scale, the likelihood of everolimus causing the liver injury in our patient was 7 (or probable) **(Table 1)**. A probable causality on this scale means that the reaction (liver injury) followed a reasonable temporal sequence after initiation of the drug and was confirmed by withdrawal of the drug.

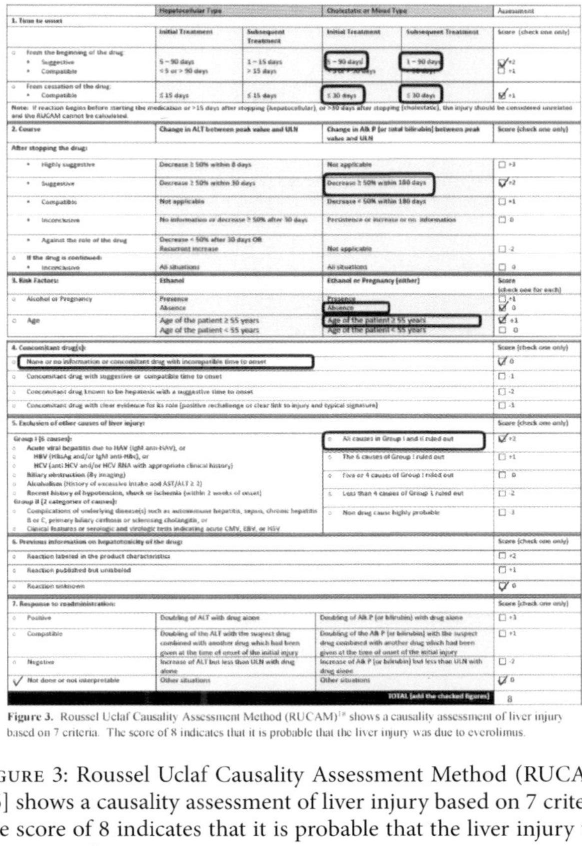

	Hepatocellular Type		Cholestatic or Mixed Type		Assessment
1. Time to onset					
	Initial Treatment	Subsequent Treatment	Initial Treatment	Subsequent Treatment	Score (check one only)
From the beginning of the drug: Suggestive / Compatible	5 – 90 days / <5 or > 90 days	1 – 15 days / > 15 days	5 – 90 days / <5 or > 90 days	1 – 90 days / > 90 days	☑ +2 / ☐ +1
From cessation of the drug: Compatible	≤ 15 days	≤ 15 days	≤ 30 days	≤ 30 days	☑ +1
Note: If reaction begins before starting the medication or >15 days after stopping (hepatocellular), or >30 days after stopping (cholestatic), the injury should be considered unrelated and the RUCAM cannot be calculated.					
2. Course	Change in ALT between peak value and ULN		Change in Alk P (or total bilirubin) between peak value and ULN		Score (check one only)
After stopping the drug:					
Highly suggestive	Decrease ≥ 50% within 8 days		Not applicable		☐ +3
Suggestive	Decrease ≥ 50% within 30 days		Decrease ≥ 50% within 180 days		☑ +2
Compatible	Not applicable		Decrease < 50% within 180 days		☐ +1
Inconclusive	No information or decrease ≥ 50% after 30 days		Persistence or increase or no information		☐ 0
Against the role of the drug	Decrease < 50% after 30 days OR Recurrent increase		Not applicable		☐ -2
If the drug is continued: Inconclusive	All situations		All situations		☐ 0
3. Risk Factors:	Ethanol		Ethanol or Pregnancy (either)		Score (check one for each)
Alcohol or Pregnancy	Presence / Absence		Presence / Absence		☐ +1 / ☑ 0
Age	Age of the patient ≥ 55 years / Age of the patient < 55 years		Age of the patient ≥ 55 years / Age of the patient < 55 years		☑ +1 / ☐ 0
4. Concomitant drug(s):					Score (check one only)
None or no information or concomitant drug with incompatible time to onset					☑ 0
Concomitant drug with suggestive or compatible time to onset					☐ -1
Concomitant drug known to be hepatoxic with a suggestive time to onset					☐ -2
Concomitant drug with clear evidence for its role (positive rechallenge or clear link to injury and typical signature)					☐ -3
5. Exclusion of other causes of liver injury:					Score (check one only)
Group I (6 causes): Acute viral hepatitis due to HAV (IgM anti-HAV), or HBV (HBsAg and/or IgM anti-HBc), or HCV (anti HCV and/or HCV RNA with appropriate clinical history); Biliary obstruction (By imaging); Alcoholism (History of excessive intake and AST/ALT ≥ 2); Recent history of hypotension, shock or ischemia (within 2 weeks of onset). Group II (2 categories of causes): Complications of underlying disease(s) such as autoimmune hepatitis, sepsis, chronic hepatitis B or C, primary biliary cirrhosis or sclerosing cholangitis, or Clinical features or serologic and virologic tests indicating acute CMV, EBV, or HSV			All causes in Group I and II ruled out		☑ +2
			The 6 causes of Group I ruled out		☐ +1
			Five or 4 causes of Group I ruled out		☐ 0
			Less than 4 causes of Group I ruled out		☐ -2
			Non drug cause highly probable		☐ -3
6. Previous information on hepatotoxicity of the drug:					Score (check one only)
Reaction labeled in the product characteristics					☐ +2
Reaction published but unlabeled					☐ +1
Reaction unknown					☑ 0
7. Response to readministration:					Score (check one only)
Positive	Doubling of ALT with drug alone		Doubling of Alk P (or bilirubin) with drug alone		☐ +3
Compatible	Doubling of the ALT with the suspect drug combined with another drug which had been given at the time of onset of the initial injury		Doubling of the Alk P (or bilirubin) with the suspect drug combined with another drug which had been given at the time of onset of the initial injury		☐ +1
Negative	Increase of ALT but less than ULN with drug alone		Increase of Alk P (or bilirubin) but less than ULN with drug alone		☐ -2
✓ Not done or not interpretable	Other situations		Other situations		☑ 0
				TOTAL (add the checked figures)	8

Figure 3. Roussel Uclaf Causality Assessment Method (RUCAM)[18] shows a causality assessment of liver injury based on 7 criteria. The score of 8 indicates that it is probable that the liver injury was due to everolimus.

FIGURE 3: Roussel Uclaf Causality Assessment Method (RUCAM) [16] shows a causality assessment of liver injury based on 7 criteria. The score of 8 indicates that it is probable that the liver injury was due to everolimus.

4. Conclusion

This case documents an association between everolimus and DILI. Use of everolimus in this post-liver transplant patient led to elevations in AST, ALT, and ALP consistent with mixed hepatocellular and cholestatic liver injury over a period of three months. In addition, the liver biopsy confirmed the finding of DILI based upon the histological characteristics, notably the presence of eosinophils, rare acidophil bodies, and focal mild portal inflammation. Finally, all other concomitant medications have been sufficiently ruled out as being the cause of DILI. The pharmacokinetic characteristics of everolimus coupled with the temporal correlation, histologic findings, and positive RUCAM and Naranjo scores point to everolimus being the likely cause of this patient's DILI. Future investigations into the factors that may have increased this patient's susceptibility should be explored.

Abbreviations

CYP3A4: Cytochrome P450 3A4
AUC: Area under the curve
DILI: Drug-induced liver injury
CNI: Calcineurin inhibitor
mTOR: Mammalian target of rapamycin
RUCAM: Roussel Uclaf Causality Assessment Method
NASH: Nonalcoholic steatohepatitis.

References

[1] Dailymed.nlm.nih.gov. (2017). *DailyMed*. online, Accessed 12 Nov. 2017, Available at: https://dailymed.nlm.nih.gov/dailymed/.

[2] T. van Gelder, L. Fischer, F. Shihab, and M. Shipkova, "Optimizing everolimus exposure when combined with calcineurin inhibitors in solid organ transplantation," *Transplantation Reviews*, vol. 31, no. 3, pp. 151–157, 2017.

[3] L. Su, N. Tam, R. Deng, P. Chen, H. Li, and L. Wu, "Everolimus-based calcineurin-inhibitor sparing regimens for kidney transplant recipients: A systematic review and meta-analysis," *International Urology and Nephrology*, vol. 46, no. 10, pp. 2035–2044, 2014.

[4] P. Ventura-Aguiar, J. M. Campistol, and F. Diekmann, "Safety of mTOR inhibitors in adult solid organ transplantation," *Expert Opinion on Drug Safety*, vol. 15, no. 3, pp. 303–319, 2016.

[5] M. Chen, J. Borlak, and W. Tong, "A Model to predict severity of drug-induced liver injury in humans," *Hepatology*, vol. 64, no. 3, pp. 931–940, 2016.

[6] Drugbank.ca. (2017). *Everolimus -DrugBank*. online, Accessed 12 Nov. 2017, Available at: https://www.drugbank.ca/drugs/DB01590.

[7] J. Klawitter, B. Nashan, and U. Christians, "Everolimus and sirolimus in transplantation-related but different," *Expert Opinion on Drug Safety*, vol. 14, no. 7, pp. 1055–1070, 2015.

[8] W. Jacobsen, N. Serkova, B. Hausen, R. E. Morris, L. Z. Benet, and U. Christians, "Comparison of the in vitro metabolism of the macrolide immunosuppressants sirolimus and RAD," *Transplantation Proceedings*, vol. 33, no. 1-2, pp. 514-515, 2001.

[9] M. Chen, A. Suzuki, S. Thakkar, K. Yu, C. Hu, and W. Tong, "DILIrank: the largest reference drug list ranked by the risk for developing drug-induced liver injury in humans," *Drug Discovery Therapy*, vol. 21, no. 4, pp. 648–653, 2016.

[10] G. W. Neff, P. Ruiz, J. R. Madariaga et al., "Sirolimus-associated hepatotoxicity in liver transplantation," *Annals of Pharmacotherapy*, vol. 38, no. 10, pp. 1593–1596, 2004.

[11] Livertox.nih.gov. (2017). *SearchLivertox Database*. online, Accessed 12 Nov. 2017, Available at: https://livertox.nih.gov/.

[12] A. Suzuki, R. J. Andrade, E. Bjornsson et al., "Drugs associated with hepatotoxicity and their reporting frequency of liver adverse events in vigibase™: unified list based on international collaborative work," *Drug Safety*, vol. 33, no. 6, pp. 503–522, 2010.

[13] K. Gutkowski, A. Chwist, and M. Hartleb, "Liver injury induced by high-dose methylprednisolone therapy: A case report and brief review of the literature," *Hepatitis Monthly*, vol. 11, no. 8, pp. 656–661, 2011.

[14] T. Hashmi, "Probable hepatotoxicity associated with the use of metformin in type 2 diabetes," *BMJ Case Reports*, vol. 2011, no. sep13 1, pp. bcr0420114092–bcr0420114092, 2011.

[15] Amlodipine, Glipizide, Metformin, Prednisone, Propranolol, & Tacrolimus. (2017). In Micromedex: Drug Interactions (Electronic version). Greenwood Village, CO:Truven Health Analytics. Retrieved September 23, 2017, from http://www.micromedexsolutions.com/.

[16] G. Danan and C. Benichou, "Causality assessment of adverse reactions to drugs—I: a novel method based on the conclusions of international consensus meetings: application to drug-induced liver injuries," *Journal of Clinical Epidemiology*, vol. 46, no. 11, pp. 1323–1330, 1993.

[17] C. A. Naranjo, U. Busto, and E. M. Sellers, "A method for estimating the probability of adverse drug reactions," *Clinical Pharmacology & Therapeutics*, vol. 30, no. 2, pp. 239–245, 1981.

Successful Stem Cell Transplantation in a Patient with Pretransplant Hepatic Inflammatory Pseudotumour

Sanjay de Mel,[1] Zarni Soe,[1] Benjamin Wong,[2] Ching Ching Ong,[3] Lynette Teo,[3] and Lip Kun Tan[4]

[1] *Department of Haematology-Oncology, National University Cancer Institute, National University Health System, 1E Kent Ridge Road, NUHS Tower Block Level 7, Singapore 119228*
[2] *Department of Pathology, National University Health System, 1E Kent Ridge Road, Singapore 119228*
[3] *Department of Diagnostic Imaging, National University Health System, 1E Kent Ridge Road, Singapore 119228*
[4] *Departments of Laboratory Medicine and Haematology-Oncology, National University Cancer Institute, National University Health System, 1E Kent Ridge Road, NUHS Tower Block Level 7, Singapore 119228*

Correspondence should be addressed to Sanjay de Mel; wspdm199@yahoo.com

Academic Editor: Carl Classen

Inflammatory pseudotumours (IPT) are rare benign neoplasms of unknown aetiology. We present a case of hepatic IPT which was incidentally discovered in a patient with relapsed B-acute lymphoblastic leukaemia (B-ALL) undergoing pretransplant workup. After investigation to exclude an infective cause she underwent a reduced intensity conditioning stem cell transplant (SCT) successfully and currently remains well and in remission. On repeat liver MRI after SCT, the IPT was seen to be resolving. To the best of our knowledge this is the first report of an adult patient with hepatic IPT successfully undergoing SCT. The reduction in size of the IPT after SCT also suggests an inflammatory rather than an infective aetiology for IPT.

1. Background

IPT are rare benign tumours which can mimic malignant neoplasms both clinically and radiologically. Historically, the terminology used to describe IPT has been diverse, mainly due to variable histological findings. It was first described in 1939 by Brunn and the term IPT was first used by Umiker and Iverson in 1954 [1]. It has been reported to be found in many different sites including the lungs, orbit, spinal cord, gastrointestinal tract, spleen, pancreas, kidney, adrenal gland, bladder, thyroid, and the retroperitoneal region [2].

The first case of IPT of the liver was described by Pack and Baker in 1953 [3]. These patients have been reported to present with fever, abdominal pain, and jaundice, sometimes leading to biliary obstruction, portal hypertension, cirrhosis, and eventually hepatic failure [4]. The key histologic finding in IPT is proliferation of spindled myofibroblast cells mixed with variable amounts of reactive inflammatory cells [4].

Radiological features of IPT are also variable and non-specific, possibly because of significant fibrosis and cellular infiltration [5]. Ultrasound can show hypo- or hyperechoic lesions with either ill-defined or well circumscribed borders [6]. These lesions often have increased vascularity during color or power Doppler examinations. CT findings are also diverse, with low, equal, or high attenuation compared with surrounding tissue having been described [6]. On MRI, IPT usually shows low signal intensity on both T1- and T2-weighted images, which may reflect the fibrotic nature of these lesions [7]. Contrast enhanced CT and MRI may show a homogenous or heterogeneous lesion. Delayed imaging often shows increasing enhancement due to the presence of fibrosis [5].

More than a hundred cases of IPT have been reported. Their aetiology is largely unknown; however, they have been postulated to be associated with inflammation, trauma, surgery, or an autoimmune process [8–10]. Treatment options remain experimental. IPT have been reported to be successfully treated by surgery, chemotherapy, and immunosuppressive therapy with rituximab in a case of orbital IPT [10–12]. There have been six cases of IPT diagnosed in patients after

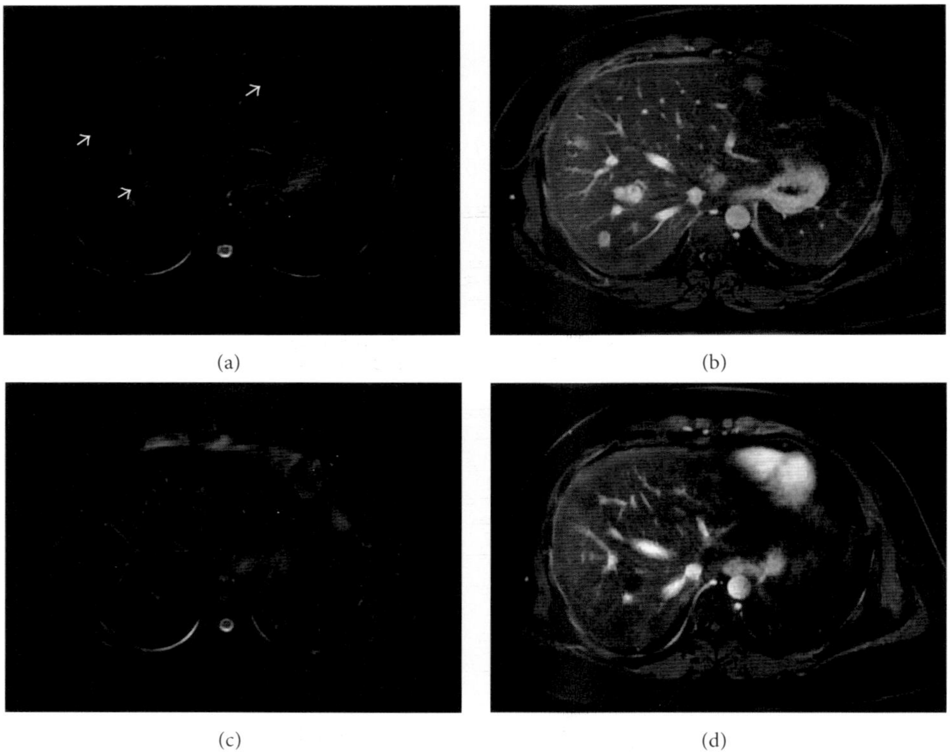

FIGURE 1: (a, b) Baseline MRI. (a) Axial T2-weighted fat saturated (T2W-FS) image shows faintly hyperintense lesions in the liver (white arrows). The liver parenchyma is hypointense and shows reduced signal in keeping with iron loading. (b) Axial delayed postcontrast T1W images show persistent delayed enhancement in the lesions (black arrows). (c, d) MRI after treatment. (c) Axial T2W-FS image shows that the lesions are isointense to the rest of the liver parenchyma which is hypointense (due to iron loading). The lesions are no longer hyperintense on the T2W-FS image. (d) Axial delayed postcontrast T1W images show that the lesions no longer show any appreciable enhancement.

haematopoietic stem cell transplant (SCT) and one case of hepatic IPT in a pediatric patient before SCT with severe congenital neutropenia [13, 14]. To the best of our knowledge, ours is the first report of hepatic IPT in an adult who was due to undergo SCT.

2. Case Report

The patient was a 25-year-old lady diagnosed with standard risk B-ALL in October 2010. She was treated with the MASPORE (Malaysia-Singapore ALL study) intermediate risk protocol. Although she did not achieve a morphologic remission after her induction therapy, the MASPORE protocol was continued and she achieved a morphologic remission as well as flow cytometric minimal residual disease (MRD) negativity in December 2012. Unfortunately her ALL relapsed in August 2014. She did not respond to the Hyper-CVAD regimen but achieved a complete remission after salvage with the FLAG-Ida protocol in November 2014. Her treatment with FLAG-Ida was complicated by neutropenic sepsis and *Escherichia coli* (*E. coli*) bacteremia which was treated with intravenous meropenem for 14 days.

She was planned for SCT from a matched unrelated donor. A routine pre-SCT transthoracic echocardiogram showed a dilated right ventricle. A magnetic resonance imaging (MRI) scan of the heart was therefore performed to further investigate the right heart pathology; this showed no significant cardiac pathology but incidentally detected multiple, bilobar hepatic lesions.

An MRI scan of the liver was therefore performed which showed multiple lesions of varying sizes throughout both lobes of the liver (Figure 1). These lesions had ill-defined margins and showed hyperintense signal on the T2-weighted fat-saturated (T2W-FS) images. They showed a target appearance, with a central core of hyperintensity and a hypointense rim on the precontrast T1-weighted (T1W) images. The lesions showed early (mainly central) arterial enhancement, with persistent enhancement on the delayed postcontrast images. The patient had no abdominal pain, icterus, or fever. Abdominal examination revealed no tenderness or clinically detectable hepatomegaly. Her liver function tests (LFT) were normal.

An ultrasound-guided liver biopsy was performed: this showed an extensive zone of cellular fibrosis with a mixed acute and chronic inflammatory infiltrate composed of eosinophils and aggregates of neutrophils (Figure 2). The zone of fibrosis merged into one of many markedly expanded portal tracts which showed oedema with a mild mixed inflammatory infiltrate. The spindle cells showed immunohistochemical reactivity with smooth-muscle actin (SMA), confirming myofibroblastic differentiation. This biopsy also showed two slender nonbranching fungal hyphae, resembling *Candida*. However, a repeat biopsy showed only cellular fibrosis accompanied by inflammatory infiltrate, with no evidence of

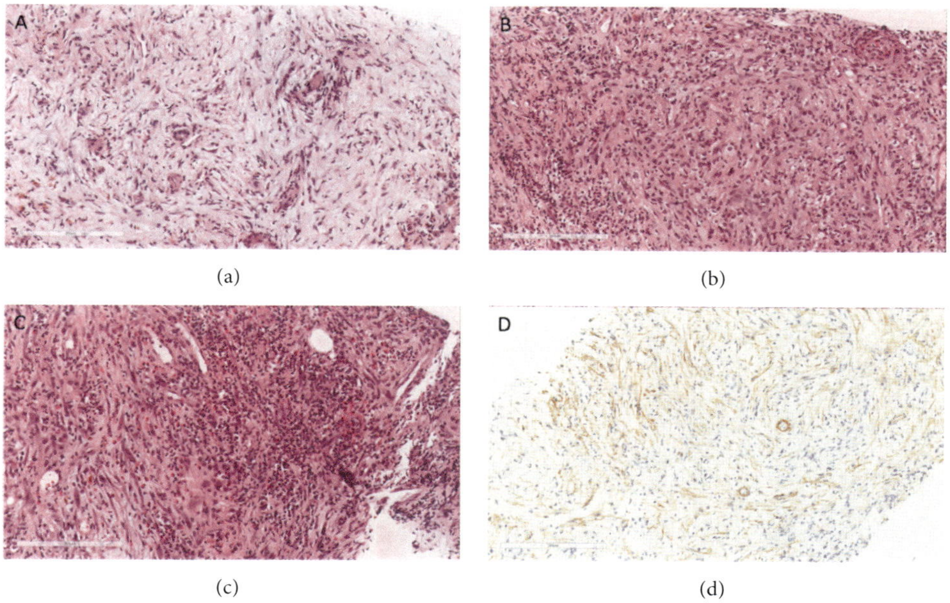

FIGURE 2: Pseudotumour histology. The H&E images (a, b, c) show a loose proliferation of fibrous tissue, accompanied by a mixed acute and chronic inflammatory infiltrate, showing entrapment of residual bile ducts and hepatic artery branches. The immunohistochemistry (d) test for smooth-muscle actin shows reactivity in spindle cells, consistent with a proliferation of myofibroblasts, as might be seen in reactive fibrosis or an inflammatory pseudotumour.

fungal organisms. It was concluded that the fungi in the first biopsy were not of clinical significance (and were possibly a contaminant).

A decision was made to proceed with SCT from a matched unrelated donor using reduced intensity conditioning (RIC): fludarabine 30 mg/m^2 for 4 days and busulfan 3.2 mg/kg for 3 days. Her graft versus host disease (GVHD) prophylaxis regimen included thymoglobulin (ATG), methotrexate, and tacrolimus. ATG was dosed at 0.5 mg/kg on D-3, 1.5 mg/kg on D-2, and 2.5 mg/kg on D-1 while methotrexate was given intravenously at 15 mg/m^2 on D+1 followed by 10 mg/m^2 on D+3, D+6, and D+11. Tacrolimus was commenced on D-3 aiming for a trough level of 8–15 μg/L. No dose adjustments to her chemotherapy were made as her LFT were normal at the point of conditioning. The CD 34+ cell dose infused was 2.76 × 10^6/kg. No prophylaxis for venoocclusive disease (VOD) was given and her LFT remained normal throughout the conditioning and recovery phases of the SCT. Apart from an episode of neutropenic fever, she had an uneventful post-stem cell infusion period with neutrophil engraftment occurring on D+26. A repeat MRI scan of the liver three months after SCT showed that the liver lesions were smaller in size and no longer hyperintense, suggesting some resolution of the inflammatory changes (Figure 1). She had no VOD or hepatic GVHD; she currently remains well and in remission with mild GVHD of the skin and a donor chimerism (CD3 lineage specific) of 98%.

3. Conclusions

The differential diagnoses for multiple hepatic lesions include a variety of infective, inflammatory, and neoplastic disorders. Pyogenic liver abscesses and disseminated fungal infection were strong considerations for our patient, especially given that she had *E. coli* bacteremia after her salvage chemotherapy. Her blood cultures were negative for bacteria and fungus while urine cultures and a chest radiograph were unremarkable.

Fangusaro et al. reported the first cases of IPT after SCT in two pediatric patients: one hepatic and one oesophageal, both treated by surgical resection [15]. All of the six reported cases of IPT after SCT were treated with surgical resection and the aetiology was thought to be SCT related immunosuppression and prior chemotherapy [13]. In contrast, a case of retroorbital IPT in a patient with systemic lupus erythematosus was successfully treated with rituximab [10]. The only reported case of IPT in a pre-SCT patient was a case of hepatic IPT in a pediatric patient with severe congenital neutropenia. Interestingly her IPT responded to granulocyte transfusion after which the SCT was successfully performed [14].

The decision of proceeding with SCT in our patient was difficult as an infective or neoplastic cause had to be excluded before subjecting her to the profound immunosuppression of SCT. The improvement of radiologic findings after SCT in our patient suggests an autoimmune or inflammatory aetiology for IPT rather than an infective cause. Another possibility is whether granulocyte colony stimulating factor (GCSF) may have contributed to the IPT; she was given GCSF following her treatment with FLAF-Ida. As she had no liver imaging before her course of FLAG-Ida we cannot be certain if the IPT was already present before her salvage therapy. Our case suggests that successful RIC SCT is possible in adult patients with IPT provided infective causes are excluded. Further studies are however required to elucidate the biology and natural history of these rare tumours.

Abbreviations

IPT: Inflammatory pseudotumour
B-ALL: B-acute lymphoblastic leukaemia
SCT: Stem cell transplant
MRI: Magnetic resonance imaging
E. coli: *Escherichia coli*
MRD: Minimal residual disease
VOD: Venoocclusive disease
GCSF: Granulocyte colony stimulating factor
GVHD: Graft versus host disease.

Competing Interests

The authors declare that they have no competing interests.

Authors' Contributions

Sanjay de Mel and Zarni Soe drafted and contributed equally to preparation of the manuscript, Benjamin Wong performed the histopathology and immunohistochemistry studies, Ching Ching Ong and Lynette Teo performed the radiologic investigations, and Lip Kun Tan conceived of the study and participated in drafting the manuscript. All authors have read and approved the final manuscript.

References

[1] W. O. Umiker and L. Iverson, "Postinflammatory tumors of the lung; report of four cases simulating xanthoma, fibroma, or plasma cell tumor," *The Journal of Thoracic Surgery*, vol. 28, no. 1, pp. 55–63, 1954.

[2] T. Fukuya, H. Honda, T. Matsumata et al., "Diagnosis of inflammatory pseudotumor of the liver: value of CT," *American Journal of Roentgenology*, vol. 163, no. 5, pp. 1087–1091, 1994.

[3] G. T. Pack and H. W. Baker, "Total right hepatic lobectomy; report of a case," *Annals of Surgery*, vol. 138, no. 2, pp. 253–258, 1953.

[4] W. Faraj, H. Ajouz, D. Mukherji, G. Kealy, A. Shamseddine, and M. Khalife, "Inflammatory pseudo-tumor of the liver: a rare pathological entity," *World Journal of Surgical Oncology*, vol. 9, article 5, 2011.

[5] S. B. Park, K.-S. Cho, K. K. Jeong et al., "Inflammatory pseudotumor (myoblastic tumor) of the genitourinary tract," *American Journal of Roentgenology*, vol. 191, no. 4, pp. 1255–1262, 2008.

[6] J. H. Lim and J. H. Lee, "Inflammatory pseudotumor of the liver ultrasound and CT features," *Clinical Imaging*, vol. 19, no. 1, pp. 43–46, 1995.

[7] M. E. Flisak, D. M. Bubris, M. C. Olson, and E. J. Zarling, "Inflammatory pseudotumor of the liver: appearance on MRI," *Clinical Imaging*, vol. 18, no. 1, pp. 1–3, 1994.

[8] M. Patnana, A. B. Sevrukov, K. M. Elsayes, C. Viswanathan, M. Lubner, and C. O. Menias, "Inflammatory pseudotumor: the great mimicker," *American Journal of Roentgenology*, vol. 198, no. 3, pp. W217–W227, 2012.

[9] L. Das Narla, B. Newman, S. S. Spottswood, S. Narla, and R. Kolli, "Inflammatory pseudotumor," *Radiographics*, vol. 23, no. 3, pp. 719–729, 2003.

[10] C. M. Escudero González, S. Rodríguez Montero, R. Martínez Pérez, C. Pastor Mañosa, M. L. Velloso Feijoo, and J. L. Marenco de la Fuente, "Resistant orbital pseudotumor treated with rituximab in a patient with systemic lupus erythematosus. A case presentation," *Reumatologia Clinica*, vol. 6, no. 4, pp. 214–216, 2010.

[11] Y. W. Kim, J. G. Lee, K. S. Kim et al., "Inflammatory pseudotumor of the liver treated by hepatic resection: a case report," *Yonsei Medical Journal*, vol. 47, no. 1, pp. 140–143, 2006.

[12] Y.-L. Tao, Z.-J. Wang, J.-G. Han, and P. Wei, "Inflammatory myofibroblastic tumor successfully treated with chemotherapy and nonsteroidals: a case report," *World Journal of Gastroenterology*, vol. 18, no. 47, pp. 7100–7103, 2012.

[13] G. Bahat, S. Kalayoglu-Besisik, S. Ozturk, I. Kilicaslan, M. Tunc, and D. Sargin, "Inflammatory pseudotumor following hematopoietic stem cell transplantation: a new case and review of the literature," *Bone Marrow Transplantation*, vol. 40, no. 10, pp. 915–918, 2007.

[14] N. Cojean, C. Blondet, L. Marcellin et al., "Successful stem cell transplantation in an infant with severe congenital neutropenia complicated by pretransplant inflammatory pseudotumor of the liver," *Bone Marrow Transplantation*, vol. 38, no. 9, pp. 641–643, 2006.

[15] J. Fangusaro, K. Klopfenstein, J. Groner, S. Hammond, and R. A. Altura, "Inflammatory myofibroblastic tumor following hematopoietic stem cell transplantation: report of two pediatric cases," *Bone Marrow Transplantation*, vol. 33, no. 1, pp. 103–107, 2004.

Tacrolimus Toxicity due to Biliary Obstruction in a Combined Kidney and Liver Transplant Recipient

Samuel Chan,[1,2] Michael T. Burke,[1,2] David W. Johnson,[1,2] Ross S. Francis,[1,2] and David W. Mudge[1,2]

[1]*Queensland Renal Transplant Service, Princess Alexandra Hospital, Brisbane, QLD, Australia*
[2]*School of Medicine, The University of Queensland, Brisbane, QLD, Australia*

Correspondence should be addressed to Samuel Chan; samuel.chan@uqconnect.edu.au

Academic Editor: David Conti

The immunosuppressant tacrolimus has a narrow therapeutic window, necessitating therapeutic drug monitoring to maintain efficacy and minimise toxicity. There are very few reports examining the impact of impaired biliary excretion on tacrolimus blood levels or toxicity. We report the case of a 26-year-old combined liver and kidney transplant recipient, who developed acute biliary obstruction leading to tacrolimus toxicity with very high blood tacrolimus levels. Despite a careful evaluation, no alternative cause was found for her acute kidney injury, and her kidney function returned to previous baseline within several days following treatment of the biliary obstruction and temporary withdrawal of tacrolimus.

1. Introduction

Tacrolimus is a calcineurin inhibitor immunosuppressant with a narrow therapeutic window [1, 2], necessitating therapeutic drug monitoring to maintain efficacy and minimise toxicity [3, 4]. It is lipophilic and insoluble in water and is a substrate for the drug efflux pump p-glycoprotein and the metabolising enzymes cytochrome P450 3A4 and cytochrome P450 3A5 [3, 4]. Metabolites are excreted primarily in bile [1]. We report the case of a recipient of a combined liver and kidney transplant with stable allograft function on tacrolimus-based immunosuppression, who developed biliary obstruction due to retained gallstones after a cholecystectomy. She rapidly developed signs of tacrolimus toxicity, predominantly central nervous system toxicity, in association with a sudden increase in her blood tacrolimus level. We postulate that the biliary obstruction led to the acute elevation of tacrolimus levels and toxicity, having excluded other possible causes.

2. Case Report

A 26-year-old female liver and kidney transplant recipient presented with a forty-eight-hour history of fever and right upper quadrant pain. She denied any recent illnesses, medication changes, or other symptoms. Her medications included tacrolimus 2.5 mg twice daily, mycophenolate mofetil 360 mg twice daily, prednisolone 7.5 mg daily, trimethoprim/sulfamethoxazole 80/400 mg daily, cholecalciferol 25 μg daily, ranitidine 150 mg twice daily, and magnesium 500 mg twice daily. Her past medical history included end-stage liver disease due to biliary atresia, which was treated with liver transplantation three years prior to presentation. She had undergone cholecystectomy two years prior to the current admission for cholelithiasis complicated by acute cholangitis. She had no other prior surgeries. Her postoperative course was uncomplicated and she made a complete recovery. She subsequently developed end-stage kidney disease due to biopsy-proven diffuse proliferative glomerulonephritis and had received kidney transplantation thirteen months prior to presentation. Her transplant was a five-human-leukocyte antigen mismatch. There were no donor specific antibodies or any antibodies present on Luminex screening. The initial therapy was standard immunosuppression at that time (tacrolimus, mycophenolate mofetil, and prednisolone). The kidney transplant course had been complicated by early delayed graft function secondary to acute

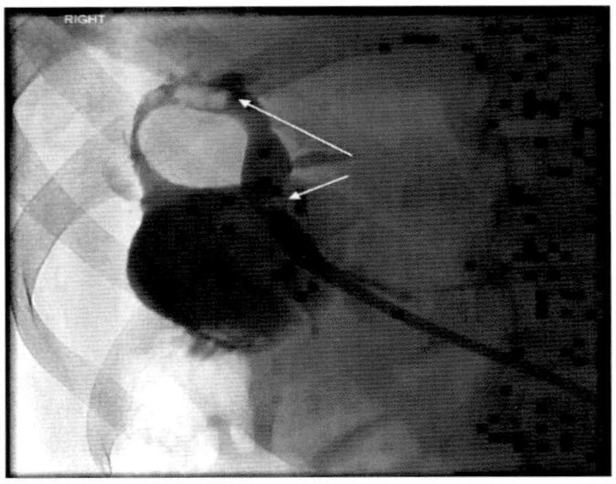

Figure 1: Cholangiogram demonstrating filling defects representative of biliary stones (arrows) present in the common bile duct.

tubular necrosis and suspected antibody-mediated rejection, with presence of peritubular capillaritis but absent C4d, which was treated successfully with a six-week course of plasma exchange. Her subsequent serum creatinine concentrations had remained stable at approximately 1.5 mg/dL.

On examination, she was febrile at 39.5°C, hypotensive with systolic blood pressure of 98 mmHg, and tachycardic at 120 beats per minute in sinus rhythm. She maintained normal oxygen saturation on room air. Her abdomen was tender in the right upper quadrant, with no palpable organomegaly or rebound tenderness. Bowel sounds were audible. There was no abnormality found on examination of her cardiovascular or respiratory systems.

Laboratory investigation demonstrated worsening graft function with a serum potassium concentration of 5.7 mmol/L, serum creatinine concentration of 2.2 mg/dL, and a trough blood tacrolimus level of 5.6 ng/mL. Her serum total bilirubin was 6.4 mg/dL, serum alkaline phosphatase was 187 U/L, gamma-glutamyl transferase was 370 U/L, alanine transaminase was 242 U/L, and aspartate transaminase was 190 U/L. Her C-reactive protein was 158 mg/L. BK virus DNA was not detected in her serum. Blood and urine cultures were sterile. Computed tomography of her abdomen and pelvis showed dilatation of the intrahepatic biliary tree within the lobar liver transplant raising the suspicion of possible biliary-enteric anastomotic stricture. Magnetic resonance cholangiopancreatography and cholangiogram revealed biliary obstruction, with intrahepatic biliary duct dilatation, due to the presence of biliary stones in the main bile duct and near the biliary-enteric anastomosis (Figure 1). The presentation was consistent with cholangitis and, hence, the patient was initially treated with fluid resuscitation with normal saline and intravenous piperacillin/tazobactam.

On admission day 2, her serum creatinine and trough blood tacrolimus concentrations rose markedly to 2.77 mg/dL and 45 ng/mL, respectively, in the absence of any new medications apart from her antibiotics (Figure 2). The immunoassay used to measure tacrolimus levels in this patient was High Performance Liquid Chromatography with tandem mass spectrometric detection. This technique is not susceptible to the interference from tacrolimus metabolites [5]. Her serum total bilirubin was 108 mg/dL, serum alkaline phosphatase was 985 U/L, gamma-glutamyl transferase was 785 U/L, alanine transaminase was 654 U/L, and aspartate transaminase was 585 U/L. She concomitantly developed nausea, vomiting, tremors, blurred vision, hypertension, and delirium without any focal neurological signs. Her tacrolimus was withheld for seven doses and then recommenced at a dose 0.5 mg twice daily (80% reduction of original dose). Tacrolimus levels progressively fell and reached a target level of 8.7 ng/mL by day 7. Her symptoms resolved by day 5. Biliary drainage was restored by day 3 via percutaneous transhepatic cholangiography.

3. Discussion

The patient described in this case report developed clinical features suggestive of acute tacrolimus toxicity, manifested by neurotoxicity, gastrointestinal upset, hypertension, and acute kidney injury, in the setting of acute biliary obstruction. The close temporal association between the rise and fall of the patient's serum tacrolimus levels and the onset and relief of her biliary obstruction strongly suggested that biliary obstruction per se led to changes in serum tacrolimus concentrations, particularly as there were no concomitant interfering medications, medication dosing errors, or preceding gastrointestinal upset. Furthermore, the associations between the rise and fall of her serum tacrolimus concentrations and the respective onsets and offsets of her nausea, vomiting, tremors, blurred vision, hypertension, delirium, and acute kidney injury suggested that these clinical manifestations represented tacrolimus toxicity. Whilst intravenous piperacillin/tazobactam may potentially interact with tacrolimus, there is minimal supporting evidence in the literature regarding this drug-drug interaction; hence, antibiotic mediated tacrolimus toxicity is an unlikely mechanism in this case.

Tacrolimus is metabolised extensively in the liver by the cytochrome P450 family enzymes (particularly CYP3A4 and CYP3A5) with approximately 95% of tacrolimus metabolites being excreted in the bile and only 2% excreted via the urine [6]. In contrast to cyclosporin, the bioavailability of tacrolimus is not appreciably reduced by the absence of bile in the intestine [7]. Consequently, biliary obstruction and/or hepatocyte dysfunction would be hypothesised to impair hepatic metabolism and biliary excretion of tacrolimus but not intestinal absorption. Whilst it has been suggested that biliary obstruction may lead to elevated serum tacrolimus levels [8], reports of this in the literature are scarce. In an experimental dog model, bile duct ligation was shown to greatly increase the area under the plasma concentration versus time curve following orally administered tacrolimus, but not following intravenously administered tacrolimus [7]. Furthermore, bile duct ligation was found to effectively increase the bioavailability of oral tacrolimus 3- to 4-fold, possibly by impaired presystemic metabolism of tacrolimus [7]. Moreover, in a single-centre, retrospective observational study of 35 liver transplant recipients, Kobuchi et al. [9] reported that postoperative biliary stricture was associated with marked intra- and interpatient variability in the tacrolimus trough level normalised dose, which was positively correlated with serum bilirubin level. These findings support the contention

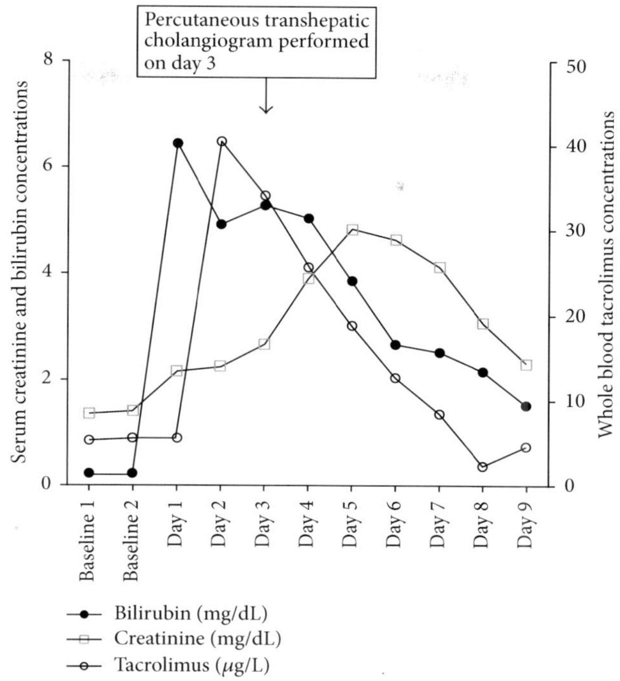

Daily tacrolimus dosage (mg)		Admission course										
	AM	2.5	2.5	2.5	0	0	0	0.5	1.5	1.5	2.5	2.5
	PM	2.5	2.5	2.5	0	0	0	0	1.5	1.5	2.5	2.5

FIGURE 2: Serum bilirubin, creatinine, and tacrolimus concentrations and total daily tacrolimus dosage throughout patient admission.

that biliary obstruction may substantially increase blood tacrolimus levels, as evidenced by this foregoing case report.

In conclusion, this case report illustrates the potential for serious elevation of blood tacrolimus levels and clinical toxicity in the presence of biliary obstruction. The diagnosis of biliary obstruction should therefore prompt clinicians to closely monitor tacrolimus blood levels and look for clinical signs of toxicity on a daily basis, with appropriate reduction of dosage when necessary. Similarly, following relief of biliary obstruction, frequent monitoring is required for several days thereafter and tacrolimus dosage may need to be increased. All clinicians (transplant and primary care) should be aware of this important clinical interaction.

Competing Interests

The authors declare that they have no competing interests.

Authors' Contributions

Samuel Chan sought patient details and drafted the manuscript. Michael T. Burke, David W. Johnson, Ross S. Francis, and David W. Mudge provided critical analysis to the paper. All authors read and approved the final manuscript.

Acknowledgments

The authors sincerely thank the patient for allowing them to publish this case report.

References

[1] T. Kino, H. Hatanaka, S. Miyata et al., "FK-506, a novel immunosuppressant isolated from a Streptomyces. II. Immunosuppressive effect of FK-506 in vitro," *Journal of Antibiotics*, vol. 40, no. 9, pp. 1256–1265, 1987.

[2] D. W. Gjertson, J. M. Cecka, and P. I. Terasaki, "The relative effects of FK506 and cyclosporine on short- and long-term kidney graft survival," *Transplantation*, vol. 60, no. 12, pp. 1384–1388, 1995.

[3] C. E. Staatz and S. E. Tett, "Clinical pharmacokinetics and pharmacodynamics of tacrolimus in solid organ transplantation," *Clinical Pharmacokinetics*, vol. 43, no. 10, pp. 623–653, 2004.

[4] J. W. Ostroff, "Post-transplant biliary problems," *Gastrointestinal Endoscopy Clinics of North America*, vol. 11, no. 1, pp. 163–183, 2001.

[5] P. J. Taylor, M. E. Franklin, C.-H. Tai, and P. I. Pillans, "Therapeutic drug monitoring of tacrolimus by liquid chromatography–tandem mass spectrometry: is it truly a routine test?" *Journal of Chromatography B*, vol. 883-884, pp. 108–112, 2012.

[6] A. Möller, K. Iwasaki, A. Kawamura et al., "The disposition of 14C-labeled tacrolimus after intravenous and oral administration in healthy human subjects," *Drug Metabolism and Disposition*, vol. 27, no. 6, pp. 633–636, 1999.

[7] H. Furukawa, O. Imventarza, R. Venkataramanan et al., "The effect of bile duct ligation and bile diversion on FK506 pharmacokinetics in dogs," *Transplantation*, vol. 53, no. 4, pp. 722–725, 1992.

[8] U. Christians, F. Braun, M. Schmidt et al., "Specific and sensitive measurement of FK506 and its metabolites in blood and urine of liver-graft recipients," *Clinical Chemistry*, vol. 38, no. 10, pp. 2025–2032, 1992.

[9] S. Kobuchi, K. Fukushima, Y. Maeda et al., "Effects of cholestasis on whole blood concentration of tacrolimus, an immunosuppressant, in living-related liver transplant recipients," *International Journal of Clinical Medicine*, vol. 4, no. 10, pp. 432–439, 2013.

Permissions

All chapters in this book were first published in CRT, by Hindawi Publishing Corporation; hereby published with permission under the Creative Commons Attribution License or equivalent. Every chapter published in this book has been scrutinized by our experts. Their significance has been extensively debated. The topics covered herein carry significant findings which will fuel the growth of the discipline. They may even be implemented as practical applications or may be referred to as a beginning point for another development.

The contributors of this book come from diverse backgrounds, making this book a truly international effort. This book will bring forth new frontiers with its revolutionizing research information and detailed analysis of the nascent developments around the world.

We would like to thank all the contributing authors for lending their expertise to make the book truly unique. They have played a crucial role in the development of this book. Without their invaluable contributions this book wouldn't have been possible. They have made vital efforts to compile up to date information on the varied aspects of this subject to make this book a valuable addition to the collection of many professionals and students.

This book was conceptualized with the vision of imparting up-to-date information and advanced data in this field. To ensure the same, a matchless editorial board was set up. Every individual on the board went through rigorous rounds of assessment to prove their worth. After which they invested a large part of their time researching and compiling the most relevant data for our readers.

The editorial board has been involved in producing this book since its inception. They have spent rigorous hours researching and exploring the diverse topics which have resulted in the successful publishing of this book. They have passed on their knowledge of decades through this book. To expedite this challenging task, the publisher supported the team at every step. A small team of assistant editors was also appointed to further simplify the editing procedure and attain best results for the readers.

Apart from the editorial board, the designing team has also invested a significant amount of their time in understanding the subject and creating the most relevant covers. They scrutinized every image to scout for the most suitable representation of the subject and create an appropriate cover for the book.

The publishing team has been an ardent support to the editorial, designing and production team. Their endless efforts to recruit the best for this project, has resulted in the accomplishment of this book. They are a veteran in the field of academics and their pool of knowledge is as vast as their experience in printing. Their expertise and guidance has proved useful at every step. Their uncompromising quality standards have made this book an exceptional effort. Their encouragement from time to time has been an inspiration for everyone.

The publisher and the editorial board hope that this book will prove to be a valuable piece of knowledge for researchers, students, practitioners and scholars across the globe.

List of Contributors

Nicolás Goldaracena and Lucas McCormack
Liver Surgery and Transplantation Unit, Hospital Alemán of Buenos Aires, Avenne Pueyrredón 1640, Buenos Aires 1118AAT, Argentina

Mariela Barreto and Gabriel Casas
Pathology Service, Hospital Alemán of Buenos Aires, Avenne Pueyrredón 1640, Buenos Aires 1118AAT, Argentina

Margarita Anders and RicardoMastai
Hepatology Service and Liver Transplantation Unit, Hospital Alemán of Buenos Aires, Avenne Pueyrredón 1640, Buenos Aires 1118AAT, Argentina

HanjayWang, Adam D. Griesemer and Jean C. Emond
Center for Liver Disease and Transplantation, Department of Surgery, Columbia University Medical Center, New York, NY 10032, USA

Benjamin Samstein
Center for Liver Disease and Transplantation, Department of Surgery, Columbia University Medical Center, New York, NY 10032, USA
New York Presbyterian Hospital/Columbia, PH Room Floor 14, Room 202, 622West 168th Street, New York, NY 10032, USA

Ronald F. Parsons
Department of Surgery, Emory University School of Medicine, Atlanta, GA 30322, USA

Jay A. Graham
Department of Surgery, Montefiore Medical Center, Bronx, NY 10467, USA

Arshad Khan, Jose Oberholzer, Ivo Tzvetanov, Raquel Garcia Roca and Enrico Benedetti
Department of Surgery, College of Medicine, University of Illinois at Chicago, Chicago, IL 60612, USA

P. Park
Department of Surgery, College of Medicine, University of Illinois at Chicago, Chicago, IL 60612, USA
Department of Surgery, Korea University Guro Hospital, 80 Guro-dong, Guro-gu, Seoul 152-703, Republic of Korea

Hoonbae Jeon
Department of Surgery, College of Medicine, University of Illinois at Chicago, Chicago, IL 60612, USA
Division of Transplantation, Department of Surgery, College of Medicine, University of Illinois at Chicago, CSB Suite 402, MC 958, 840 SouthWood Street, Chicago, IL 60612, USA

Ron C. Gaba
Department of Radiology, College of Medicine, University of Illinois at Chicago, Chicago, IL 60612, USA

Cristiano Piangatelli, Claudia Cristiani and Ilaria Valentini
Division of Anaesthesia and Resuscitation, Department of Emergency, Ospedali Riuniti, Via Conca 71, 60020 Ancona, Italy

Lucia Faloia
Department of Emergency, Anesthesia and Resuscitation Unit, Universit`a Politecnica delleMarche, Via Conca 71, 60020 Ancona, Italy

Marco Vivarelli
Department of Liver Surgery and Transplantation, Ospedali Riuniti, Via Conca 71, 60020 Ancona, Italy

Akira Umemura, Hiroyuki Nitta, Akira Sasaki, Takeshi Takahara, Yasushi Hasegawa and Go Wakabayashi
Department of Surgery, Iwate Medical University, 19-1 Uchimaru, Morioka 020-8505, Japan

Annie K. Hung and Eugene E. Lee
Department of Internal Medicine, California Pacific Medical Center, San Francisco, CA 94115, USA

Jennifer Guy
Department of Hepatology, California Pacific Medical Center, San Francisco, CA 94115, USA

Caroline M. Behler
Department of Hematology Oncology, California Pacific Medical Center, San Francisco, CA 94115, USA

Marina Moguilevitch and Carlene Broderick
Department of Anesthesiology, Montefiore Medical Center, Albert Einstein College of Medicine, Bronx, NY 10463, USA

Emanuele Felli, Giovanni Vennarecci, Marco Colasanti, Roberto Santoro, Edoardo deWerra, Andrea Scotti, Mirco Burocchi, Giovanni B. Levi Sandri, Alessandra Campanelli, Pasquale Lepiane and Giuseppe M. Ettorre
Digestive and Transplant Liver SurgeryUnit, S. Camillo Hospital, Piazza Carlo Forlanini 1, 00151 Rome, Italy

Hui-Hui Tan, Jason Pik-Eu Chang and Chee-Kiat Tan
Liver Transplant Service, Department of Gastroenterology and Hepatology, Singapore General Hospital, Singapore 169608

Hoe-NamLeong
Department of Infectious Diseases, Singapore General Hospital, Singapore 169608

Boon-Huan Tan
Defence Science Organisation, Singapore 118230

Lynette Lin-Ean Oon and Kiat-Hon Lim
Department of Pathology, Singapore General Hospital, Singapore 169608

Kim-Diêp Dang-Tran and Valérie Chabbert
Service de Radiologie Générale, Centre Hospitalier Universitaire Rangueil, 1 avenue du Professeur Jean Poulhés, TSA 50032, 31059 Toulouse Cedex 9, France

Hervé Rousseau and Phillippe Otal
Service de Radiologie Générale, Centre Hospitalier Universitaire Rangueil, 1 avenue du Professeur Jean Poulhés, TSA 50032, 31059 Toulouse Cedex 9, France
Université Paul Sabatier, 31059 Toulouse, France

Fabrice Dédouit
Service de Radiologie Générale, Centre Hospitalier Universitaire Rangueil, 1 avenue du Professeur Jean Poulhés, TSA 50032, 31059 Toulouse Cedex 9, France
Service de Médecine Légale, Centre Hospitalier Universitaire Rangueil, 1 avenue du Professeur Jean Poulhés, 31059 Toulouse Cedex 4, France

Laure Esposito
Department of Nephrology and Organ Transplantation, CHU Rangueil, TSA 50032, 31059 Toulouse Cedex 9, France

Lionel Rostaing and Nassim Kamar
Department of Nephrology and Organ Transplantation, CHU Rangueil, TSA 50032, 31059 Toulouse Cedex 9, France
Université Paul Sabatier, 31059 Toulouse, France
INSERM U1043, IFR-BMT, CHU Purpan, 31059 Toulouse, France

Céline Guilbeau-Frugier
Service d'Anatomo-Pathologie, Centre Hospitalier Universitaire Rangueil, 1 avenue du Professeur Jean Poulhés, 31059 Toulouse Cedex 4, France
Université Paul Sabatier, 31059 Toulouse, France

Saravanan Ramamoorthy
Department of Anesthesiology, Penn State Hershey Medical Center, 500 University Drive, H187 Hershey, PA 17033-0850, USA

Shachi Patel, Piotr K. Janicki and Dmitri Bezinover
Department of Anesthesiology, Penn State Hershey Medical Center, Hershey, PA-17033, USA

Eric Bradburn
Department of Surgery, Penn State Hershey Medical Center, Hershey, PA-17033, USA

Zakiyah Kadry, Tadahiro Uemura and Riaz Ali Shah
Department of Transplant Surgery, Penn State Hershey Medical Center, Hershey, PA-17033, USA

PedroW. Baron, Thomas Amankonah, Arputharaj H. Kore, Arvand Elihu and Michael E. de Vera
Transplantation Institute, Loma Linda University Medical Center, 25865 Barton Road, Suite 101, Loma Linda, CA 92354, USA

Robert F. Cubas
Department of Surgery, Loma Linda University Medical Center, 25865 Barton Road, Suite 101, Loma Linda, CA 92354, USA

Mia C. N. Perez
Departments of Pathology and Laboratory Medicine, Loma Linda University Medical Center, 25865 Barton Road, Suite 101, Loma Linda, CA 92354, USA

Vinaya C.Maddukuri
Division of Hepatology, Carolinas Medical Center, 1000 Blythe Boulevard, Charlotte, NC 28203, USA

Mark W. Russo
Division of Hepatology, Carolinas Medical Center, 1000 Blythe Boulevard, Charlotte, NC 28203, USA
Transplant Center, Carolinas Medical Center, 3rd Floor Annex building, Charlotte, NC 28203, USA

Courtney D. Stephenson
Department of Obstetrics and Gynecology, Carolinas Medical Center, 1000 Blythe Boulevard, Charlotte, NC 28203, USA

Lon Eskind
Department of Surgery, Carolinas Medical Center, 1000 Blythe Boulevard, Charlotte, NC 28203, USA

William A. Ahrens
Department of Pathology, Carolinas Medical Center, 1000 Blythe Boulevard, Charlotte, NC 28203, USA

Preston Purdum
Carolinas Digestive Health Associates, Charlotte, NC 28211, USA

Naoya Kanogawa, Tatsuo Kanda, Masato Nakamura, TatsuoMiyamura, Shin Yasui, Makoto Arai, HitoshiMaruyama, Keiichi Fujiwara and Osamu Yokosuka
Department of Gastroenterology and Nephrology, Chiba University, Graduate School of Medicine, 1-8-1 Inohana, Chuo-ku, Chiba 260-8677, Japan

Masayuki Ohtsuka and Masaru Miyazaki
Department of General Surgery, Chiba University, Graduate School of Medicine, Chuo-ku, Chiba 260-8677, Japan

Makio Shozu
Department of Reproductive Medicine, Chiba University, Graduate School of Medicine, Chuo-ku, Chiba 260-8677, Japan

Shigeto Oda
Department of Emergency and Critical Care Medicine, Chiba University, Graduate School of Medicine, Chuo-ku, Chiba 260-8677, Japan

Xu-Yong Sun, Ke Qin, Jian-Hui Dong, Hai-Bin Li, Liu-Gen Lan, Ying Huang, Song Cao and Zhuang-Jiang Li
Guangxi Key Laboratory of Transplant Medicine, Institute of Transplant Medicine, 303 Hospital of People's Liberation Army, Nanning 530021, China

Yinka K. Davies
Division of Gastroenterology, Hepatology, and Nutrition, Department of Pediatrics, School of Medicine, Stanford University, Stanford, CA 95762, USA

Cynthia J. Tsay
Yale University, New Haven, CT 06510, USA

Dario V. Caccamo
Department of Pathology, Sutter Medical Center, Sacramento, CA 95816, USA

Kathleen M. Cox, Ricardo O. Castillo and Kenneth L. Cox
Division of Gastroenterology, Hepatology, and Nutrition, Department of Pediatrics, School of Medicine, Stanford University, Stanford, CA 95762, USA
Department of Pediatrics, Lucile Packard Children's Hospital, Stanford University, Palo Alto, CA 94304, USA

Cuneyt Kayaalp, Sezai Yilmaz and Emrah Otan
Inonu University, Liver Transplantation Institute, 44280 Malatya, Turkey

Erdem Kinaci
Inonu University, Liver Transplantation Institute, 44280 Malatya, Turkey
Istanbul Training and Research Hospital, Department of General Surgery, 34098 Istanbul, Turkey

Rachael Leek, Erika Aldag, Iram Nadeem and Vikraman Gunabushanam
Department of Abdominal Transplant, Aurora St. Luke's Medical Center, Milwaukee, WI, USA

Ajay Sahajpal
Department of Abdominal Transplant, Aurora St. Luke's Medical Center, Milwaukee, WI, USA
University ofWisconsin School of Medicine and PublicHealth, Madison, WI 53726, USA

David J. Kramer
University of Wisconsin School of Medicine and Public Health, Madison, WI 53726, USA
Department of Critical Care, Aurora St. Luke's Medical Center, Milwaukee, WI, USA

Thomas J. Walsh
Weill Cornell Medicine, Cornell University and New York Presbyterian Hospital, New York, NY, USA

E. Jakobovich
Kaplan Medical Center, Rehovot, Israel

B. Koplewitz
Department of Medical Imaging, Hadassah Hebrew University Medical Center, Jerusalem, Israel

E. Marva
Central Laboratory, Ministry of Health, Jerusalem, Israel

E. Granot
Hebrew University, Hadassah Medical School, Jerusalem, Israel

Rita Jermyn and Julia Shin
Division of Heart Failure, Department of Cardiology, Montefiore Medical Center, Albert Einstein College of Medicine, Bronx, NY, USA

Eiei Soe, Milan Kinkhabwala and Paul J. Gaglio
Division of Hepatology, Department of Gastroenterology, Montefiore Medical Center, Albert Einstein College of Medicine, Bronx, NY, USA

David D'Alessandro and William Jakobleff
Department of Cardiothoracic Surgery, Montefiore Medical Center, Albert Einstein College of Medicine, Bronx, NY, USA

Daniel Schwartz
Department of Pathology, Montefiore Medical Center, USA

Jorge Herrador Benito, M. G. Zunzarren, T. Pozancos de Simón, L. Tortolero, R. Latorre Fragua and E. Lobo
Department of General and Digestive Surgery, Ram´on y Cajal Hospital, Cra. Colmenar Km 9, 1, 28034 Madrid, Spain

J. Nuño
Liver Transplantation Unit, Department of General and Digestive Surgery, Ram´on y Cajal Hospital, Cra. Colmenar Km 9, 1, 28034 Madrid, Spain

Adam T. Hauch, Joseph F. Buell, Parisha Bhatia, Mary Killackey, Bob Saggi and Anil S. Paramesh
Tulane Transplant Institute, Tulane University School of Medicine, 1415 Tulane Avenue, HC-5, New Orleans, LA 70112, USA

Margit McGowan
Department of Hematology and Oncology, Tulane University School of Medicine, New Orleans, LA 70112, USA

Eleanor Lewin
Department of Pathology, Tulane University School of Medicine, New Orleans, LA 70112, USA

Nathan J. Shores, Luis A. Balart and Martin Moehlen
Department of Gastroenterology, Section of Hepatology, Tulane University School of Medicine, New Orleans, LA 70112, USA

Marina Moguilevitch and Ellise Delphin
Department of Anesthesiology, Montefiore Medical Center, Albert Einstein College of Medicine, Bronx, NY 10463, USA

Christopher M. Moore, Anne K. Bartels and David H. Van Thiel
Section of Hepatology, Rush University Medical Center, Chicago, IL 60612, USA

Ihab Lamzabi and Shriram Jakate
Section of Pathology, Rush University Medical Center, Chicago, IL 60612, USA

Shweta Yemul Golhar and Michael S. Green
Department of Anesthesiology, Drexel University College of Medicine/Hahnemann University Hospital, Philadelphia, PA, USA

Stephen Guy
Department of Surgery, Drexel University College of Medicine/Hahnemann University Hospital, Philadelphia, PA, USA

Sonia Radunz, Carmen Kirchner, Jürgen Treckmann, Andreas Paul and Fuat H. Saner
Department of General, Visceral, and Transplantation Surgery, Essen University Hospital, 45122 Essen, Germany

Fahri YetiGir
General Surgery Department, Atat¨urk Research and Training Hospital, Turkey
Liver Transplantation Institute, Inonu University, Malatya, Turkey

Cuneyt Kayaalp and Sezayi Yilmaz
Liver Transplantation Institute, Inonu University, Malatya, Turkey

S. Murad Dogan
Liver Transplantation Institute, Inonu University, Malatya, Turkey
General Surgery Department, ˙Izmir Research and Training Hospital, Turkey

Ruslan Mamedov
Liver Transplantation Institute, Inonu University, Malatya, Turkey
Azerbaijan Medical University, Baku, Azerbaijan

Juliet A. Emamaullee
Department of Surgery, University of Southern California, Los Angeles, CA, USA

Klaudia Nowak, Marla Beach and Julinor Bacani
Department of Anatomic Pathology, University of Alberta, Edmonton, AB, Canada

A. M. James Shapiro
Department of Surgery, University of Alberta, Edmonton, AB, Canada

M. I. Montenovo and R. Bakthavatsalam
Division of Transplantation, Department of Surgery, University of Washington, Seattle, WA, USA

F. G. Jalikis and B. Hoch
Department of Anatomic Pathology, University of Washington, Seattle, WA, USA

Lampros Kousoulas, MichaelWinkler, Frank Lehner, Nicolas Richter, Juergen Klempnauer and Fabian Helfritz
Department of General, Visceral and Transplant Surgery, HannoverMedical School, Carl-Neuberg-Street 1, 30625 Hanover, Germany

Kristina Imeen Ringe
Institute of Radiology, Hannover Medical School, Carl-Neuberg-Street 1, 30625 Hanover, Germany

Sushrut Trakroo
Department of Surgery, Temple University Hospital, Philadelphia, PA 19140, USA

Kamran Qureshi
Section of Gastroenterology and Hepatology, Temple University Lewis Katz School of Medicine, Philadelphia, PA 19140, USA

Tanima Jana, Jorge D. Machicado and Giovanni E. Davogustto
Department of Internal Medicine, University of Texas Medical School at Houston, Houston, TX 77030, USA

Jen-Jung Pan
Division of Gastroenterology, Hepatology and Nutrition, Department of Internal Medicine, University of Texas Medical School at Houston, Houston, TX 77030, USA

Pablo Serrano Rodriguez, David Allen Gerber and Chirag Sureshchandra Desai
Department of Surgery, Division of Abdominal Transplant Surgery, The University of North Carolina at Chapel Hill, ChapelHill, NC 27599, USA

Alfred Sidney Barritt IV
Division of Gastroenterology and Hepatology, The University of North Carolina at Chapel Hill, Chapel Hill, NC 27599, USA

R. Kula, M. Melter, J. Kunkel, C. Dörfler, S. Alikadic, B. Knoppke and R. Zant
KUNO University Children's Hospital, Regensburg, Germany

Napatt Kanjanahattakij, Kamolyut Lapumnuaypol and Sanna Fatima
Department of Internal Medicine, Einstein Medical Center, Philadelphia, PA, USA

Eyob Feyssa
Department of Transplantation, Einstein Medical Center, Philadelphia, PA, USA

Caroline Protin, Dmitri Bezinover and Thomas Verbeek
Department of Anesthesia and Perioperative Medicine, Penn State Health Milton S. Hershey Medical Center, Hershey, PA, USA

Zakiyah Kadry
Department of Surgery, Penn State HealthMilton S. HersheyMedical Center, Hershey, PA, USA

FlorianWolfgang Rudolf Vondran, Wolfgang Knitsch, Juergen Klempnauer, Hueseyin Bektas and Frank Lehner
Department of General, Visceral and Transplant Surgery, Hannover Medical School, 30625Hannover, Germany

Carsten Schumacher and Kai Johanning
Department of Anaesthesiology and Intensive Care Medicine, Hannover Medical School, 30625 Hannover, Germany

Björn Hartleben
Institute of Pathology, Hannover Medical School, 30625 Hannover, Germany

Olaf Wiesner
Department of Respiratory Medicine, Hannover Medical School, 30625 Hannover, Germany

Elmar Jaeckel and Michael Peter Manns
Department of Gastroenterology, Hepatology and Endocrinology, Hannover Medical School, 30625 Hannover, Germany

Lucas Souto Nacif, Estrella Bianca de Mello, Rafael Soares Pinheiro, Rodrigo Bronze de Martino, Wellington Andraus and Luiz Carneiro D'Albuquerque
Liver and Gastrointestinal Transplant Division, Department of Gastroenterology, 05403-900 São Paulo, Brazil

Fabiana Roberto Lima
Department of Pathology, University of São Paulo School of Medicine, 05403-900 São Paulo, Brazil

Serena Patel and Shirley M. Tsunoda
University of California (UC) San Diego, Skaggs School of Pharmacy and Pharmaceutical Sciences, USA

Michel H. Mendler
UC San Diego, Department of Medicine, Division of Hepatology, USA

Mark A. Valasek
UC San Diego, Department of Pathology, USA

Sanjay de Mel and Zarni Soe
Department of Haematology-Oncology, National University Cancer Institute, National University Health System, 1E Kent Ridge Road, NUHS Tower Block Level 7, Singapore 119228

Benjamin Wong
Department of Pathology, National University Health System, 1E Kent Ridge Road, Singapore 119228

Ching Ching Ong and Lynette Teo
Department of Diagnostic Imaging, National University Health System, 1E Kent Ridge Road, Singapore 119228

Lip Kun Tan
Departments of Laboratory Medicine and Haematology-Oncology, National University Cancer Institute, National University Health System, 1E Kent Ridge Road, NUHS Tower Block Level 7, Singapore 119228

Samuel Chan, Michael T. Burke, David W. Johnson, Ross S. Francis and David .W Mudge
Queensland Renal Transplant Service, Princess Alexandra Hospital, Brisbane, QLD, Australia
School of Medicine, The University of Queensland, Brisbane, QLD, Australia

Index